T0201224

THE BIOSTATISTICS
OF AGING

THE BIOSTATISTICS OF AGING

From Gompertzian Mortality to an Index of Aging-Relatedness

GILBERTO LEVY
Rio de Janeiro, Brazil

BRUCE LEVIN
Department of Biostatistics
Columbia University
New York, NY

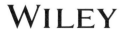

Published by John Wiley & Sons, Inc., Hoboken, New Jersey
Published simultaneously in Canada

For general information on our other products and services or for technical support, please contact our
Customer Care Department within the United States at (800) 762-2974, outside the United States at
(317) 572-3993 or fax (317) 572-4002.

Wiley also publishes its books in a variety of electronic formats. Some content that appears in print may
not be available in electronic formats. For more information about Wiley products, visit our web site at
www.wiley.com.

Library of Congress Cataloging-in-Publication Data:

Levy, Gilberto, author.
   The biostatistics of aging : from Gompertzian mortality and to an index of aging-relatedness /
Gilberto Levy, Bruce Levin.
      pages cm
   Includes bibliographical references and index.
   ISBN 978-1-118-64585-7 (cloth)
1. Aging–Statistical methods.   2. Mortality–Statistical methods.   3. Life spans (Biology)
I. Levin, Bruce (Bruce A.), 1948– author.   II. Title.
   QH529.L48 2013
   571.8'78–dc23

2013034339

Printed in the United States of America

10 9 8 7 6 5 4 3 2 1

To my parents Menache and Norma Levy
G.L.

To my wife Betty
B.L

The decay of vitality with age is a biological fact most recognize in themselves and none fail to recognize in others; but the biometry of the subject is a difficult undertaking.
Greenwood, M. and Irwin, J. O. (1939). The biostatistics of senility. *Human Biology*, **11**, 1–23.

CONTENTS

PREFACE AND ACKNOWLEDGMENT

The purpose of this book is to describe a new quantitative method to examine the relative contributions of genetic factors and lifetime exposures to rates of mortality and disease incidence in a population. The book is highly multidisciplinary. The theoretical foundations of the work presented here involve the fields of statistics, evolutionary biology, demography, and epidemiology and should be of interest to those in these fields. Moreover, in its applications the work is broadly relevant to medicine, aging, and public health. Researchers and practitioners in these areas are also target audiences. We expect readers to comprise a spectrum from the more mathematically inclined to the more biologically inclined, though of course there will be readers who have expertise in both domains. This made the choice of level of presentation especially difficult. We chose to tilt the balance in favor of reaching a wide audience, at the cost of possibly making some (though hopefully not all) of the material in a field seem basic for an expert in that field. We also endeavored to make the book more widely appealing by keeping the denser mathematical material in a separate section in Chapter 2 and in a few appendices, and by providing summary pictures and statements after a series of mathematical results and at the end of some elaborate arguments. We bring the results and arguments from different areas of knowledge together starting in Section 2.2.1, and we hope the reader's forbearance will be rewarded with some interesting synergies.

On a personal note, we have enjoyed collaborating on this project immensely and have learned a great deal from each other. From one perspective, the statistical modeling required was of the most precious kind as it derived from careful evolutionary and causal thinking, leading inexorably to consideration of one special model, rather than a plethora of them. From another perspective, the evolutionary arguments benefited from giving them a sound statistical underpinning and the clarity that mathematics can bring to an argument. In the interchange of ideas, we could hardly have had more fun.

The book greatly benefited from an illustrative application of the proposed method using data from the Israeli Ischemic Heart Disease (IIHD) study (Section 4.5). This was possible thanks to a collaboration with Uri Goldbourt, Ph.D., of the Division of Epidemiology and Preventive Medicine at the Sackler Faculty of Medicine of Tel Aviv University. The IIHD study collected mortality information on more than 10,000 subjects over a 43-year follow-up period (1963–2006), and Dr. Goldbourt has been involved with the study for nearly half a century. We deeply appreciate his invaluable help and responsiveness and are grateful for his graciousness in allowing us to report some of our analytic results from these data here.

GILBERTO LEVY
Rio de Janeiro

BRUCE LEVIN
New York

1

INTRODUCTION

The so-called aging-related diseases currently constitute a major public health concern, and their importance only tends to increase with the increase in absolute and relative numbers of older people in the population. The qualification "aging-related" is commonly used in the medical literature for diseases or disorders in a wide range of categories (e.g., neurodegeneration, cardiovascular, metabolic, neoplasia) and affecting virtually every organ system. In addition to *aging-related*, other terms that are often used with the same meaning are *age-related*, *age-dependent*, and *age-associated*. Although usually no formal definition is given, these terms are generally employed as referring to diseases whose age-specific point incidence rates (or, briefly, "incidence") increase with increasing age.

However, some authors have drawn a fundamental distinction among these terms. While considerations about the relation between disease and aging go back a long way (Blumenthal, 2003), perhaps one of the earliest discussions specifically pointing to that terminological distinction is to be found in Kohn (1963), who noted, "it is useful to make two categories of the bad things that happen to people with increasing age— basic aging processes and age-related diseases, and to consider that the latter may be conditioned by, or dependent on, the former." He then distinguished between a category of diseases that shows an increasing incidence with increasing age and a category that shows "a less clear-cut, age-related increase in incidence." Two decades later, Kohn (1982) proposed that age-related diseases could be categorized in three ways: diseases that are normal aging processes themselves, diseases in which the

The Biostatistics of Aging: From Gompertzian Mortality to an Index of Aging-Relatedness,
First Edition. Gilberto Levy and Bruce Levin.
© 2014 John Wiley & Sons, Inc. Published 2014 by John Wiley & Sons, Inc.

incidence increases with increasing age, and diseases that have more serious consequences the older the affected persons. The more precise distinction that is most relevant to this work was given by Brody and Schneider (1986), who described two
classes of "chronic diseases and disorders of old age" as follows: "Age-dependent diseases and disorders are defined as those whose pathogenesis appears to involve the
normal aging of the host. Mortality and morbidity from age-dependent diseases
and disorders (e.g. coronary artery disease and Alzheimer's disease) increase exponentially. Age-related diseases and disorders, on the other hand, have a temporal relationship to the host but are not necessarily related to aging processes. They occur at a
specific age and then decline in frequency or continue at less than an exponential rate
of increase (e.g. multiple sclerosis and amyotrophic lateral sclerosis)."[1]

Particularly relevant to this work, Brody and Schneider (1986) suggested that the
group of diseases related to the aging process is characterized by an exponential
increase in age-specific incidence or mortality rates, as opposed to "less than an
exponential rate of increase." However, they did not provide a basis rooted in biological
or statistical principles for that notion. Similarly, Kohn (1963) had considered,
without justification from first principles, that an exponential increase in cause
(disease)-specific (DS) mortality rates with age "is characteristic of deaths due to basic
age-related processes and suggests the extent to which a disease is related to such processes." Brody and Schneider (1986) illustrated such notion by plotting DS mortality
rates by age for cardiovascular disease and cancer, representing the groups with and
without exponential increase in age-specific rates, respectively (Fig. 1.1).

In the context of a meta-analysis of dementia prevalence, Ritchie and Kildea (1995)
distinguished between an "ageing-related disorder" ("caused by the ageing process
itself") and an "age-related disorder" ("occurring within a specific age range"). Thus,
they suggested that one category had a causal relation to the aging process and the
other did not (labeled "ageing-related" and "age-related," respectively), as Brody
and Schneider (1986) had done before but instead labeling the first category "age-
dependent." As an example that this distinction continues to provoke and underlie
the debate about the relation between diseases and aging in the twenty-first century,
even if the causality notion is not always explicitly conveyed, Blumenthal (2003)
offered the following "note on terminology" in his article titled "The aging-disease
dichotomy: true or false?": "In this essay I have used the term aging-associated disease
rather than age-related disease. This choice is to emphasize that the primary focus here
has been on diseases with age at onset in the senescent period of the life span, the
oldest old, rather than through progressive periods of the total life span."[2]

Yet, in a sense, the relation between diseases and aging has eluded medical thinking. While employing separate terms or categories for qualitatively different relations
between diseases and aging seems warranted, it may not be clear under which

---

[1] Reproduced from *Journal of Chronic Diseases*, **39**, Brody, J. A. and Schneider, E. L., Diseases and
disorders of aging: An hypothesis, pages 871–876, Copyright 1986, with permission from Elsevier.
[2] Reproduced from *The Journals of Gerontology Series A: Biological Sciences and Medical Sciences*, **58**,
Blumenthal, H. T., The aging–disease dichotomy: True or false? pages M138–M145, Copyright 2003, with
permission from Oxford University Press.

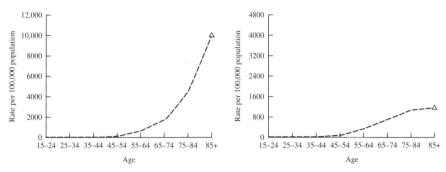

FIGURE 1.1 Cause (disease)-specific mortality rates by age for cardiovascular disease (left) and all cancers (right), data from the United States, 1978 (reproduced from *Journal of Chronic Diseases*, **39**, Brody, J. A. and Schneider, E. L., Diseases and disorders of aging: An hypothesis, pages 871–876, Copyright 1986, with permission from Elsevier).

category a disease falls given how its incidence increases with age. On the other hand, diseases considered to be in the same category may show different rates of increase in incidence rates with age. This may be seen as reflecting the fact that the aforementioned distinction arises from an underlying relation on a continuous scale, which therefore might better be considered using a quantitative approach. Although the authors quoted in the preceding text have attempted to clarify the meaning of aging-relatedness, the quantification of aging-relatedness has not been addressed at all in the medical, biostatistical, epidemiological, or demographic literature. *Hence, we aimed to develop an index of aging-relatedness, as a means of quantifying and elucidating the underlying meaning of aging-relatedness.*

Since the increase of mortality rates with age is an expression of aging at the population level, the notion of aging-relatedness applies as well, and perhaps even more naturally, to mortality. Medawar (1955) distinguished between a personal measure of aging, which "purports to measure a process that takes place in the life history of an individual animal," and a statistical or actuarial measure of aging, "which is founded upon the mortality of a population of individuals and which bears only indirectly upon the changes that occur within the lifetime of anyone." The assumed relevance of the mortality experience of a population to the physiological process of aging of its members is reflected in other authors' definitions of aging or senescence. For instance, Maynard Smith (1962) stated, "Ageing processes may be defined as those which render individuals more susceptible as they grow older to the various factors, intrinsic or extrinsic, which may cause death." Similarly, Comfort (1979, p. 21) stated, "Senescence shows itself as an increasing probability of death with increasing chronological age: the study of senescence is the study of the group of processes, different in different organisms, which lead to this increase in vulnerability." More recent statements include Kirkwood's (1985): "The pattern of mortality experienced by human populations serves to illustrate what is most commonly understood by the term *aging*. Following the attainment of sexual maturity and a peak of vitality which occurs early in adulthood, a long period of progressive deterioration takes place during which individuals become increasingly likely to die." Or Finch's (1990, p. 5): "Senescence is mainly used to describe age-related changes in an organism that adversely affect its vitality and functions, but most importantly, increase the mortality rate as a function of time." The implicit assumption in all these authors' definitions—that the pattern of age at death (or schedule of age-specific mortality rates) in a population parallels functional changes in the organism—is supported by experimental research with a variety of organisms (Austad, 2001).

Consistent with this premise, the index of aging-relatedness that we propose in this book is based on the schedule of age-specific mortality rates at a given point in time, through the use of time-to-event population-based data. Likewise, the index of aging-relatedness as applied to specific diseases is based on age-specific incidence rates or DS and age-specific mortality rates. The terms *aging-related* and *aging-relatedness* are used in this work without reference to the terminological distinctions in the preceding text. Indeed, developing a quantitative index of aging-relatedness would turn these distinctions moot. This is also to say that no claim of causality in the sense expressed by Brody and Schneider (1986) and Ritchie and Kildea (1995) is made in connection with the proposed index of aging-relatedness. Rather, in Chapters 2 and 3, we develop an extensive theoretical framework for the proposed index of aging-relatedness involving the statistical theory of extreme values and the evolutionary theory of aging, both of which rest on solid ground. We start by considering the biological basis of the Gompertz survival distribution, which is precisely characterized by the exponentially increasing hazard rate referred to by Kohn (1963) and Brody and Schneider (1986) and has long played a central role in demography for describing the survival time of human populations. The theoretical framework then includes (i) original mathematical results on the asymptotic behavior of the minimum of time-to-event random variables, extending those of the classical statistical theory of extreme values (Section 2.1.2); (ii) an account of the Gompertz pattern of mortality in human populations, using those results on the statistical theory of extreme values and arguments based on the evolutionary theory of aging (Section 2.2.1); and (iii) the development of the sufficient and component causes model of causation in epidemiology into an evolution-based model of causation, relevant to mortality and aging-related diseases of complex etiology (Section 3.2). While these are necessary steps toward devising the proposed index of aging-relatedness, each stands on its own as a theoretical contribution.

The index of aging-relatedness is presented in Chapter 4. The evolution-based model of causation provides the motivation for a statistical model for describing mortality and incidence of aging-related diseases of complex etiology involving a mixture of the Gompertz and Weibull distributions. This creates a framework for interpreting the index of aging-relatedness, which is defined as a parameter of this model (Sections 4.1 and 4.2). We describe the estimation procedures for obtaining the index and present an illustrative application to a real set of data (Sections 4.4 and 4.5). Although the overall presentation of this book proceeds from Gompertzian mortality to the index of aging-relatedness, we originally set out to develop an index of aging-relatedness. As we considered the theoretical basis for various proposals and found the mixture model index especially appealing from a theoretical viewpoint, the scope of the work widened considerably—while remaining in essence a medically motivated quantitative/statistical pursuit—to involve other disciplines such as demography, epidemiology, evolutionary biology, and population genetics. With this widening scope came a deeper reach. Even as our motivation was at first sight purely conceptual, a practical biomedical and public health relevance of the index arises from its interpretation, in a special sense, in terms of genetic and environmental contributions to mortality or disease incidence in a population. As a consequence, despite an ostensibly narrow initial aim, there are widespread implications of our theoretical framework and the index of aging-relatedness. These are discussed in Chapter 5. In its implications, the work presented in this book is additionally relevant to the fields of gerontology and geriatrics (Sections 5.3 and 5.4), as well as any medical specialty whose practitioners deal with aging-related diseases, but the most direct and practical implications are for public health (Sections 5.5 and 5.6) now and into the future.

2

AN ACCOUNT OF GOMPERTZIAN MORTALITY THROUGH STATISTICAL AND EVOLUTIONARY ARGUMENTS

While several statistical models of age-specific mortality rates have been developed, including those based on the Weibull and logistic distributions, the most widely applied to mortality data in demography and gerontology has been the Gompertz model. Benjamin Gompertz was a nineteenth-century British mathematician and actuary who observed that the death rate in humans within a certain range of adult ages increased geometrically as age increased arithmetically (Gompertz, 1825). Thus, the Gompertz equation was developed based on empirical human mortality observations to describe an exponential relation between age-specific mortality rates and age:

$$h_G(x) = \lambda e^{\theta x}, \tag{2.1}$$

where $h_G(x)$ is the hazard function (also called hazard rate function, instantaneous death rate, or force of mortality) for the Gompertz model, $\lambda > 0$ is a parameter denoting the initial mortality rate (at birth or another arbitrary age), and θ is an exponential rate parameter. The parameter λ has also been called the vulnerability parameter, while θ has been called the rate of aging or Gompertz parameter (Carey, 1999; Sacher, 1977). The derivative of Equation 2.1,

$$h'_G(x) = \theta \lambda e^{\theta x} = \theta h_G(x), \tag{2.2}$$

shows that the rate of change of the Gompertz hazard function at a given age is proportional to the value of the hazard function at that age. For $\theta > 0$, $h_G(x)$ is a

The Biostatistics of Aging: From Gompertzian Mortality to an Index of Aging-Relatedness,
First Edition. Gilberto Levy and Bruce Levin.
© 2014 John Wiley & Sons, Inc. Published 2014 by John Wiley & Sons, Inc.

monotonically increasing function of x, and for $\theta < 0$, $h_G(x)$ is monotonically decreasing. For $\theta = 0$, $h_G(x)$ reduces to the constant hazard function of the exponential distribution. By taking the logarithm of both sides of Equation 2.1, we obtain

$$\log h_G(x) = \log \lambda + \theta x, \tag{2.3}$$

which shows that when there is a good fit of the Gompertz distribution to mortality data, a plot of the log of the mortality rates by age (a semilog plot) follows a closely linear relation with slope θ and intercept $\log \lambda$.

In contrast, the Weibull distribution was developed by the Swedish engineer Waloddi Weibull, in the context of modeling the strength of materials (Weibull, 1939, 1951). Similar to the role played by the Gompertz distribution in demography, the Weibull distribution plays a prominent role in reliability theory, which applies to the failure of mechanical devices (Barlow and Proschan, 1981, p. 73; Rausand and Høyland, 2004, pp. 37–41). While the Gompertz equation describes an exponential relation between age-specific mortality (or failure) rates and age, the Weibull hazard function describes a power relation:

$$h_W(x) = \alpha\gamma x^{\gamma-1}, \tag{2.4}$$

where $\alpha > 0$ and $\gamma > 0$ are parameters. The shape of the Weibull hazard function depends on the value of γ, which is known as the shape parameter, while α^{-1} is a scale parameter. In addition to reliability theory, the Weibull distribution is widely used in parametric survival analysis, since the Weibull hazard function can take a variety of forms, depending on the value of the shape parameter γ, and summary statistics can be easily obtained (Collett, 2003, pp. 154–155). The derivative of Equation 2.4,

$$h'_W(x) = \alpha\gamma(\gamma-1)x^{\gamma-2} = \frac{\gamma-1}{x} h_W(x), \tag{2.5}$$

shows that the rate of change of the Weibull hazard function at a given age is proportional to the hazard function at that age divided by the age. For $\gamma > 1$, $h_W(x)$ is a monotonically increasing function of x, and for $0 < \gamma < 1$, $h_W(x)$ is monotonically decreasing. For $\gamma = 1$, the Weibull hazard function reduces to the hazard function of the exponential distribution. Hence, the exponential distribution is a special case of both the Gompertz and the Weibull distributions. The log of Equation 2.4,

$$\log h_W(x) = \log(\alpha\gamma) + (\gamma-1)\log x, \tag{2.6}$$

shows that when there is a good fit of the Weibull distribution to mortality or failure data, a plot of the log of the rates by the log of age (a log-log plot) follows a closely linear relation with slope $\gamma - 1$ and intercept $\log(\alpha\gamma)$.

Figure 2.1 shows plots of the Gompertz and Weibull hazard functions by age in the same graph, accompanied by the corresponding semilog and log-log plots in two other graphs. In semilog plots, the Gompertz hazard function is represented by a straight line

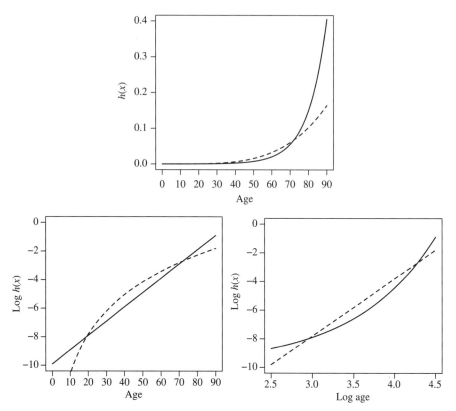

FIGURE 2.1   Plots of the Gompertz (solid line) and Weibull (dashed line) hazard functions by age, with parameter values $\lambda = 5e - 5$, $\theta = 0.10$, $\alpha = 5e - 10$, and $\gamma = 5.0$. The lower left panel is a semilog plot of the two hazard functions, and the lower right panel is a log-log plot.

and the Weibull hazard function is represented by a curved line with a logarithmic shape. Conversely, in log-log plots, the Weibull hazard function is represented by a straight line and the Gompertz hazard function is represented by a curved line with an exponential shape. Semilog plots of mortality rates are most commonly used in demography and will be employed in the data analysis presented in Section 4.5.

Although the Gompertz equation was empirical, Gompertz (1825) considered a priori reasons why it should hold: "If the average exhaustions of a man's power to avoid death were such that at the end of equal infinitely small intervals of time, he lost equal portions of his remaining power to oppose destruction which he had at the commencement of those intervals, then at the age x his power to avoid death, or the intensity of his mortality might be denoted by aq^x, a and q being constant quantities." In a paper presented to the International Statistical Congress in 1860 and reprinted in 1871 in the *Journal of the Institute of Actuaries* after his death in 1865 (see Hooker (1965) for a biographical note), Gompertz (1871) further elaborated on the "physiological" basis of his law of mortality using an analogy with an air pump. He introduced this speculation with the often-quoted sentence, "And contemplating on this law of mortality, I endeavoured to enquire if there could be any physical cause for its existence." Since then, despite the long-standing use of the Gompertz distribution in demography, there has been no satisfactory biological explanation of its relatively good fit to human mortality data, notably for deaths occurring between about 10–15 and 90 years old (see Section 2.2.2). Even though several researchers in the fields of biochemistry, radiation biology, and gerontology began looking for a biological explanation for Gompertz's "law of mortality" early in the twentieth century (Olshansky and Carnes, 1997), the way in which the Gompertz model is generally regarded—as empirical rather than based on biological principles—has not substantially changed. This is reflected in relatively recent statements such as Finch's (1990, pp. 15–16), "The Gompertz model is empirical and is not based on any principle or law that requires a particular relationship between mortality rate parameters and age," and Williams' (1999), "Despite its many decades of usage, this model is based entirely on intuition and data-fitting, rather than inference from biological principles."

As posited by Beard (1959), "A satisfying basis for a law of mortality would be a formula that, starting from some fundamental concepts about the biological ageing process, led to a distribution of deaths by age which was comparable with observational data." The phrase, *starting from some fundamental concepts about the biological aging process*, underscores to us what has been lacking from most, if not all, proposed explanations of the Gompertz pattern of mortality. In our view, the evolutionary theory of aging currently provides such fundamental concepts about the biological aging process, inasmuch as genes correspond to a fundamental level of biological causation and evolutionary biology is *the* discipline underlying our understanding of how biological processes have come to be what they are. Some theories accounting for Gompertzian mortality, such as Strehler and Mildvan's (1960) and Sacher and Trucco's (1962), may be regarded as even more fundamental because they draw inspiration from, or rely on analogies with, physicochemical processes. In this respect, these authors were preceded by Brownlee (1919), who was one of the first to explore a relation between basic biology and the life table. However, at the strictly biological level, these theories refer to physiological processes; Strehler and Mildvan's (1960) and Sacher and Trucco's (1962) biological reasoning involves homeostatic systems, which tend to bring the organism to a relatively stable equilibrium through regulatory biochemical and cellular mechanisms.

Another group of explanations for Gompertzian mortality relies on analogies with mechanical devices and uses the tools of system reliability theory, which includes the statistical theory of extreme values. An example in this group is Gavrilov and Gavrilova's (2001) reliability theory of aging and longevity. Even as they acknowledge that "organisms prefer to die according to the Gompertz law, while technical devices typically fail according to the Weibull law," Gavrilov and Gavrilova's (2001) theory tries to explain this dichotomy by taking into account the initial flaws and redundancy of biological systems (created by self-assembly) as contrasted with technical devices (created by external assembly). It is important to note that in subsuming biological aging under a more general aging process applying to both living organisms and inanimate matter (Gavrilov and Gavrilova, 2004), one may be led to bypass considerations unique to the biological aging process. Some have used the tools of system reliability theory while additionally pursuing a specific biological reasoning. For instance, Abernethy (1979) thoroughly employed the statistical theory of extreme values to account for Gompertzian mortality; his theory involves biological "components" identified with "minimal subsets of cells such that every subset is demonstrably vital for survival" (e.g., a critical mass of heart muscle). Abernethy (1998) later developed a more detailed account, in large part by making the biological processes explicit, but the biological considerations in his theory are at the cellular level, rather than at the more fundamental level of genetic causes, and only briefly touch on evolutionary theory.

For more comprehensive reviews of the search for an explanation for Gompertzian mortality, see Economos (1982) and Olshansky and Carnes (1997). In this chapter, we offer an account of the Gompertz pattern of mortality through the statistical theory of extreme values (Section 2.1) and biological evolution (Section 2.2). Our use of extreme value theory depends fundamentally on some original results presented in Section 2.1.2. In Chapter 3, we consider departures from the Gompertz model and account for those departures by further developing the theoretical framework in this chapter into an evolution-based model of causation—at which point the contribution of the Weibull distribution to a proposed survival mixture model of the Gompertz and Weibull distributions will be justified. *In a real sense, this book is about appreciating the distinctions between the Gompertz and Weibull models for human mortality and disease incidence, how those distinctions can be predicted to arise on the basis of the statistical theory of extreme values as driven by the evolution-based model of causation, and the considerably challenging data analytic problem of estimating the degree to which each model contributes to the overall pattern of events.*

2.1 THE STATISTICAL THEORY OF EXTREME VALUES

The statistical theory of extreme values concerns the distribution of the maximum, the minimum, or another extreme order statistic derived from an *initial* or *parent distribution*. The probability that an observation from a probability density function (p.d.f.) $f(x)$ falls at or short of x is given by definition by the cumulative distribution function (c.d.f.), or simply distribution function, $F(x)$. The probability that n independent observations from the initial distribution all fall at or short of x is $F^n(x)$. This is the same as the probability that the maximum among n independent observations is no greater than x, so that $F^n(x)$ is the distribution function of the maximum (Gumbel, 1954). Similarly, the distribution function of the minimum is $1 - [1 - F(x)]^n$. If the independent observations come from n different initial distributions $F_i(x)$ for $i = 1, \ldots, n$, the distribution functions of the maximum and minimum are given, respectively, by $\prod_{i=1}^{n} F_i(x)$ and $1 - \prod_{i=1}^{n} [1 - F_i(x)]$. Thus, it is evident that the distribution of the maximum or minimum depends not only on the initial distribution but also on n. Throughout this section, $F(x)$ will refer to an initial or parent distribution, and n will denote the number of observations from the initial distribution. The aforementioned expressions underlie the *exact* statistical theory of extreme values.

Asymptotic extreme value theory concerns the *limiting* distribution of an extreme order statistic as n tends to infinity. It has found widespread application in areas of engineering such as reliability theory, aeronautics, and naval engineering and in the study of extreme climatological phenomena (e.g., floods, droughts, maxima and minima of atmospheric pressures and temperatures) (Gumbel, 1954, 1958). As n tends to infinity, it is clear that for any fixed value of x, $\lim_{n\to\infty} F^n(x) = 0$ or 1 if, respectively, $F(x) < 1$ or $F(x) = 1$. That is, the limiting distribution of the maximum is degenerate. Therefore, a possible nondegenerate limiting distribution must be found as the distribution of some sequence of transformed or "reduced" values that depend on n but not on x (Kotz and Nadarajah, 2000, p. 5). When the observations are independent and identically distributed (i.i.d.) with some initial distribution function, the results from *classical* extreme value theory have established that there are only three possible types of nondegenerate limiting distributions of the maximum (and the minimum), which have been called Fréchet-type, Weibull-type, and Gumbel-type (Coles, 2001, pp. 46–47; Kotz and Nadarajah, 2000, pp. 3–4).[1]

For the purpose of our application, we will be interested in the asymptotic extreme value theory for the minimum, hence the focus of what follows. Let $X_1, X_2, ..., X_n$ be i.i.d. random variables with distribution function $F(x)$ and denote their minimum by $W_n = \min\{X_1, X_2, ..., X_n\}$. To obtain a nondegenerate limiting distribution of the minimum, the extreme value is normalized through a linear transformation with coefficients that depend on n. An initial distribution function $F(x)$ is said to belong to the *minimum domain of attraction* of a nondegenerate asymptotic distribution if there exist sequences of normalizing coefficients $a_n > 0$ and b_n $(n = 1, 2, ...)$ such that $\lim_{n\to\infty} [1 - F(a_n x + b_n)]^n = 1 - G(x)$, where $G(x)$ is the limiting distribution of the shifted and scaled minimum $W_n^* = (W_n - b_n)/a_n$ (de Haan, 1976). Of the three possible types of $G(x)$,

$$G_1(x) = \begin{cases} 1 - \exp[-(-x)^{-\rho}] & x < 0, \rho > 0 \\ 1 & x \geq 0 \end{cases} \quad \text{(Fréchet-type)}, \qquad (2.7)$$

$$G_2(x) = \begin{cases} 0 & x < 0 \\ 1 - \exp(-x^\rho) & x \geq 0, \rho > 0 \end{cases} \quad \text{(Weibull-type)}, \qquad (2.8)$$

$$G_3(x) = 1 - \exp(-e^x) \quad -\infty < x < \infty \quad \text{(Gumbel-type)}, \qquad (2.9)$$

---

[1] These three types were obtained by Fréchet (1927) and by Fisher and Tippett (1928), using the so-called stability postulate, which means the following for the maximum: Consider N samples, each of size n, taken from the same population, for a total of Nn observations. In each sample of size n, there is a largest value. The largest of the N largest values from the N samples is also the largest value of the Nn observations. Therefore, the distribution of the largest value in a sample of size Nn should be the same as the distribution of the largest value in a sample of size n, except for a linear transformation (Gumbel, 1954, p. 21, 1958, pp. 157–162). The stability postulate for the maximum is written as $H^N(x) = H(a_N x + b_N)$, and Fisher and Tippett (1928) arrived at three solutions of this functional equation. The Gumbel-type distribution is obtained by taking $a_N = 1$, and the Fréchet-type and Weibull-type distributions are obtained by taking $a_N \neq 1$ (Kotz and Nadarajah, 2000, pp. 5–6).

where ρ is a shape parameter, only the Weibull-type and Gumbel-type limiting distributions are relevant to time-to-event random variables, since $G_1(x)$ is confined to the negative axis and cannot arise as the limiting distribution of the minimum of non-negative random variables (Barlow and Proschan, 1981, p. 229). The lower endpoint of an initial distribution in the minimum domain of attraction of $G(x)$, denoted $\alpha(F) = \inf\{x : F(x) > 0\}$, is required to be $-\infty$ for $G_1(x)$, while $\alpha(F)$ for $G_2(x)$ must be finite. Although the support of limiting distribution $G_3(x)$ extends from $-\infty$ to ∞, there is no requirement that $\alpha(F)$ be $-\infty$ (Galambos, 1987, pp. 58–59).

As indicated earlier, the "Weibull-type" and "Gumbel-type" nomenclature can be used for the limiting distribution of either the maximum or the minimum. The Weibull-type distribution of the minimum is the Weibull distribution itself, characterized by a power hazard function (Eq. 2.4) and corresponding survival function of the form $S(x) = \exp(-\alpha x^\gamma)$, where $\alpha > 0$ and $\gamma > 0$ are parameters. The Gumbel-type distribution of the minimum has an exponential hazard function. As we show in the succeeding text (Eqs. 2.19 and 2.20), when restricted to the positive half line, it becomes the Gompertz distribution, also with exponential hazard function (Eq. 2.1) and survival function of the form $S(x) = \exp[-(\lambda/\theta)(e^{\theta x} - 1)]$, where $\lambda > 0$ and θ are parameters.

In order to use the asymptotic distributions (Eqs. 2.8 and 2.9) in practice, we need to pass back and forth between the observed minimum W_n and the shifted and scaled minimum $W_n^* = (W_n - b_n)/a_n$. For any given number w and large positive integer n, let $w_n^* = (w - b_n)/a_n$. Then,

$$P[W_n \leq w] = P\left[W_n \leq a_n w_n^* + b_n\right] = P\left[\frac{W_n - b_n}{a_n} \leq w_n^*\right] = P\left[W_n^* \leq w_n^*\right]. \quad (2.10)$$

Thus, the Weibull-type and Gumbel-type approximations to the distributions of W_n are

$$P[W_n \leq w] \approx G_2\left(w_n^*\right) = 1 - \exp\left[-\left(\frac{w - b_n}{a_n}\right)^\rho\right] \quad w \geq b_n, \rho > 0 \quad \text{(Weibull-type)}, \quad (2.11)$$

$$P[W_n \leq w] \approx G_3\left(w_n^*\right) = 1 - \exp\left[-e^{(w - b_n)/a_n}\right] \quad -\infty < w < \infty \quad \text{(Gumbel-type)}, \quad (2.12)$$

where $\rho > 0$ is a shape parameter. The constant b_n is often viewed as the lower terminus parameter of the approximating Weibull distribution on the right-hand side of Equation 2.11, in which case b_n may be written μ_n or simply as μ when n is fixed in an application. Similarly, the centering constant b_n in Equation 2.12 may be viewed as a location parameter μ_n or μ for the approximating Gumbel distribution. In either approximation, a_n is often viewed as a scale parameter σ_n or σ of the approximating distribution. The Weibull-type and Gumbel-type limiting distributions of the minimum are related by the fact that if X has a Weibull-type distribution of the minimum, $Y = \log(X - \mu)$ has a Gumbel-type distribution of the minimum (Kotz and Nadarajah, 2000, pp. 3–4).

For the application described in Sections 2.2 and 3.2, we will want to use a nonzero lower endpoint w_0 of the parent distribution. To accommodate this shift of origin, we consider the *residual lifetime after* w_0, $R_n = W_n - w_0$. For the Weibull-type distribution, we obtain from Equation 2.11 the survival function

$$P[W_n > w] \approx \exp\left[-\left(\frac{w - b_n}{a_n}\right)^{\rho}\right], \quad w \geq b_n. \tag{2.13}$$

Galambos (1987, p. 58) shows that the values of the lower terminus constants can be chosen as $b_n = \alpha(F)$ and the scaling constants can be chosen as $a_n = \sup\{x : F(x) \leq (1/n)\} - \alpha(F)$. With $b_n = \alpha(F) = w_0$ and letting $\alpha_n = a_n^{-\rho}$ and $\gamma = \rho$, we can write

$$P[W_n > w] \approx \exp\left[-\left(\frac{w - b_n}{a_n}\right)^{\rho}\right] = \exp[-\alpha_n(w - w_0)^{\gamma}], \tag{2.14}$$

so that $P[W_n - w_0 > w - w_0] \approx \exp[-\alpha_n(w - w_0)^{\gamma}]$ or with $w' = w - w_0$,

$$P[W_n - w_0 > w'] \approx \exp(-\alpha_n w'^{\gamma}). \tag{2.15}$$

This shows that $R_n = W_n - w_0$ has an approximate Weibull distribution, because the right-hand side of Equation 2.15 has the form of a scaled Weibull survival function.

For the Gumbel-type distribution, from Equation 2.12, the survival function is

$$P[W_n > w] \approx \exp\left[-e^{(w - b_n)/a_n}\right], \quad -\infty < w < \infty. \tag{2.16}$$

If we let $\theta_n = 1/a_n$ and $\lambda_n = (1/a_n)\exp(-b_n/a_n)$, we can write Equation 2.16 as

$$P[W_n > w] \approx \exp\left(-\frac{\lambda_n}{\theta_n} e^{\theta_n w}\right). \tag{2.17}$$

Then, the hazard function for the approximating distribution is

$$-\frac{d}{dw}\log\left[\exp\left(-\frac{\lambda_n}{\theta_n} e^{\theta_n w}\right)\right] = \frac{d}{dw}\left(\frac{\lambda_n}{\theta_n} e^{\theta_n w}\right) = \lambda_n e^{\theta_n w}, \tag{2.18}$$

which shows that the Gumbel-type distribution, like the Gompertz distribution, has an exponential hazard function. When we restrict attention to the minimum of time-to-event variables, W_n is positive with probability 1, so without loss of generality, we may condition on the event $[W_n > 0]$. Using the same Gumbel-type approximation for the unit probability $P[W_n > 0]$ in the denominator of the conditioning expression, we can insure that the approximation reflects the fact that $P[W_n > w] = 1$ for $w = 0$ by writing

$$P[W_n > w] = P[W_n > w | W_n > 0] = \frac{P[W_n > w]}{P[W_n > 0]} \approx \frac{\exp\left[-(\lambda_n/\theta_n)e^{\theta_n w}\right]}{\exp\left[-(\lambda_n/\theta_n)e^{\theta_n 0}\right]}$$

$$= \exp\left[-\frac{\lambda_n}{\theta_n}\left(e^{\theta_n w} - 1\right)\right], \tag{2.19}$$

which has the form of a Gompertz survival function. More generally, if the initial distribution has lower terminus $w_0 > 0$, then without loss of generality, we may condition on the event $[W_n > w_0]$ and insure that the approximation reflects $P[W_n > w] = 1$ for $w = w_0$ by writing

$$P[W_n > w] = P[W_n > w | W_n > w_0] \approx \frac{\exp\left[-(\lambda_n/\theta_n)e^{\theta_n w}\right]}{\exp\left[-(\lambda_n/\theta_n)e^{\theta_n w_0}\right]} = \exp\left[-\frac{\lambda_n}{\theta_n}\left(e^{\theta_n w} - e^{\theta_n w_0}\right)\right]$$

$$= \exp\left\{-\frac{\lambda_n}{\theta_n}e^{\theta_n w_0}\left[e^{\theta_n(w-w_0)} - 1\right]\right\} = \exp\left[-\frac{\lambda_n'}{\theta_n}\left(e^{\theta_n w'} - 1\right)\right], \qquad (2.20)$$

where $\lambda_n' = \lambda_n e^{\theta_n w_0}$ (i.e., the hazard rate at w_0) and $w' = w - w_0$. Thus, for initial distributions in the Gumbel minimum domain of attraction, the distribution of $R_n = W_n - w_0$ may be approximated by the Gompertz distribution with parameters $\lambda_n' = \lambda_n e^{\theta_n w_0}$ and θ_n, because Equation 2.20 has the form of a Gompertz survival function. We will exhibit explicit choices of a_n and b_n, or equivalently λ_n and θ_n, in Section 2.1.2.

An arbitrary initial distribution, even after suitable standardization, will not necessarily have a nondegenerate limiting distribution of the maximum or the minimum, which is to say that some distributions do not belong to the maximum or minimum domain of attraction of any of the three possible limiting distributions. A discrete distribution such as the Poisson distribution provides an example—there do not exist any constants such that the distribution of W_n^* converges to anything but the degenerate distribution at 0 (David and Nagaraja, 2003, p. 296). Examples of survival distributions in the minimum domain of attraction of the Weibull-type distribution are the exponential and gamma distributions, while the lognormal distribution is an example of a survival distribution in the minimum domain of attraction of the Gumbel-type distribution. The same initial distribution may belong to the minimum domain of attraction of one limiting distribution and the maximum domain of attraction of another limiting distribution. This is the case for the exponential and gamma distributions, which belong to the maximum domain of attraction of the Gumbel-type distribution (Kotz and Nadarajah, 2000, p. 59). With respect to the minimum domains of attraction of the Weibull-type and Gumbel-type limiting distributions, we briefly present some known results in Section 2.1.1. These results provide a theoretical background for the original results then given in Section 2.1.2.

2.1.1 Background to Results

For the i.i.d. case, Gnedenko (1943) derived necessary and sufficient conditions for an initial distribution to be in the minimum and maximum domain of attraction of each of the three types of limiting distributions. Gnedenko's (1943) result for the Gumbel-type distribution was admittedly not obtained in satisfactory form and was improved by de Haan (1970) (David and Nagaraja, 2003, pp. 298–299; Galambos, 1987, pp. 53–59). Still, the necessary and sufficient condition for an initial distribution to be in the domain of attraction of the Gumbel-type distribution is difficult to verify, and a simpler sufficient condition obtained by von Mises (1936) is most useful and widely applied (Barlow and Proschan, 1981, p. 253; David and Nagaraja, 2003, pp. 299–300). We give here, respectively, the necessary and sufficient condition for an initial distribution to be in the minimum domain of attraction of the Weibull-type distribution and the von Mises sufficient condition for an initial distribution to be in the minimum domain of attraction of the Gumbel-type distribution, in a form that is appropriate for time-to-event distributions (Barlow and Proschan, 1981, pp. 240–243).

Theorem 1. (Barlow and Proschan, 1981, p. 241). A distribution $F(x)$ belongs to the minimum domain of attraction of $G_2(x) = 1 - \exp(-x^\rho), \; x \geq 0, \rho > 0$, iff

(a) There exists x_0 such that $F(x_0) = 0$ and $F(x_0 + \varepsilon) > 0$ for all $\varepsilon > 0$.

(b)

$$\lim_{t \downarrow 0} \frac{F(xt + x_0)}{F(t + x_0)} = x^\rho \quad \text{for all } x > 0. \tag{2.21}$$

Theorem 2. (von Mises condition; Barlow and Proschan, 1981, p. 243). Let the distribution $F(x)$ be absolutely continuous with a differentiable density function $f(x)$. Let there exist x_0 such that $F(x_0) = 0$ and $F(x_0 + \varepsilon) > 0$ for all $\varepsilon > 0$, and let

$$\lim_{x \downarrow x_0} \frac{d}{dx} \left[\frac{1}{\phi'(x)} \right] = 0, \quad \text{where } \phi(x) = -\log F(x). \tag{2.22}$$

Then, $F(x)$ belongs to the minimum domain of attraction of $G_3(x) = 1 - \exp(-e^x)$.

Defining $\phi(x) = -\log F(x)$, we have $\phi'(x) = -f(x)/F(x)$ and $1/\phi'(x) = -F(x)/f(x) = (S(x) - 1)/f(x) = 1/h(x) - 1/f(x)$, where $S(x) = 1 - F(x)$ and $h(x) = f(x)/S(x)$ are, respectively, the survival and hazard functions of the initial distribution. Hence, Equation 2.22 can also be expressed in the equivalent form

$$\lim_{x \downarrow x_0} \frac{d}{dx} \left[\frac{-F(x)}{f(x)} \right] = \lim_{x \downarrow x_0} \frac{-f(x)^2 + f'(x)F(x)}{f(x)^2} = \lim_{x \downarrow x_0} \left[-1 + \frac{f'(x)F(x)}{f(x)^2} \right] = 0$$

$$\Rightarrow \lim_{x \downarrow x_0} \left[\frac{f'(x)F(x)}{f(x)^2} \right] = 1. \tag{2.23}$$

Note from Equation 2.23 that $f'(x)$ must eventually become positive as x approaches $\alpha(F) = x_0$ from above in order for the von Mises sufficient condition for the minimum to hold. Thus, $f(x)$ increases in x in a right-neighborhood of $\alpha(F)$, and since $S(x)$

is nonincreasing, the hazard function $h(x) = f(x)/S(x)$ increases in the same right-neighborhood. In the case of the maximum, Galambos and Obretenov (1987, Theorem 3) showed that assuming a nondecreasing hazard function in a left-neighborhood of the upper endpoint of the initial distribution, the von Mises condition for the maximum is both necessary and sufficient. We give here the analogous result for the minimum:

Theorem 3. (Galambos and Obretenov, 1987). Let $N(A) = \{x : \alpha(F) < x < A\}$ be a right-neighborhood of $\alpha(F)$. If there is an $A > \alpha(F)$ such that, on $N(A)$, both $f(x)$ and $f'(x)$ exist, $f'(x) > 0$, and $\phi'(x)$ is nondecreasing, then the von Mises condition (Eq. 2.22) is both necessary and sufficient for $F(x)$ to be in the minimum domain of attraction of the Gumbel-type limiting distribution.

A nondecreasing $\phi'(x)$ implies

$$\phi''(x) = -\frac{d^2}{dx^2} \log F(x) = \frac{d}{dx}\left[\frac{-f(x)}{F(x)}\right] = \frac{-F(x)f'(x) + f(x)^2}{F(x)^2} \geq 0,$$

which is to say, from $(d^2/dx^2)\log F(x) \leq 0$, that any $F(x)$ satisfying this assumption of Theorem 3 is log-concave in a right-neighborhood of $\alpha(F)$. In the next section, we provide an example of a function meeting the von Mises condition for which this assumption does not hold.

When the parent distributions for independent $X_1, X_2, \ldots, X_n$ are not identical, Juncosa (1949) showed that the class of limiting distributions for the minimum is much wider than the three limits for the i.i.d. case. Notwithstanding, we present one of Juncosa's (1949) results for the nonidentically distributed case in which the limiting distribution is the Weibull-type distribution of the minimum. Here, X_k for $k = 1, 2, \ldots, n$ are independent random variables, each with distribution function from the same family of distributions; that is, $F_k(x) = F(\alpha_k x + \beta_k)$, where $\{\alpha_k > 0\}$ and $\{\beta_k\}$ are sequences of constants. In particular, we consider the scale family $F_k(x) = F(\alpha_k x)$ where $F(x)$ has lower endpoint at 0.

Theorem 4. (Juncosa, 1949, Theorem 7, p. 614). Let $F(x)$ be a c.d.f. with $F(0) = 0$ and $F(x) > 0$ for $x > 0$. Suppose that for $x > 0$, there exists a positive number ρ such that $\lim_{t \downarrow 0} F(xt)/F(t) = x^\rho$. Suppose further that $\sum \alpha_k^\rho = \infty$ and $\alpha_n = o\left(\sum_{k=1}^n \alpha_k^\rho\right)$. Then for any $\varepsilon > 0$, there exist $\{a_n\}$ and a number N such that $F(\alpha_k a_n x) < \varepsilon$ for $n > N$ and $k \leq n$, and such that

$$\lim_{n \to \infty} \prod_{k=1}^n [1 - F(\alpha_k a_n x)] = \exp(-x^\rho). \tag{2.24}$$

Galambos (1987, chapter 3) reviewed the results for situations in which the assumption of independent random variables is replaced by less restrictive assumptions, covering stochastic models such as exchangeable random variables, stationary sequences of random variables (including m-dependence and "mixing"), and the so-called E_n-sequence. The results pertain to what new types of limiting distribution are obtained for the extremes under these less restrictive dependence assumptions and what restrictions lead to the same types of limiting distribution as in the i.i.d. case. Gumbel (1958, p. 164) anticipated many of these results: "the distribution of extreme values depends only on the properties of the initial distribution for large [or small] values of the variate where the influence of interdependence may vanish. Therefore, the asymptotic distribution of extremes may still be valid for interdependent observations." We focus on the E_n-sequence here as its relevance to our application, in combination with the results in the next section, will be described in Section 2.2.1. The definition of an E_n-sequence in the subsequent text and the ensuing comments follow Galambos (1987, pp. 211–212).

For a given sequence $X_1, X_2, \ldots, X_n$ of random variables, a set E_n of so-called exceptional pairs of subscripts (i, j), $i < j$, is defined as follows. We place (i, j) into the set E_n if it is not reasonable to assume (or if it fails to hold) that as x_n tends to $\max[\alpha(F_i), \alpha(F_j)]$, $P[X_i < x_n, X_j < x_n]$ is asymptotically $F_i(x_n) F_j(x_n)$, where as before $\alpha(F) = \inf\{x : F(x) > 0\}$ and $F_t(x)$ denotes the distribution function of X_t. Thus, from this definition, if the subscripts $(i_1, i_2, \ldots, i_k)$ are such that no pairs from them are contained in E_n, the events $\{X_{i_t} < x_n\}, t = 1, \ldots, k$, are pairwise asymptotically independent as x_n tends to the largest of $\alpha(F_t)$. Then, $X_1, X_2, \ldots, X_n$ constitute an E_n-sequence if three assumptions are satisfied:

(i) If the subscripts $i(k) = (i_1, i_2, \ldots, i_k)$ contain no pairs from the set E_n, then the difference

$$d_{i(k)}(x_n) = P[X_{i_1} < x_n, X_{i_2} < x_n, \ldots, X_{i_k} < x_n] - \prod_{t=1}^{k} F_{i_t}(x_n) \qquad (2.25)$$

is negligible compared to either of the terms as $x_n \to \sup_{t \geq 1} \alpha(F_t)$.

(ii) If there is exactly one pair (i_s, i_m) among the components of $i(k) = (i_1, i_2, \ldots, i_k)$ that belongs to the set E_n, then

$$P[X_{i_1} < x_n, X_{i_2} < x_n, \ldots, X_{i_k} < x_n] \leq \eta_k P[X_{i_s} < x_n, X_{i_m} < x_n] \prod_{\substack{t=1 \\ t \neq m, s}}^{k} F_{i_t}(x_n), \qquad (2.26)$$

where η_k is a constant.

(iii) The number N of the elements of the set E_n is of smaller order of magnitude than n^2, or $N(n) = o(n^2)$.

Note that no assumption was made, in the definition of either the set E_n or the E_n-sequence, that $X_1, X_2, \ldots, X_n$ are identically distributed. If $(i_1, i_2, \ldots, i_k)$ contains no pairs of the set E_n, it is assumed in (i) that pairwise independence can be extended to independence. If $(i_1, i_2, \ldots, i_k)$ contains exactly one pair of the set E_n, assumption (ii) is less strict than asymptotic independence, because the constant η_k can be arbitrarily large. Then, if $(i_1, i_2, ..., i_k)$ contains more than one pair of E_n, there is no assumption on the interdependence of $(X_1, X_2, ..., X_n)$. This is to say that if we consider a subset of the original set of random variables that contains at least two pairs about which we could not accept asymptotic independence, this subset can have an arbitrary structure. Galambos (1987, pp. 211–212) lastly argues that assumption (iii) is "a natural one," because the number of all pairs of the subscripts 1, 2, ..., n is $\binom{n}{2} = (n^2 - n)/2$, which is of the order of n^2. Thus, assumption (iii) only requires that the number of elements of the set E_n be of smaller order of magnitude than the maximum possible number. Then, for an E_n-sequence, the following result shows that, under minor assumptions, the extreme value distributions coincide with those in the i.i.d. case if $X_1, X_2, ..., X_n$ are identically distributed:

Theorem 5. (Galambos, 1987, pp. 212–213). Let X_1, X_2, ..., X_n be an E_n-sequence. Let x_n be such that as $n \to +\infty$,

$$\sum_{j=1}^{n} F_j(x_n) \to a \quad 0 < a < +\infty. \tag{2.27}$$

Let us assume that there is a constant K such that for all j and n, $nF_j(x_n) \leq K$. Let, finally,

$$\lim_{n \to +\infty} \sum_{(i,j) \in E_n} P[X_i < x_n, X_j < x_n] = 0. \tag{2.28}$$

Then, as $n \to +\infty$,

$$\lim P[W_n < x_n] = 1 - e^{-a}. \tag{2.29}$$

In particular, if $F_j(x) = F(x)$ for all j, then the theory of the classical extreme value theory for the i.i.d. case applies to W_n.

2.1.2   Original Results

In this section, we present some useful results on the asymptotic behavior of the minimum of time-to-event random variables that, to our knowledge, have not appeared in the extreme value theory literature. Detailed proofs are provided in Appendix A. In the following, we express Equation 2.22 in a form that only involves the survival function. From $\phi(x) = -\log[1 - S(x)]$,

$$\phi'(x) = \frac{S'(x)}{1 - S(x)} = \frac{S'(x)/S(x)}{[1 - S(x)]/S(x)} = \frac{S(x)}{1 - S(x)} \frac{d}{dx} \log S(x), \tag{2.30}$$

$$\frac{d}{dx}\left[\frac{1}{\phi'(x)}\right] = \frac{1}{S(x)}\left\{-1 - \frac{1 - S(x)(d^2/dx^2)\log S(x)}{[(d/dx)\log S(x)]^2}\right\}. \tag{2.31}$$

Since $S(x_0) = 1$, the limit of the expression in Equation 2.31 as $x \to x_0$ is equal to 0 if and only if

$$\lim_{x\downarrow x_0} \frac{[1-S(x)](d^2/dx^2)[-\log S(x)]}{[(d/dx)\log S(x)]^2} = 1.\qquad(2.32)$$

By re-expressing the left-hand side in Equation 2.32 as $\lim_{x\downarrow x_0}[1-S(x)]$ $[S'(x)^2 - S(x)S''(x)]/S'(x)^2$, we notice that if $S'(x_0)$ and $S''(x_0)$ are finite, and $S'(x_0) \neq 0$, this limit is 0, in which case Equation 2.32 does not hold. Hence, if the conditions of Theorem 2 hold, $S'(x)$ evaluated at x_0 must be 0. Generally, we prove the following corollary of the von Mises condition for the minimum:

Corollary to Theorem 2. Let the survival function $S(x)$ be infinitely differentiable at $x = x_0$ and assume that $S(x_0) = 1$ and $S(x) < 1$ for $x > x_0$. If $S(x)$ satisfies the von Mises sufficient condition for an initial distribution to be in the minimum domain of attraction of the Gumbel-type limiting distribution, then all its derivatives at x_0 are equal to 0; that is, $S(x)$ is infinitely differentiable or C^∞ at x_0 but is not analytic there.

From this corollary, the von Mises condition for the minimum implies that the survival function $S(x)$ has all derivatives at x_0 equal to 0. This is to say that $S(x)$ (hence $F(x)$ too) is "infinitely flat" at the lower endpoint of the distribution, which we will also refer to simply as *flat*. Under certain assumptions, the converse is true as well; that is, if $F(x)$ is flat at the lower endpoint of the distribution, then the von Mises condition for the minimum is met.

Theorem 6. (Converse of the Corollary to Theorem 2). Let $F(x)$ be a c.d.f. that is C^∞ in a right-neighborhood of x_0 with $F(x_0) = 0$ and $F(x) > 0$ for $x > x_0$. Let $\phi(x) = -\log F(x)$ and define $\psi(x) = -1/\phi'(x)$. Assume that the limit of $\phi'(x)$ exists and equals $-\infty$ as $x \to x_0$, so that $\psi(x) \to 0$ as $x \to x_0$. Assume further that $\psi'(x)$ is continuous at x_0, so that $\lim_{x\downarrow x_0}\psi'(x)$ exists and equals $\psi'(x_0) = \lim_{x\downarrow x_0}(\psi(x)-\psi(x_0))/(x-x_0)$. If $F(x)$ has all derivatives at $x = x_0$ equal to 0, then $\lim_{x\downarrow x_0}\psi'(x) = 0$; that is, the von Mises sufficient condition for $F(x)$ to be in the minimum domain of attraction of the Gumbel-type limiting distribution holds.

Remark 2.1. The function $\psi(x)$ plays an important role in determining what choices of constants a_n and b_n can be used for approximating the distribution of W_n with Gumbel-type limiting distributions. For the simplest illustration, let $F(x)$ satisfy the conditions of Theorem 2, let $b_n = F^{-1}(1/n)$, and let $a_n = \psi(b_n)$. We now show that $W_n^* = (W_n - b_n)/a_n$ has a limiting Gumbel-type distribution. Let w^* be a fixed constant. We have $P[W_n^* > w^*] = P[W_n > a_n w^* + b_n] = P[X_i > a_n w^* + b_n$ for each $i]$, so

$$P[W_n^* > w^*] = [1 - F(a_n w^* + b_n)]^n = \left[1 - \frac{F(a_n w^* + b_n)}{nF(b_n)}\right]^n.\qquad(2.33)$$

Thus, $P\left[W_n^* > w^*\right] \to \exp\left(-e^{w^*}\right)$ as $n \to \infty$ if we have that $F(a_n w^* + b_n)/$ $F(b_n) = e^{w^*} + o(1)$. But taking logarithms and applying a Taylor expansion around b_n,

$$\log F(a_n w^* + b_n) - \log F(b_n) = \phi(b_n) - \phi(b_n + a_n w^*) = -\phi'(b_n + t a_n w^*) a_n w^* \quad (2.34)$$

for some number $0 < t < 1$, so that

$$\log F(a_n w^* + b_n) - \log F(b_n) = \frac{a_n w^*}{\psi(b_n + t a_n w^*)}, \quad (2.35)$$

and with another Taylor expansion to write

$$\psi(b_n + t a_n w^*) = \psi(b_n) + \psi'(b_n + t' t a_n w^*) t a_n w^* \quad (2.36)$$

for some other number $0 < t' < 1$, we have

$$\log F(a_n w^* + b_n) - \log F(b_n) = \frac{a_n w^*}{a_n + \psi'(b_n + t' t a_n w^*) t a_n w^*}$$

$$= \frac{w^*}{1 + \psi'(b_n + t' t a_n w^*) t w^*} = w^* + o(1), \quad (2.37)$$

since $\psi'(x) \to 0$ by the von Mises condition.

We assumed the continuity of $\psi'(x)$ at x_0 in Theorem 6 in order to rule out certain pathological cases that also violate the assumptions of Theorem 3. The following provides an example of a function $\psi(x)$ for which $F(x_0) = 0$, $F(x) > 0$ for $x > x_0$, and $F(x)$ is flat at $x = x_0 = 0$, but for which the assumption that $\lim_{x \downarrow x_0} \psi'(x)$ exists is not true:

$$\psi(x) = x^2 \left[x + \sin^2\left(\frac{1}{x}\right)\right]. \quad (2.38)$$

To show that, we obtain an upper bound for $F(x)$ as follows:

$$\phi(x) = \int_x^\infty \frac{1}{\psi(u)} du = \int_x^\infty \frac{du}{u^2[u + \sin^2(1/u)]} \geq \int_x^\infty \frac{du}{u^2[u+1]} \geq \frac{1}{2} \int_x^\infty \frac{du}{u^2} + \text{const}$$

$$= \frac{1}{2} \left(\frac{-1}{u}\right)\bigg|_x^1 + \text{const} = \frac{1}{2x} + \text{const}, \quad (2.39)$$

in which case

$$F(x) = \exp[-\phi(x)] \leq k \exp\left(-\frac{1}{2x}\right), \quad (2.40)$$

with $k > 0$. We show that this implies that $F(x)$ is flat at 0 through the following argument: $F(0) = 0$, so by induction, assuming $F^{(j)}(0) = 0$ for $j = 0, \ldots, r$,

$$\frac{F^{(r+1)}(0)}{(r+1)!} = \lim_{x \downarrow 0} \frac{F(x)}{x^{r+1}} \geq 0, \tag{2.41}$$

but also

$$\lim_{x \downarrow 0} \frac{F(x)}{x^{r+1}} \leq k \lim_{x \downarrow 0} \frac{e^{-1/2x}}{x^{r+1}} = 0. \tag{2.42}$$

Then, from Equations 2.41 and 2.42,

$$\frac{F^{(r+1)}(0)}{(r+1)!} = \lim_{x \downarrow 0} \frac{F(x)}{x^{r+1}} = 0 \Rightarrow F^{(r+1)}(0) = 0, \tag{2.43}$$

which shows that $F(x)$ is flat at 0. But $\lim_{x \downarrow 0} \psi'(x)$ does not exist, because

$$\psi'(x) = x^2 \left[1 + \sin\left(\frac{2}{x}\right)\left(-\frac{1}{x^2}\right) \right] + \left[x + \sin^2\left(\frac{1}{x}\right) \right] 2x$$

$$= 3x^2 + 2x \sin^2\left(\frac{1}{x}\right) - \sin\left(\frac{2}{x}\right) \tag{2.44}$$

and the term $\sin(2/x)$ does not have a limit as $x \to 0$. For Equation 2.38, Figure 2.2 shows plots of $\psi(x)$, $\phi(x)$, $F(x)$, and their derivatives, with numerical integration used for $\phi(x)$, $F(x)$, and $F'(x) = f(x)$, focusing on the behavior of these functions close to 0. The widely wobbling behavior of $\psi'(x)$ close to 0 accounts for the fact that the right-hand limit of $\psi'(x)$ at $x_0 = 0$ does not exist, while this is not the case for $\psi(x)$, which approaches 0 as $x \to 0$.

We also show that Equation 2.38 divided by 6,

$$\psi(x) = \frac{x^2[x + \sin^2(1/x)]}{6}, \tag{2.45}$$

provides an example of a function for which the assumption in Theorem 3 of a nonde-creasing $\phi'(x)$ on $N(A)$ does not hold, with a c.d.f. $F(x)$ satisfying the following properties:

   (i) $F(0) = 0$, $F(x) > 0$ for $x > 0$, and F is flat at 0;
  (ii) $F''(x) = f'(x) > 0$ in a right-neighborhood of 0; but
 (iii) F is not log-concave in a right-neighborhood of 0 or, equivalently, any of the following:
    (a) $\phi'(x)$ is not nondecreasing in any neighborhood of 0;
    (b) $\phi''(x) < 0$ infinitely often in any neighborhood of 0;
    (c) $\psi(x)$ is not nondecreasing in any neighborhood of 0;
    (d) $\psi'(x) < 0$ infinitely often in any neighborhood of 0.

Property (i) follows as before (Eqs. 2.39 through 2.43), since the constant 1/6 does not affect the argument. For property (ii), write

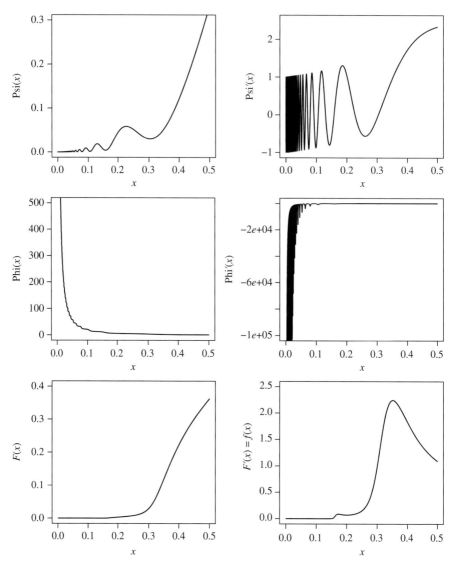

FIGURE 2.2 Example for which the assumption of Theorem 6 that the right-hand limit of $\psi'(x)$ at the lower endpoint of the distribution exists does not hold.

$$F(x) = \exp\left[-\int_x^\infty \frac{1}{\psi(u)}\,du\right] \tag{2.46}$$

so that

$$F'(x) = \exp\left[-\int_x^\infty \frac{1}{\psi(u)}\,du\right]\frac{d}{dx}\left[-\int_x^\infty \frac{1}{\psi(u)}\,du\right] = \frac{F(x)}{\psi(x)}, \tag{2.47}$$

and differentiating again, and using the previous expression for $F'(x)$,

$$F''(x) = \frac{\psi(x)F'(x) - F(x)\psi'(x)}{\psi(x)^2} = \frac{\psi(x)F(x)/\psi(x) - F(x)\psi'(x)}{\psi(x)^2} = \frac{F(x)}{\psi(x)^2}[1 - \psi'(x)].$$

(2.48)

Therefore, $F''(x) > 0$ in a right-neighborhood of 0 iff $\psi'(x) < 1$. But

$$\psi'(x) = \frac{3x^2 + 2x\sin^2(1/x) - \sin(2/x)}{6},$$

(2.49)

and we notice that for $x < 1$,

$$3x^2 + 2x\sin^2\left(\frac{1}{x}\right) \le 3x^2 + 2x < 5,$$

(2.50)

while $-\sin(2/x)$ is never greater than 1. Hence, the numerator in Equation 2.49 is less than 6, so that $\psi'(x) < 1$ and thus $F''(x) > 0$ for any $x < 1$. For property (iii), we only need to show that $\psi'(x)$ takes negative values infinitely often as x approaches 0. Let i take on integer values $i = 1, 2, 3, \ldots$ and consider values of x given by

$$x = \frac{4}{(4i + 1)\pi} \Rightarrow \frac{2}{x} = \frac{(4i + 1)\pi}{2} \Rightarrow \sin\left(\frac{2}{x}\right) = 1.$$

(2.51)

Then, for such values of x,

$$\psi'(x) = \frac{3x^2 + 2x\sin^2(1/x) - 1}{6},$$

(2.52)

which is less than 0 because

$$x = \frac{4}{(4i + 1)\pi} \le \frac{4}{5\pi} < \frac{1}{3}$$

(2.53)

and so $3x^2 + 2x\sin^2(1/x) - 1 < 3(1/3)^2 + 2(1/3) - 1 = 0$.

The examples in Equations 2.38 and 2.45 demonstrate that the assumptions of Theorems 3 and 6 are not trivial from a mathematical point of view. Although $F(x)$ and $F'(x) = f(x)$ are apparently smooth close to 0 in Figure 2.2 (lower panel), the wobbling behavior of $\psi(x)$, $\phi(x)$, and their derivatives close to 0 indicates that periodic irregularities also occur for $F(x)$ and $F'(x) = f(x)$, even if we cannot observe them in the presented plots. Despite the nontrivial mathematical meaning of the assumptions of Theorems 3 and 6, such irregular behavior in a neighborhood of the lower endpoint would make the initial distribution functions corresponding to Equations 2.38 and 2.45 less plausible for biological phenomena in general and our application in particular, as we will describe starting in Section 2.2.1.

Henceforth in this section, we take the lower endpoint of the initial distribution to be 0; that is, $\alpha(F) = x_0 = 0$. Assuming that $F(0) = 0$, $F(x) > 0$ for $x > 0$, and that $F(x)$ has infinitely many right derivatives at 0, we define:

(i) F is *infinitely flat at 0* iff

$$F^{(p)}(0) = 0 \quad \text{for all positive integers } p. \tag{2.54}$$

(ii) F is *slowly varying at 0* iff

$$\lim_{t \downarrow 0} \frac{F(xt)}{F(t)} = 1 \quad \text{for all } x \text{ in a neighborhood of 1.} \tag{2.55}$$

(iii) F is *regularly varying at 0* with exponent ρ iff

$$\lim_{t \downarrow 0} \frac{F(xt)}{F(t)} = x^\rho \quad \text{for all } x \text{ in a neighborhood of 1.} \tag{2.56}$$

Any regularly varying $F(x)$ can be written as

$$F(x) = x^\rho L(x), \tag{2.57}$$

where $L(x)$ is slowly varying, because if $F(x)$ is regularly varying and $L(x) = F(x)/x^\rho$, then

$$\lim_{t \downarrow 0} \frac{L(xt)}{L(t)} = \lim_{t \downarrow 0} \frac{F(xt)}{x^\rho t^\rho} \frac{t^\rho}{F(t)} = \frac{1}{x^\rho} \lim_{t \downarrow 0} \frac{F(xt)}{F(t)} \frac{x^\rho}{x^\rho} = 1. \tag{2.58}$$

We illustrate these definitions with the following prototypical examples of an infinitely flat function, a slowly varying function, and a regularly varying function with exponent ρ:

$$F(x) = e^{-1/x} \quad 0 < x < \infty \quad \text{(infinitely flat at 0),} \tag{2.59}$$

$$F(x) = -\frac{1}{\log x} \quad 0 < x < e^{-1} \quad \text{(slowly varying at 0),} \tag{2.60}$$

$$F(x) = -\frac{x^\rho}{\log x} \quad 0 < x < x^* \quad \text{(regularly varying at 0),} \tag{2.61}$$

where x^* is such that $F(x^*) = 1$. Define $F(0) = 0$ in each case. For the prototype of flat function (Eq. 2.59), Figure 2.3 shows plots of $\psi(x)$, $\phi(x)$, $F(x)$, and their derivatives, focusing on their behavior close to 0. Since the assumptions of Theorems 3 and 6 hold in relation to Equation 2.59, these plots provide a contrast with those in Figure 2.2. Figure 2.4 shows plots of the three prototypes (Eqs. 2.59–2.61) giving a visual sense of their behavior close to 0. In the next results, we provide a different way to see that the Gumbel-type distribution of the minimum arises from initial time-to-event distributions that are flat at the lower endpoint of the distribution.

The necessary and sufficient condition for an initial distribution to be in the minimum domain of attraction of the Weibull-type distribution (Eq. 2.21) becomes, for $x_0 = 0$,

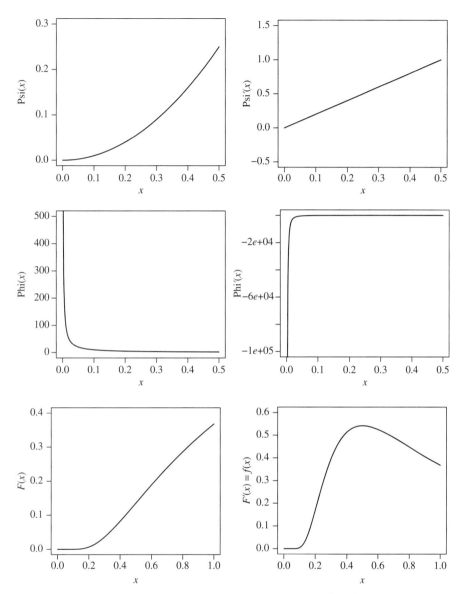

FIGURE 2.3 Prototype of flat function; plots of $\psi(x)=x^2$, $\psi'(x)=2x$, $\phi(x)=1/x$, $\phi'(x)=-1/x^2$, $F(x)=e^{-1/x}$, and $F'(x)=f(x)=e^{-1/x}/x^2$ (compare to Fig. 2.2).

$$\lim_{t\downarrow 0}\frac{F(xt)}{F(t)}=x^\rho \quad \text{for some } \rho \text{ with } 0<\rho<\infty. \tag{2.62}$$

This is to say, from Equation 2.56, that an initial distribution $F(x)$ in the minimum domain of attraction of the Weibull-type distribution is regularly varying at 0 with exponent $0<\rho<\infty$. Thus, by showing that such regularly varying $F(x)$ cannot have all derivatives

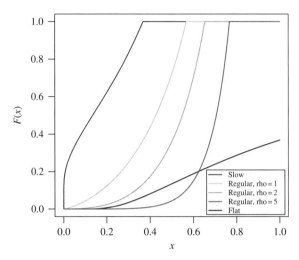

FIGURE 2.4 Plots of the prototypes of infinitely flat, slowly varying, and regularly varying functions at 0; for regularly varying function, we use values of the exponent $\rho = 1$, 2, and 5.

equal to 0 at $x = 0$, that is, there exists some integer i such that $F^{(i)}(0) \neq 0$, we will be proving that a c.d.f. in the minimum domain of attraction of the Weibull-type distribution cannot be flat at 0. It follows that if an initial distribution is flat at 0 and has a nondegenerate limiting distribution of the minimum, the limiting distribution cannot be the Weibull-type; hence, the initial distribution must be in the minimum domain of attraction of the Gumbel-type distribution. To do this, we start with a c.d.f. $F(x)$ that is infinitely differentiable in a right-neighborhood of the lower endpoint at $x = 0$ and define $L(x) = F(x)/x^\rho$. We prove the proposition that if $F(x)$ is flat at 0, $L(x)$ must be flat at 0 too. Then, we prove that if $L(x)$ is slowly varying at 0 with $L(0) = 0$ and $L(x) > 0$ for $x > 0$, $L(x)$ is not flat at 0. By combining these results, we obtain the conclusion that a regularly varying $F(x)$ cannot be flat at 0. We formally state the results:

Proposition. Let $F(x)$ be a c.d.f. that is C^∞ in a right-neighborhood of 0 with $F(0) = 0$ and $F(x) > 0$ for $x > 0$. For $x > 0$, define $L(x) = F(x)/x^\rho$ for some positive constant ρ. Suppose $F(x)$ has all derivatives at $x = 0$ equal to 0. Then, the right-hand limits at $x = 0$ of $L(x)$ and all its derivatives exist and equal 0.

Theorem 7. Assume $L(x)$ is slowly varying at 0 with $L(0) = 0$ and $L(x) > 0$ for $x > 0$. Then, $L'(0) = \infty$; hence, $L(x)$ is not flat at 0.

Remark 2.2. The definition of slowly and regularly varying functions at 0 stems from the notion of regular variation at infinity introduced by Karamata (1930), which has found many applications in probability theory and the statistical theory of extreme values (Feller, 1966, pp. 268–272; de Haan and Ferreira, 2006, app. B). A representation theorem: function $Z(x)$ is slowly varying at infinity iff it is of the form

$$Z(x) = \alpha(x) \exp\left[\int_1^x \frac{\varepsilon(u)}{u} du\right], \tag{2.63}$$

where $\varepsilon(x)$ is continuous with $\varepsilon(x) \to 0$ and $\alpha(x) \to c$ $(0 < c < \infty)$ as $x \to \infty$ (Feller, 1966, pp. 272–276; Karamata, 1930, 1933; Korevaar et al., 1949). Using the change of variable involving the reciprocal of x, we obtain the analogous representation for $L(x)$ slowly varying at 0, $L(x) = a(x) \exp\left[\int_x^1 (g(u)/u) du\right]$, where $g(x) = \varepsilon(1/x)$ is continuous with $g(x) \to 0$ and $a(x) = \alpha(1/x) \to c$ $(0 < c < \infty)$ as $x \to 0$ (Polfeldt, 1970; Qualls and Watanabe, 1972). We note, however, that there is an arbitrariness in the choice of the upper limit of integration, since it does not affect the behavior of $L(x)$ near 0. We thus write the representation for $L(x)$ with the upper limit of integration given by some constant ω,

$$L(x) = a(x) \exp\left[\int_x^\omega \frac{g(u)}{u} du\right], \tag{2.64}$$

where $g(x)$ is continuous for $x > 0$ with $g(x) \to 0$ and $a(x) \to c$ $(0 < c < \infty)$ as $x \to 0$. Any function $L(x)$ that is slowly varying at 0 with $L(0) = 0$ must have $g(x)$ satisfying

(i) $g(0) = 0$, (ii) $(g(x)/x) \to -\infty$ as $x \to 0$, and (iii) $\int_x^\omega (g(u)/u) du \to -\infty$ as $x \to 0$.

Any $g(x)$ satisfying (i)–(iii) approaches 0 more slowly than $-x^p/(-\log x)^q$ or even $-x^p$, where $p \neq 0$ (i.e., $g(x)$ cannot contain a power of x). Functions satisfying (i)–(iii) are, for example,

$$g(x) = \frac{-[\log(-\log x)]^p}{(-\log x)^q} \quad \text{for } p \geq 0 \text{ and } 0 < q \leq 1. \tag{2.65}$$

As an explicit example, consider taking $p = 0$ and $q = 1$ in Equation 2.65, giving $g(x) = 1/\log x$, and taking $a(x) = 1$. Then, from Equation 2.64,

$$L(x) = a(x) \exp\left[\int_x^\omega \frac{g(u)}{u} du\right] = \exp\left[\int_x^\omega \frac{1}{u \log u} du\right] = \exp\left[-\int_x^\omega \frac{du}{u(-\log u)}\right]$$

$$= \exp\left[\int_{-\log x}^{-\log \omega} \frac{1}{v} dv\right] = \exp\left[\log v \big|_{-\log x}^{-\log \omega}\right] = \frac{\text{const}}{-\log x}. \tag{2.66}$$

The prototypical example (Eq. 2.60) corresponds to const $= -\log \omega = 1 \Rightarrow \omega = 1/e$.

To summarize the previous results for the i.i.d. case, if the initial distribution of i.i.d. time-to-event random variables is flat at the lower endpoint of the distribution, under some reasonable smoothness assumptions, the limiting distribution of the minimum is the Gumbel-type distribution, and under other assumptions, it cannot

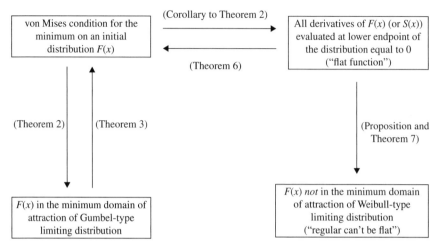

FIGURE 2.5 Diagram summarizing results on the asymptotic behavior of the minimum of time-to-event random variables for the i.i.d. case, starting from the von Mises sufficient condition for the minimum (Theorem 2). Other arrows represent the relations established by corollary to Theorem 2 ("von Mises implies flat"), Theorem 6 ("flat implies von Mises"), Theorem 3 ("von Mises also necessary"), and the combination of the proposition ("if regular is flat, slow must be flat too") and Theorem 7 ("slow can't be flat"). The results involve different assumptions; for example, in Theorem 6, we assume that the limit of $\phi'(x)$ exists and equals $-\infty$ as $x \to x_0$ and $\psi'(x)$ is continuous at x_0, where $\psi(x) = -1/\phi'(x)$ and $\phi(x) = -\log F(x)$, and in Theorem 3, we assume a nondecreasing $\phi'(x)$ in a right-neighborhood of the lower endpoint of the distribution.

belong to the minimum domain of attraction of the Weibull-type distribution. Given the different assumptions, we consider these results complementary. Figure 2.5 diagrammatically presents these results.

The theorems summarized in Figure 2.5 do not explicitly convey the quality of the asymptotic approximation by the Gumbel/Gompertz distribution to the exact distribution of the minimum. Suppose we were to obtain the exact c.d.f. of the minimum of n i.i.d. random variables whose parent distribution is a flat function, and compare that graphically to the approximating Gompertz distribution obtained with an appropriate choice of a_n and b_n. We do that here in two ways, but we note initially that in the following graphs, as well as in several graphs from the data analysis in Section 4.5, the functions are plotted over abscissas 10 years older than the values actually used to obtain the ordinate from the functions. We do this because, for reasons that will become clear in this and the next chapter, we analyze the *residual* lifetime after age 10 years, yet we wish to plot the graphs in terms of actual age. Thus, if $f(t)$ denotes a function for residual lifetime $t > 0$, the graphs display a plot of $(x, f(x-10))$ in terms of actual age $x > 10$.

First, we start with a given flat initial distribution and obtain the exact and approximating Gompertz distribution of the minimum for $n = 100$, 500, and 1000 (Fig. 2.6). To concentrate the density functions for the minimum in the age range

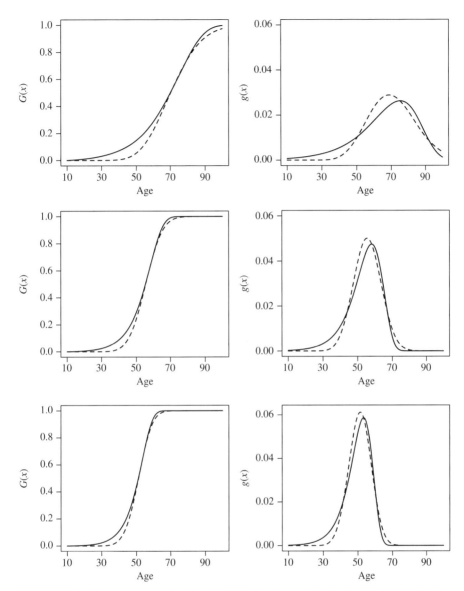

FIGURE 2.6 Gompertz approximation (solid line) and exact distribution (dashed line) of the minimum of i.i.d. random variables, whose parent distribution is a fixed scaled prototype flat function, for $n = 100$, 500, and 1000 (first, second, and third rows of graphs, respectively). Column of graphs at the left gives the c.d.f. and at the right gives the p.d.f. See text for details.

10–90 years, we used a scaled version of the prototype flat distribution, namely, $F(x) = e^{-300/x}$. For the Gompertz approximation, we used $b_n = 300/\log n$ and $a_n = 300/(\log n)^2$ from the Lemma in Appendix A (see also Remark A.1). We can see in Figure 2.6 that the quality of the approximation improves with increasing n and is reasonably good for $n = 500$ and 1000. Second, we fix the approximating Gompertz distribution of the minimum and obtain the corresponding parameters for an extended version of the prototype flat initial distribution containing scale and shape parameters, from which we then obtain the exact distribution of the minimum for $n = 100$, 500, and 1000 (Fig. 2.7). To make this illustration relevant to our application, we use estimates of the Gompertz parameters λ and θ from our data analysis in Section 4.5 (first column in Table 4.5). The initial flat distribution is given by $F(x) = e^{-(\sigma/x)^{\rho}}$, where $\sigma > 0$ and $\rho > 0$ are the scale and shape parameters, respectively. (The reader may check that $F(x)$ is flat with $\psi(x) = (x^{\rho+1})/(\rho\sigma^{\rho})$.) For given λ and θ, we obtain σ and ρ from $\rho = [\log (\theta/\lambda)]/\log n$ and $\sigma = (\log n)^{1/\rho}[\log (\theta/\lambda)]/\theta$. As can be seen in Figure 2.7, the quality of the approximation in this case is already reasonably good for $n = 100$. Upon careful inspection, one can also see that the approximation improves with increasing n as the exact distribution moves slightly toward the fixed approximation.

We next present results that show that we can somehow relax the requirement of identical initial distributions and still obtain the Gumbel-type and Weibull-type limiting distributions of the minimum. First, we present two results with respect to the Gumbel-type distribution of the minimum, which refer to initial distributions from a family of flat functions at 0 obtained by incorporating scale and shape parameters into our prototype example of a flat function (Eq. 2.59). Then, we complement Juncosa's (1949) result regarding the scale parameter of a family of initial distributions in the minimum domain of attraction of the Weibull-type distribution (Theorem 4) with a result regarding the shape parameter.

Theorem 8. Let $F_i(x) = \exp[-(\sigma_i/x)^{\rho}] = \exp(-\tau_i/x^{\rho})$ for $i = 1, 2, \ldots$, where $\sigma_i > 0$ is a scale parameter, $\tau_i = \sigma_i^{\rho} > 0$, and $\rho > 0$ is a shape parameter, such that $F_i(0) = 0$, $F_i(x) > 0$ for $x > 0$, and $\psi_i'(x) \to 0$ as $x \to 0$ for all i (von Mises condition), where $\psi_i(x) = -1/\phi_i'(x)$ and $\phi_i(x) = -\log F_i(x)$. Assume that, after reordering indices if necessary, there exists a function $\tau : [0,1] \to \Re^{+}$, which is nondecreasing and continuous except possibly for countably many jumps, such that for each n, $\tau_i = \tau(i/n)$ for $i = 1, 2, \ldots, n$. Let $G(\tau)$ denote the induced c.d.f. for τ, such that for any measurable function v,

$$\int_0^1 v(\tau(u))du = \int_{\tau(0)}^{\infty} v(\tau)dG(\tau).$$ Assume further that the support of $G(\tau)$ has lower endpoint equal to $\tau_0 > 0$ with $g(\tau_0) = G'(\tau_0) \neq 0$ for continuous τ or $dG(\tau_0) \neq 0$ for discrete τ. Then, there exist constants a_n and b_n such that with $W_n = \min\{X_1, X_2, \ldots, X_n\}$ and independent $X_i \sim F_i$, we have, for any fixed w^*,

$$P[W_n > a_n w^* + b_n] \to \exp(-e^{w^*}) \text{ as } n \to \infty. \tag{2.67}$$

Theorem 9. Let $F_i(x) = \exp[-(\sigma_i/x)^{\rho_i}] = \exp(-\tau_i/x^{\rho_i})$, where $\sigma_i > 0$ is a scale parameter and $\rho_i > 0$ is a shape parameter with $\tau_i = \sigma_i^{\rho_i}$ for $i = 1, 2$, such that $F_i(0) = 0$, $F_i(x) > 0$ for $x > 0$, and the von Mises condition holds, that is, $\psi_i'(x) \to 0$ as $x \to 0$, where $\psi_i(x) = -1/\phi_i'(x)$ and $\phi_i(x) = -\log F_i(x)$. Suppose we have a proportion n_i/n of n independent observations from $F_i(x)$, and assume

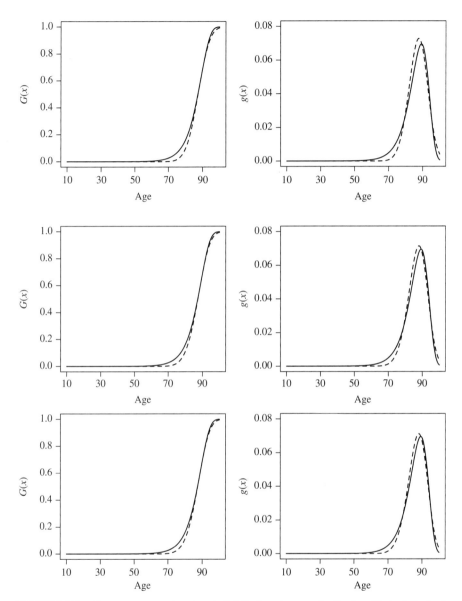

FIGURE 2.7 Gompertz approximation (solid line) and exact distribution (dashed line) of the minimum of i.i.d. random variables, whose parent distribution is the prototype flat function with scale and shape parameters corresponding to the parameters of a fixed Gompertz approximation, for $n = 100$, 500, and 1000 (first, second, and third rows of graphs, respectively). Column of graphs at the left gives the c.d.f. and at the right gives the p.d.f. See text for details.

$$\#\{k : X_k \sim F_1(x)\}/n \to p_1 \text{ as } n \to \infty \text{ and } p_1 > 0. \tag{2.68}$$

Let the normalizing coefficients be $b_n = F_1^{-1}(1/n)$ and $a_n = \psi_1(b_n)$. Then, if $\rho_2 > \rho_1$, with $W_n = \min\{X_1, X_2, \ldots, X_n\}$, we have

$$P[W_n > a_n w^* + b_n] \to \exp\left(-p_1 e^{w^*}\right) \text{ as } n \to \infty; \tag{2.69}$$

that is, the limiting distribution of $W_n^* = (W_n - b_n)/a_n$ is a member of the general two-parameter family of extreme value distributions with survival function $\exp\left[-(\lambda/\theta)e^{\theta w^*}\right]$, whose conditional distribution given that $W_n > 0$ is a member of the general two-parameter family of Gompertz distributions with hazard function of the exponential form.

Theorem 10. Let $F_i(x) = x^{\rho_i}L(x)$ for $i = 1, 2$, where $L(x)$ is slowly varying at 0 and $\rho_i > 0$ is a shape parameter. Suppose we have a proportion n_i/n of n independent observations from $F_i(x)$, and assume

$$\#\{k : X_k \sim F_1(x)\}/n \to p_1 \text{ as } n \to \infty \text{ and } p_1 > 0. \tag{2.70}$$

Let a_n be such that $F_1(a_n) = 1/n$; that is, $a_n = F_1^{-1}(1/n)$. Then, if $\rho_2 > \rho_1$, with $W_n = \min\{X_1, X_2, \ldots, X_n\}$, we have

$$P[W_n > a_n x] \to \exp(-p_1 x^{\rho_1}) \text{ as } n \to \infty; \tag{2.71}$$

that is, the limiting distribution of W_n/a_n is a member of the general two-parameter family of Weibull distributions with survival function $\exp(-\alpha x^\gamma)$ and power hazard function.

Theorems 8–10, along with Theorem 4 (Juncosa, 1949), extend the results for the i.i.d. case summarized in Figure 2.5 to the nonidentically distributed case. While Theorems 4 and 8 allow for infinitely many values of the scale parameter, the results of Theorems 9 and 10 refer to two values of the shape parameter ρ but are readily generalizable to any finite number of shape parameters. A result analogous to Theorem 10 can be obtained if, under the framework of the i.i.d. case, we take the initial distribution to be a finite mixture of regularly varying functions with different shape parameters. That is, $F(x) = \sum_{i=1}^{j} p_i F_i(x)$, where p_i is the mixing proportion for component distribution $F_i(x) = x^{\rho_i}L(x)$, where $L(x)$ is slowly varying at 0 and $\rho_i > 0$ is a shape parameter. Then, the following development shows that Equation 2.21 holds with $\rho = \min(\rho_i)$, in which we use rank notation such that $\min(\rho_i) = \rho_{(1)} < \rho_{(2)} < \cdots < \max(\rho_i)$ and $p_{(1)}, p_{(2)}, \ldots, p_{(j)}$ are the mixing proportions corresponding to the shape parameters $\rho_{(1)}, \rho_{(2)}, \ldots, \rho_{(j)}$, respectively:

$$\lim_{t\downarrow 0}\frac{F(xt)}{F(t)} = \lim_{t\downarrow 0}\frac{\sum_{i=1}^{j}p_{i}F_{i}(xt)}{\sum_{i=1}^{j}p_{i}F_{i}(t)} = \lim_{t\downarrow 0}\frac{\sum_{i=1}^{j}p_{i}x^{\rho_{i}}t^{\rho_{i}}L(xt)}{\sum_{i=1}^{j}p_{i}t^{\rho_{i}}L(t)}$$

$$= \lim_{t\downarrow 0}\frac{x^{\rho_{(1)}}t^{\rho_{(1)}}\left[p_{(1)}L(xt) + p_{(2)}x^{\rho_{(2)}-\rho_{(1)}}t^{\rho_{(2)}-\rho_{(1)}}L(xt) + \cdots + p_{(j)}x^{\rho_{(j)}-\rho_{(1)}}t^{\rho_{(j)}-\rho_{(1)}}L(xt)\right]}{t^{\rho_{(1)}}\left[p_{(1)}L(t) + p_{(2)}t^{\rho_{(2)}-\rho_{(1)}}L(t) + \cdots + p_{(j)}t^{\rho_{(j)}-\rho_{(1)}}L(t)\right]}$$

$$= x^{\rho_{(1)}}\lim_{t\downarrow 0}\frac{p_{(1)}L(xt) + p_{(2)}x^{\rho_{(2)}-\rho_{(1)}}t^{\rho_{(2)}-\rho_{(1)}}L(xt) + \cdots + p_{(j)}x^{\rho_{(j)}-\rho_{(1)}}t^{\rho_{(j)}-\rho_{(1)}}L(xt)}{p_{(1)}L(t) + p_{(2)}t^{\rho_{(2)}-\rho_{(1)}}L(t) + \cdots + p_{(j)}t^{\rho_{(j)}-\rho_{(1)}}L(t)}$$

$$= x^{\rho_{(1)}}\lim_{t\downarrow 0}\frac{\left[p_{(1)} + p_{(2)}x^{\rho_{(2)}-\rho_{(1)}}t^{\rho_{(2)}-\rho_{(1)}} + \cdots + p_{(j)}x^{\rho_{(j)}-\rho_{(1)}}t^{\rho_{(j)}-\rho_{(1)}}\right]L(xt)}{\left[p_{(1)} + p_{(2)}t^{\rho_{(2)}-\rho_{(1)}} + \cdots + p_{(j)}t^{\rho_{(j)}-\rho_{(1)}}\right]L(t)}$$

$$= x^{\rho_{(1)}}\lim_{t\downarrow 0}\frac{L(xt)}{L(t)}\lim_{t\downarrow 0}\frac{p_{(1)} + p_{(2)}x^{\rho_{(2)}-\rho_{(1)}}t^{\rho_{(2)}-\rho_{(1)}} + \cdots + p_{(j)}x^{\rho_{(j)}-\rho_{(1)}}t^{\rho_{(j)}-\rho_{(1)}}}{p_{(1)} + p_{(2)}t^{\rho_{(2)}-\rho_{(1)}} + \cdots + p_{(j)}t^{\rho_{(j)}-\rho_{(1)}}}$$

$$= x^{\rho_{(1)}}\lim_{t\downarrow 0}\frac{L(xt)}{L(t)} = x^{\rho_{(1)}}. \tag{2.72}$$

Overall, as we will fundamentally employ them for the purpose of our application, the results for the nonidentically distributed case can be summarized as follows: (i) if the initial distributions belong to a certain family of functions that are infinitely flat at the lower endpoint of the distribution, the limiting distribution of the minimum is the Gumbel-type distribution, and (ii) if the initial distributions belong to a family of functions that are regularly varying at the lower endpoint of the distribution with exponent $0 < \rho < \infty$, the limiting distribution of the minimum is the Weibull-type distribution. We note, however, that the observations from the initial distributions are assumed to be independent. In Sections 2.2.1 and 3.2, we will argue that the requirement of independence can also be relaxed for our application based on the definition of an E_n-sequence and Theorem 5.

As in the i.i.d. case, we illustrate the quality of the approximating Gumbel/Gompertz distribution in the nonidentically distributed case based on Theorem 8 (Fig. 2.8 and Fig. 2.9). Again, we use the extended prototype flat function with $\tau_i = \sigma_i^{\rho}$, such that the family of initial distributions is $F_i(x) = e^{-(\sigma_i/x)^{\rho}} = e^{-(\tau_i/x^{\rho})}$ for $i = 1, 2, ..., n$. For this illustration, the parameters τ_i are arrayed in a uniform grid in the interval $[\tau_0, \tau_1]$ with midpoint τ_m. Similar to the illustration for the i.i.d. case (Fig. 2.7), we obtain τ_m and ρ from the estimates of the Gompertz parameters λ and θ from our data analysis (first column in Table 4.5) and take $\tau_0 = \tau_m - 0.1\tau_m$ and $\tau_1 = \tau_m + 0.1\tau_m$, for $n = 100$, 500, and 1000. In Figure 2.8, we use the normalizing coefficients a_n and b_n for the Gompertz approximation from Theorem 8 (see proof and Remark A.3 in Appendix A). These plots show that the quality of the approximation is not very good,

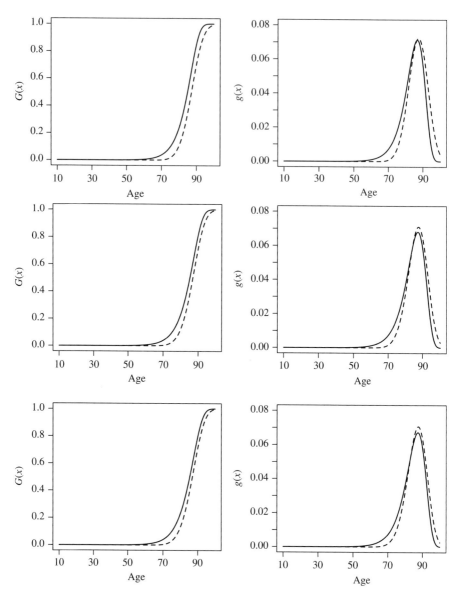

FIGURE 2.8 Gompertz approximation (solid line) and exact distribution (dashed line) of the minimum of nonidentically distributed random variables, whose parent distributions belong to a family of flat functions, for $n = 100,\ 500,$ and 1000 (first, second, and third rows of graphs, respectively). Normalizing coefficients a_n and b_n for the Gompertz approximation are from Theorem 8. Column of graphs at the left gives the c.d.f. and at the right gives the p.d.f. See text for details.

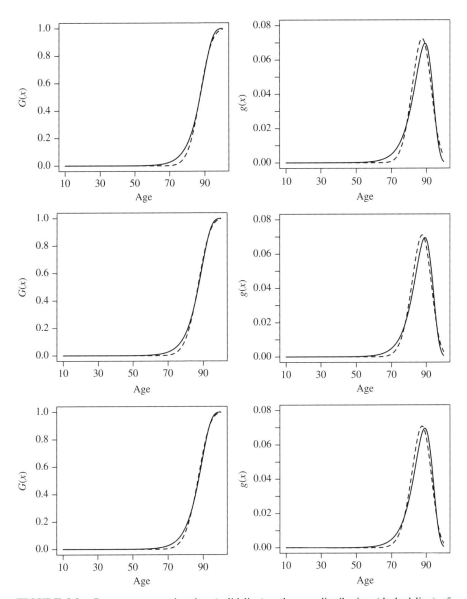

FIGURE 2.9 Gompertz approximation (solid line) and exact distribution (dashed line) of the minimum of nonidentically distributed random variables, whose parent distributions belong to a family of flat functions, for $n = 100$, 500, and 1000 (first, second, and third rows of graphs, respectively). Normalizing coefficients a_n and b_n for the Gompertz approximation are as in the i.i.d. case. Column of graphs at the left gives the c.d.f. and at the right gives the p.d.f. See text for details.

even though it gradually improves with increasing n. This is not in contradiction to the result of Theorem 8 since, as an asymptotic theorem, it does not say how accurate the approximation is in any finite setting. In Figure 2.9, we instead use the normalizing coefficients from the i.i.d. case evaluated at τ_m and ρ for each n (see Remark A.1). In this case, the quality of the approximation is already reasonably good for $n = 100$. A justification for the appropriateness and much better quality of this approximation is given in Remark A.6, while in Remark A.5, we explain why the exact distributions in Figure 2.8 and Figure 2.9 are almost indistinguishable from those in the i.i.d. case (Fig. 2.7).

2.2 THE EVOLUTIONARY THEORY OF AGING

Some authors have made a distinction between the terms *aging* and *senescence*. For instance, Medawar (1952) stated: "It will be convenient to use the seventeenth century word *senescence* to stand for the deterioration that accompanies ageing, and to leave ageing itself to stand for merely growing old." In his book, Finch (1990, p. 5) also chose to use the term *senescence*, because the term *aging* is generally used to describe changes that occur during "the passage of physical time," which may have "little or no adverse effect on vitality or lifespan." Consistent with that, Carnes et al. (1996) stated, "In simple terms, aging is the passage of clock time and senescence is the passage of biological time." In this book, no such distinction between aging and senescence is made; that is, the term *aging* is used in the same sense as the term *senescence* in some authors' use and in several quotations in this section. Rose (1991, pp. 18–19) listed reasons in favor of using the term *senescence* with the restrictive connotation of deterioration but considered that "this would be at variance with the overwhelming precedent of American biological research, in which the term *senescence* is rarely used compared with the term *aging*, and both have an association with deterioration." We additionally make the choice of not drawing a distinction between these terms because on the evolutionary view taken here, as we will discuss in the following text, aging is nonadaptive and therefore intrinsically associated with deterioration. Thus, the need to invoke aging as the mere passage of time does not arise, except in those instances in which the term *chronological aging* would be used anyway.

Researchers have advanced a strikingly large number of theories to explain aging. Indeed, Medvedev (1990) counted and tried to classify more than 300 theories of aging. A useful approach to broadly categorizing theories of aging is to take into account their level of explanation (Mayr, 1961). Austad (2001) delineated two levels of explanation as follows: "One category of aging theory seeks to answer the question of why the aging of biological organisms exists at all…. Another distinct group of theories addresses how, that is, by what mechanistic processes, aging proceeds." He labeled these two levels "ultimate theories" and "proximate mechanisms," respectively. Starting with this broad categorization, we further classify theories of aging as summarized in Figure 2.10. We will focus here on ultimate theories and, in particular, the evolutionary theory of aging. We note that although ultimate theories can provide a rationale for specific proximate mechanisms, ultimate theories are not generally

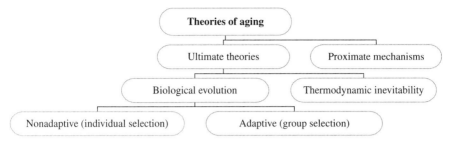

FIGURE 2.10   Classification of theories of aging.

inconsistent with any proposed proximate mechanism of aging, as the levels of explanation are different (Le Bourg, 1998). However, as will become clear in this section,
the evolutionary theory of aging implies that there is no reason to expect universality
across species or uniqueness within species for a biochemical mechanism of aging
(Rose and Graves, 1989).

Among ultimate theories, two categories can be distinguished. A first category,
which Austad (2001) named "thermodynamic inevitability" theories, includes several
theories that posit implicitly or explicitly that aging is an inevitable consequence of
the physical nature of matter. These theories, such as the reliability theory of aging
(Gavrilov and Gavrilova, 2001, 2006), have also been referred to as wear-and-tear
theories of aging and are purported to apply to living organisms in a similar way
as to mechanical devices. According to these theories, the aging process occurs
because of "the many physical and chemical factors that tend to move physical
systems towards high values of entropy: oxidation, metal fatigue, cracks due to
mechanical stress, accumulation of combustion byproducts, and so on" (Rose,
1991, p. 100). One major problem with these theories is that they predict that aging
should be observed universally among living organisms, which has not been shown to
be the case, as we will discuss later in this section. Another problem is the fundamental
dissimilarity between living organisms and mechanical devices, in that mechanical
devices represent static systems in which the same material is continuously present,
while living organisms are open systems in constant exchange with the environment
(Williams, 1957). We note that the evolutionary theory of aging does not dismiss the
possible contribution of wear-and-tear mechanisms to the aging of living organisms,
even if from an evolutionary perspective the accumulation of wear and tear is neither a
necessary nor sufficient explanation (Rose, 1991, p. 102).

The second category of ultimate theories includes theories that attribute aging to
biological evolution. The earliest evolutionary theory of aging, proposed by the nineteenth-century German biologist August Weismann, was predicated on the notion that
aging was somehow adaptive or beneficial and on the concept of group selection,
which refers to natural selection acting at the level of populations or species
(as opposed to the classical form of individual selection) (Rose, 1991, pp. 4–7).
Weismann's theory involves (i) the idea that the elderly age so that they may die
and leave room and resources for the young, who otherwise could not reproduce,

and (ii) the existence of programmed death or "a specific death-mechanism designed by natural selection to eliminate the old, and therefore wornout, members of a population" (Williams, 1957). Weismann's theory has many problems, starting with the assumption of a predominance of group selection over individual selection, which would mean that "selection for advantage to the species or group was more effective than selection among individuals within the group for the reproductive advantages of a longer life" (Kirkwood, 1985). In addition, it is not consistent with the fact that organisms in the wild are most often killed before aging becomes manifest, by accident, predation, and infectious disease (Medawar, 1952). Therefore, as aging is rarely observed in wild populations, there is no opportunity for a mechanism to terminate life to evolve (Kirkwood, 1985; Williams, 1957). Lastly, there is something circular about Weismann's theory in that, as noted by Comfort (1979, p. 11), it "assumes what it sets out to explain, that the survival of an individual decreases with increasing age."

A later evolutionary theory of aging based on the classical form of individual selection was able to reconcile evolution with the idea that aging is nonadaptive. At first sight, the existence of aging seems paradoxical from the evolutionary perspective of individual selection, because natural selection acting on individuals supposedly causes the evolution of increased, not decreased, fitness. The central idea of the current evolutionary theory of aging was initially articulated most explicitly in two publications by Peter B. Medawar (Medawar, 1946, 1952). Medawar (1952) made his argument starting from a theoretical potentially immortal and ever-reproducing population (i.e., its members do not deteriorate with increasing age and their rate of reproduction does not change with age). He argued that the older the members of this theoretical population are, the fewer there will be of them, not because they become more vulnerable with increasing age, but simply because they are exposed for a longer time to the hazard of suffering an accidental death. Then, older individuals make progressively less contribution in terms of reproduction to the next generation, showing "how it must be that the force of natural selection weakens with increasing age—even in a theoretically immortal population, provided only that it is exposed to real hazards of mortality" (Medawar, 1952).

Based on Medawar's (1952) argument and premised on the existence of genes whose effects tend to occur at a given age (*age-specific genetic effects*), the central idea of the evolutionary theory of aging can be stated as follows: (i) The force of natural selection acting on age-specific genetic effects declines with adult age, because the reproductive contribution to the next generation decreases with increasing adult age. (ii) Aging then results from the accumulation of deleterious mutations with late age-specific effects, as such mutations encounter little or no negative selection. Since natural selection is the source of adaptation, the resilience of organisms declines as natural selection fades away, leading to the progressive deterioration of physiological function with increasing age (Kirkwood, 1985; Rose and Mueller, 1998). Importantly, the age-specificity of genetic effects is not defined by when a gene is expressed at the molecular level, but when it affects survival and fecundity (Partridge and Barton, 1993). Moreover, the notion of natural selection acting on age-specific genetic effects implies the existence of age classes that might vary in the intensity of selection acting upon them. This is not the case, for example, for species that reproduce by fission (e.g., bacteria) and show no distinction between soma and germ lines.[2] We will further address this last point as we discuss comparative biology studies later in this section.

It is important to realize that the evolutionary theory of aging, as elaborated by Medawar (1946, 1952), does not require the preexistence of reproductive aging (i.e., decreasing rate of reproduction with age) or a postreproductive period. According to the evolutionary theory of aging, the weakening of natural selection with increasing age occurs during evolutionary history due to the hazards of an accidental or extrinsic death, which reduces the reproductive output of older individuals merely because there are fewer of them—since the longer one lives, the longer one is subject to suffering an accidental death. This is enough to justify the accumulation of late-onset deleterious genetic mutations in the population, which in turn accounts for the evolution of increasing mortality with age as well as reproductive aging.

Moreover, we note that there may be a distinction between menopause in human females and the gradual process of reproductive aging in human males and in other sexually reproducing species. An evolutionary explanation for menopause, as suggested by Williams (1957), involves the notion that it may be more advantageous with respect to fitness for females to care for their existing children than to have more children at the risk of dying during pregnancy or in childbirth. In that case, while reproductive aging is nonadaptive (i.e., it results from a failure of selection against late-onset deleterious mutations), menopause would be adaptive. Indeed, Williams (1957) considered that menopause "may have arisen as a reproductive adaptation to a life-cycle already characterized by senescence, unusual hazards in pregnancy and childbirth, and a long period of juvenile dependence." He then adds, "If so, it is improper to regard menopause as a part of the aging syndrome." The evidence for and against Williams's (1957) hypothesis is not conclusive, and variants of this explanation have been proposed, particularly along the lines of the "grandmother hypothesis," which relates the labor of older postmenopausal women to the successful childbearing of their daughters and the chances of survival of their grandchildren (Austad, 1994; Hawkes et al., 1998; Kirkwood, 1999, chapter 11; Rogers, 2003). More recently, although he acknowledged that the evolutionary explanation of menopause was still best considered unresolved, Williams (1999) added another reason for viewing menopause as a special human adaptation: that it is an event with "reliably expressed hormonal and histological changes" and that occurs in a relatively narrow age range.

Starting with Fisher's (1930) work, "The Genetical Theory of Natural Selection," and mostly through the works of Hamilton (1966) and Charlesworth (1994), population genetics has provided the evolutionary theory of aging with a mathematically explicit basis. Fisher (1930, pp. 22–27) described a quantity that he called "the Malthusian parameter of population increase," partly based on the ideas from the life table: "In order to obtain a distinct idea of the application of Natural Selection to all stages in the life-history of an organism, use may be made of the ideas developed in the

---

[2] The concept of soma and germ lines originated in August Weismann's germ plasm theory (Kirkwood and Cremer, 1982). In multicellular sexually reproducing species, germ cells are those that transmit heritable information (i.e., the gametes), and somatic cells are those that carry out other body functions.

actuarial study of human mortality." Fisher (1930, pp. 24–25) additionally introduced the notion of a table of reproduction, analogous to the life table, giving rates of reproduction at each age. The Malthusian parameter is given by the only real number solution for m in the following equation:

$$\int_0^\infty e^{-mx}l(x)b(x)dx = 1, \tag{2.73}$$

where $l(x)$ is the probability of survival from birth to age x (i.e., the survival function) and $b(x)$ is the instantaneous birth rate (or rate of reproduction) at age x.[3] Equation 2.73 is called the Euler–Lotka equation, because its derivation traces back to the work of Leonhard Euler (1707–1783) and Alfred Lotka (1880–1949) (Charlesworth, 2000). If we consider the analogue of the Euler–Lotka equation for discrete age classes,

$$\sum_{x=1}^\infty e^{-mx}l(x)b(x) = 1, \tag{2.74}$$

this equation provides a means for calculating m if the set of age-specific birth rates and death rates (from which the probability of survival to age x can be obtained) are known for all ages.

The Euler–Lotka equation was originally developed for describing population growth (Lotka, 1907, 1913). Because of the negative sign in the exponent of e^{-mx}, m is positive for a population increasing in size and negative for a population decreasing in size; for a constant population size, m is 0.[4] Two assumptions are implicitly made in connection with the Euler–Lotka equation. First, it is assumed that the age-specific birth and death rates in the population are constant. A population with constant age-specific birth and death rates eventually attains a stable age distribution, and in this state, the population size will increase or decrease at a constant rate. Thus, m represents the instantaneous rate of increase in population size *after the population has achieved a stable age distribution* (Lotka, 1922). Second, implicit in the Euler–Lotka equation is the assumption that the rate of growth of the population is proportional to the population size at any given moment, which results in an exponentially increasing population. However, the assumption of exponential growth implies an unrestricted environment without competition for limited resources such as food (density-independent case) (Charlesworth, 1973; Roff, 2008). In a situation of competition for limited resources (density-dependent case), which is more realistic for the growth of natural populations, other models of population growth such as the logistic equation may be more appropriate (Crow and Kimura, 1970, pp. 22–25; Hairston et al., 1970).

---

[3] The use of $l(x)$ for the survival function follows Fisher (1930) and is consistent with actuarial life-table notation.

[4] As explained by Rose (1991, p. 8), an intuitive way of understanding the Euler–Lotka equation is to look at the equality to 1 at the right-hand side of the equation as representing the absence of population growth or constant population size. Then, for positive m, the Euler–Lotka equation conveys what "pressure" reducing population size, represented by the exponential in the integral, would have to be used to eliminate the expected population growth due to the reproductive output of each individual in the population.

A distinction must be made between the context in which the Euler–Lotka equation was developed and its use by Fisher (1930). In the study of population growth, the Euler–Lotka equation is relevant to the whole population of individuals. The quantity equivalent to Fisher's Malthusian parameter was originally called the "natural rate of increase" of the population and denoted r (Lotka, 1907, 1913).[5] Although he does not make it initially obvious, Fisher (1930) uses the Malthusian parameter in reference to a specific genotype or "each conceivable genotype" in the population (Hairston et al., 1970). This is made clear, for instance, in the following: "The Malthusian parameter will in general be different for each different genotype, and will measure the fitness to survive of each" (Fisher, 1930, p. 46). One can conceive of Fisher's (1930) use of the Euler–Lotka equation as referring to *a hypothetical subpopulation of individuals* with a particular genotype. Analogously, if we imagine an asexually reproducing population consisting of many clones, each with different life history traits, the Euler–Lotka equation applies to each clone separately and the Malthusian parameter measures the absolute fitness of each (Charlesworth, 2000; Stearns, 1992, pp. 20–25). Following Fisher's (1930) intention, the Euler–Lotka equation is used in population genetics for the genetic analysis of sexually reproducing populations or, as put by Stearns (1992, p. 24), for "analyzing the marginal effect of a gene substitution with impact on birth and death rates in a sexually outcrossing population." Importantly, the assumption of exponential growth is less restrictive or unrealistic in this context, because "The exponential growth referred to is not that of a population but the rate of spread of an allele with marginal effects on a life history. Gene frequencies can change in populations with constant numbers of organisms" (Stearns, 1992, p. 25).

In Medawar's (1952) seminal contribution, there is the suggestion that another quantity proposed by Fisher (1930, pp. 27–30) and holding a relation to the Euler–Lotka equation, the reproductive value function, might be an appropriate measure of the intensity of selection on genes acting at a given age. The reproductive value was introduced as a measure of the relative extent to which an individual of age a, in a population with stable age distribution, contributes to the ancestry of the future population. It is given by

$$v(a) = \frac{e^{ma}}{l(a)} \int_a^\infty e^{-mx} l(x) b(x) dx. \tag{2.75}$$

Note that by using the Euler–Lotka equation, $v(0) = (e^{m0}/l(0)) \int_0^\infty e^{-mx} l(x) b(x) dx = 1$.

That is, the reproductive value at age 0 takes the value of unity, which shows that the reproductive value of an individual of age a is measured relative to that of a newborn child. Medawar's (1952) association of the reproductive value with the intensity of

[5] Many names have been used for r: "It has been called the true, the real, the incipient, the inherent, and the intrinsic rate of increase or of natural increase…" (Caughley and Birch, 1971). Taylor et al. (1974) suggested that the most appropriate name was "ultimate rate of increase," "because it correctly emphasizes that r is the value attained when the life history parameters are constant and the stable age distribution is realized."

selection on genes acting at a given age apparently followed from Fisher's (1930, p. 29) comment: "It is probably not without significance in this connexion that the death rate in Man takes a course generally inverse to the curve of reproductive value." However, Hamilton (1966) gave reasons why the use of the reproductive value in this sense was not appropriate. (The reproductive value turned out to be an important quantity in the related field of life history theory.)

Hamilton's (1966) work, titled "The moulding of senescence by natural selection," is credited with providing "the beginning of rigorous thought on the evolution of senescence" (Williams, 1999). Hamilton (1966) proposed that a measure of the intensity of selection on genes acting at a given age, or *the force of natural selection*, be based on the Malthusian parameter. Implicitly assuming that the Malthusian parameter was an appropriate measure of fitness, in the sense of accurately predicting the effect of selection on gene frequencies, he proceeded to derive the effect on the Malthusian parameter of changes in survival at a given age. Hamilton (1966) used the analogue of the Euler–Lotka equation for discrete age classes and expressed the survival function as $l(x) = p(0)$ $p(1)p(2) \cdots p(x-1)$, where $p(x)$ gives the proportion of population members who have already reached age x who then reach age $x + 1$. Then, by implicit differentiation, he obtained the partial derivative of m with respect to the logarithm of $p(x)$ at a given age a, based on the rationale that "genetic effects on survival probabilities are more likely to be additive on a log scale" (Charlesworth, 1994, p. 191):

$$\frac{\partial m}{\partial \log p(a)} = \frac{\sum_{x=a+1}^{\infty} e^{-mx}l(x)b(x)}{\sum_{x=1}^{\infty} xe^{-mx}l(x)b(x)}. \tag{2.76}$$

In Appendix B, we present the derivation of Equation 2.76. Hamilton (1966) similarly derived the analogous equation representing the effect on m of changes in fertility at a given age. For our purposes, we will restrict our attention here to Equation 2.76 or Hamilton's equation for the force of natural selection on mortality.

The partial derivative of m with respect to $\log p(a)$ is taken as a measure of the force of natural selection acting on a mutation that reduces survival at age a, because it purportedly captures the change in fitness induced by a change in survival probability at that age. As mutations are constantly arising, one can think of the force of natural selection as a measure of how fast a new mutation will be fixed or lost in a population (Promislow et al., 2006). Note that the denominator in the right-hand side of Equation 2.76 does not depend on the age a; the expression in the denominator is a measure of generation time or "the mean age of the mothers of a set of new-born individuals in a population with a stable age-distribution" (Charlesworth, 1994, p. 30). Then, the effect on m of a change in survival probability at age a changes with age as follows: once reproduction has started, so that the $b(x)$ values in the numerator are greater than 0, the effect on m of changes in survival at a given age decreases with age, because fewer positive terms are included in the sum in the numerator. Once a reaches the last age at which $b(x)$ is greater than 0, or the last age at reproduction in the population, the effect on m of changes in survival becomes 0, remaining at that value for all subsequent ages. Hamilton's (1966) work thus formally showed that the

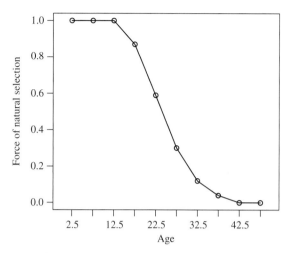

FIGURE 2.11   Force of natural selection on a mutation that affects survival at a given age, for the population of the United States about 1940; dots give the values of the force of natural selection at midpoints of 5-year age intervals (redrawn from Charlesworth and Williamson (1975)).

force of natural selection acting on a mutation that reduces survival (at a given age) decreases with age starting at the earliest age at reproduction in the population and reaching 0 at the end of reproduction in the population, as had been proposed by Medawar (1946, 1952). Figure 2.11 illustrates this using data from the U.S. population about 1940 (from Charlesworth and Williamson (1975)). In this graph, the force of natural selection is actually calculated based on a quantity determining the probability of survival of a mutant gene in a random-mating population with overlapping generations, denoted u; the y-axis is the partial derivative of u with respect to $\log p(a)$, which for these data closely follows the partial derivative of m in Equation 2.76. The use of u is favored by Charlesworth and Williamson (1975) because it "has a more direct relation with the effectiveness of natural selection."

Charlesworth (1994) has thoroughly tested Hamilton's (1966) assumption that m predicts the effect of selection on gene frequencies, in the course of extensive work in theoretical population genetics pertaining to evolution in age-structured populations, defined as "populations whose members are not born into distinct generations, and where fertility and survival are functions of age" (Charlesworth, 1994, p. xi). According to Charlesworth (2000), there was no obvious guarantee that the use of m as a measure of fitness would produce accurate results when modeling "a sexually reproducing diploid population in which each parent produces a mixture of genotypes, especially as changes in genotype frequencies induced by selection must cause continual changes in age structure." Overall, his theoretical work has shown that the differences among genotypes in the Malthusian parameter can be used only as approximate predictors of the rate of change of allele frequency under selection, although the approximation is very good if selection is weak (Charlesworth, 2000). In general, this has been viewed as supporting Hamilton's (1966) assumption as a reasonable working assumption for the study of the evolution of aging (Rose, 1991, pp. 15–16).

Hamilton's (1966) formalization of the evolutionary theory of aging has also been qualified with respect to the fact that it focuses on fertility alone, represented by $b(x)$ in Equation 2.76, to explain age-specific selective pressure on mortality. Lee (2003) offered a formal theory that extends Hamilton's (1966) work by incorporating selection due to transfers of food and care in social species (e.g., parental care and help from others such as older siblings or grandparents in humans). This extended theory explains postreproductive survival in terms of fitness gains through continued investment in children and grandchildren, or the so-called intergenerational transfers. As stated by Williams (1957), "The term *post-reproductive* needs clarification with respect to man. ...Any individual, of whatever age, who is caring for dependent offspring is acting in a way that promotes the survival of his own genes and is properly considered a part of the breeding population." Lee's (2003) theory is relevant to our work in that it suggests that Hamilton's equation (Eq. 2.76), by not taking into account transfers in social species, underestimates the force of natural selection at human adult ages and, parallel to that, underestimates the age at which the force of natural selection effectively reaches 0 (see Fig. 2.11). In particular, as we will argue in the next section in relation to the extreme dependence of human offspring, the rate of the initial decline in the force of natural selection after the earliest age at reproduction in the population must be extremely slow.[6]

Another explanation that has been offered for postreproductive human survival involves positive pleiotropy, as described by Mueller and Rose (1996): "One of the more puzzling features of the evolutionary analysis of aging is that the force of natural selection drops long before the comparable period of rapid decline in adult survivors. This may be due to alleles that are selected because of early beneficial effects that have pleiotropic beneficial effects at some later ages, though not all. Then, for example, middle-aged humans that are surviving better than expected on the evolutionary theory can be explained as the beneficiaries of the action of natural selection at earlier ages. The effects of this type of pleiotropy should fade with age, at adult ages farther and farther away from early adulthood."[7] The term *pleiotropy* generally refers to the production by a single gene of two or more phenotypic effects and will be

---

[6] The notion in Lee's (2003) theory of evolutionary gains through continued investment in children and grandchildren is relevant to the "grandmother hypothesis" (Rogers, 2003). Indeed, a footnote in Medawar's (1952) work sounds reminiscent at once of both the notion of evolutionary gains through intergenerational transfers and the grandmother hypothesis. Referring to the sentence "In the post-reproductive period of life, the direct influence of natural selection has been reduced to zero," he notes: "The word 'direct' is important. Grandparents, though no longer fertile, may yet promote (or impede) the welfare of their grandchildren, and so influence the mode of propagation of their genes. A gene for grandmotherly indulgence should therefore prevail over one for callous indifference, in spite of the fact that the gene is propagated *per procurationem* and not by the organism in which its developmental effect appears. Selection for grandmotherly indulgence I should describe as 'indirect,' and the indirect action of selection becomes important whenever there is any degree of social organization."

[7] Reproduced from *Proceedings of the National Academy of Sciences of the United States of America*, **93**, Mueller, L. D. and Rose, M. R., Evolutionary theory predicts late-life mortality plateaus, pages 15249–15253, Copyright 1996, with permission from the National Academy of Sciences, USA.

encountered again in the following text in the form of *antagonistic pleiotropy*. Positive pleiotropy will also be invoked in Section 2.2.2 in relation to the deceleration of the increase in mortality rates at late ages.

Extensive empirical work on the evolutionary theory of aging has been conducted, involving experimental and comparative biology studies (Rose, 1991, chapters 3 and 5). Among experimental studies, the most striking evidence has come from tests of the prediction that experimentally changing the force of natural selection in laboratory populations should give rise to changes in patterns of aging. According to Hamilton's (1966) work, a decrease in the force of natural selection only occurs after the earliest age at reproduction in the population. If this age is postponed by the intervention of an experimenter, then the force of natural selection will remain at full intensity for a longer part of an organism's lifetime and, over a large number of generations, this should lead to a postponement of aging (Rose, 1991, p. 50). Experimental studies conducted by different investigators have supported this prediction, as well as the reverse prediction that decreasing the force of natural selection at later ages accelerates aging. For instance, in experiments using the fruit fly *Drosophila melanogaster*, the period of intense natural selection was prolonged by delaying reproduction, which was accomplished by discarding eggs laid by younger flies and only allowing older flies to reproduce. After many generations, delayed reproduction led to postponed aging as indicated by greater survival among those bred under delayed-reproduction condition compared to those bred normally (Luckinbill et al., 1984; Rose, 2004; Rose and Charlesworth, 1981).

Another prediction of the evolutionary theory of aging concerns the comparative biology method (i.e., studies using comparisons across species): "The theory regards senescence as an evolved characteristic of the soma. We should find it wherever a soma has been evolved, but not elsewhere" (Williams, 1957). In general, comparative biology studies have not refuted this prediction; many species that lack a separation of the soma (e.g., prokaryotes, some sea anemones, some protozoa) do not seem to exhibit aging, while species with a clear distinction between soma and germ lines, including all vertebrates, exhibit aging (Rose, 1991, pp. 84–91). More recently, the requirement for species expected to age has been refined as follows: "The critical requirement for the evolution of ageing is that there be a distinction between a parent individual and the smaller offspring for which it provides. If the organism breeds by dividing equally into identical offspring, then the distinction between parent and offspring disappears, the intensity of selection on survival and reproduction will remain constant and individual ageing is not expected to evolve" (Partridge and Barton, 1993).[8] Therefore, although organisms that reproduce by fission, like bacteria, lack a distinction between soma and germ lines, they can still exhibit aging if cell division is asymmetrical (e.g., damaged cell components can be partitioned differentially to one of the two products of fission) (Rose et al., 2007).

Age-specific genetic effects can be either beneficial or deleterious at a given age, or involve both beneficial and deleterious effects at different ages (Rose, 1991, p. 70).

---

[8] Reproduced from *Nature*, **362**, Partridge, L. and Barton, N. H., Optimally, mutation and the evolution of ageing, pages 305–311, Copyright 1993, with permission from Macmillan Publishers Ltd.

This distinction is related to the two main population genetic mechanisms that have been proposed to underlie the evolutionary outcome of aging: mutation accumulation and antagonistic pleiotropy. Mutation accumulation is defined as the passive accumulation of mutations with late deleterious effects, *passive* because they have no effect in early life and have deleterious effects only when selection is weak or absent in late life (Medawar, 1952). Antagonistic pleiotropy, elaborated in detail by Williams (1957), is defined as the active fixation of mutations with early beneficial effects and late deleterious effects, because they have beneficial effects in early life when selection is intense and deleterious effects when selection is weak or absent.[9] The proposed mechanisms of mutation accumulation and antagonistic pleiotropy have also been submitted to scrutiny by experimental and comparative biology studies. While these studies have provided empirical evidence for the action of both mutation accumulation and antagonistic pleiotropy in the evolution of aging (Rose and Charlesworth, 1980; Rose, 1991, chapters 4 and 5), it is not currently clear which of the two mechanisms plays a more important role, especially as they may operate simultaneously (Charlesworth, 2000).

The evolutionary theory of aging can also be understood in the broader context of life history theory (or life history evolution) (Roff, 2002; Stearns, 1976, 1992). Life history theory pertains to the features of a life cycle, such as how fast the organism grows, when it matures, how many times it gives birth, how many offspring it has, and how long it lives. These features of a life cycle define the "life history traits," including age-specific birth and death rates (Stearns, 1992, p. 10). One of the main theoretical techniques used in the study of life history evolution is optimality theory or evolutionary optimization theory. Optimality theory assumes that natural selection leads to the establishment of a life history that maximizes fitness, subject to a set of constraints among the life history traits in question. Constraints can be intrinsic constraints of physiology or extrinsically imposed by the environment (Charlesworth, 1990; Partridge and Barton, 1993). A constrained relationship among life history traits leads to trade-offs, which exist when a fitness benefit through a change in one life history trait is linked to a fitness cost through a change in another life history trait. For example, a fitness benefit through increased current reproduction may have a cost in decreased current or future survival or decreased future reproduction (Stearns, 1992, p. 14).

---

[9] Medawar (1952) described mutation accumulation as follows: "There is a constant feeble pressure to introduce new variants of hereditary factors into a natural population, for 'mutation,' as it is called, is a recurrent process. Very often such factors lower the fertility or viability of the organisms in which they make their effects apparent; but it is arguable that, if only they make them apparent late enough, the force of selection will be too attenuated to oppose their establishment and spread." Although he did not elaborate on it, as Williams (1957) thoroughly did, Medawar (1952) also suggested the operation of antagonistic pleiotropy in the evolution of aging: "It is not good enough to say that what happens to very old animals hardly matters and that what happens to youngsters matters a great deal. For the degree to which anything may matter varies in a predictable way with age, and the selective advantage or disadvantage of a hereditary factor is rather exactly weighted by the age in life at which it first becomes eligible for selection. A relatively small advantage conferred early in the life of an individual may outweigh a catastrophic disadvantage withheld until later."

The evolutionary explanation of aging can be framed in optimality theory terms as late survival sacrificed for enhanced early reproduction (Kirkwood and Rose, 1991). More generally, aging evolves as part of an optimal life history because of deleterious side effects late in life of processes that are favorable early on (Partridge and Barton, 1993). Since the force of natural selection is weaker at older ages compared to younger ages, which is to say that natural selection favors traits that appear earlier rather than later, the optimal life history includes aging as a by-product of beneficial early traits. The disposable soma theory is an optimality account of aging in which allocation of resources to reproduction is done at the cost of somatic repair mechanisms (i.e., there is a trade-off between the allocation of resources to reproduction and to repair of somatic damage and hence survival) (Kirkwood and Rose, 1991; Partridge and Barton, 1993). According to the disposable soma theory, it is the mortality due to extrinsic hazards (i.e., accident, predation, and infectious disease) that makes it not worthwhile to invest in better maintenance to preserve somatic functions: high mortality due to extrinsic hazards in the wild during evolutionary history has meant that there was more to gain in fitness by investing resources in reproduction than in the repair of somatic damage (Kirkwood and Rose, 1991). This clearly resonates with the central role that the "real hazards of mortality" plays in Medawar's (1952) account of the evolution of aging, as described earlier. This reasoning also leads to the prediction of a relationship between the impact of extrinsic hazards of death during evolutionary history and the rate of aging; higher externally imposed death rates of adults are expected to cause evolution of higher rates of aging (Partridge and Barton, 1996; Williams, 1957).

The optimality account of aging, in particular the disposable soma theory, has come to be often equated with antagonist pleiotropy (Partridge and Barton, 1993). However, the disposable soma theory accounts for aging at a different level than the population genetic mechanisms of mutation accumulation and antagonistic pleiotropy (Kirkwood and Rose, 1991). Two factors contribute to the blurring of the distinction between the disposable soma theory and antagonistic pleiotropy. First, although Williams (1957) did not originally propose pleiotropic effects specifically involving the trade-off of survival for fecundity (i.e., the nature of the gene actions was not specified), more recent renditions of antagonistic pleiotropy have referred particularly to these trade-offs.[10] Second, although under optimality theory the outcome of aging could in principle be reached by fixation of genes with an effect on fitness at only one age, the optimality account of aging is often developed in terms of genes with effects on survival and fertility at different ages (i.e., pleiotropic effects) (Partridge and Barton, 1993). As emphasized by Kirkwood and Austad (2000), the disposable soma theory focuses on physiological mechanisms, as opposed to the general pattern of gene action invoked by antagonistic pleiotropy.

Given the unexplained observation of longer survival of human females compared to human males, which is strikingly consistent across countries and time periods

---

[10] Williams (1957) gave as a hypothetical example of antagonistic pleiotropy a mutation "that has a favorable effect on the calcification of bone in the developmental period but which expresses itself in a subsequent somatic environment in the calcification of the connective tissue of arteries."

(Austad, 2006), Kirkwood (1999, chapter 13; 2010) suggested an evolutionary explanation for why women live longer within the framework of the disposable soma theory. He claimed that women are "less disposable than men," hence worth greater investment in somatic maintenance, due to their exclusive role in gestation and breast-feeding and their generally greater contribution to child raising; the biological effects on longevity of this difference in disposability would be brought about through the actions of sex hormones, particularly testosterone. Based on the grandmother hypothesis, as described previously, females can also be seen as "less disposable" due to the special importance of grandmothers in the genus Homo and close ancestors for the survival of their grandchildren (Hawkes, 2003; Hawkes et al., 1998). Lahdenperä et al. (2004) investigated the fitness benefits of prolonged human female postreproductive life span using multigenerational data from Finland and Canada during the eighteenth and nineteenth centuries. Controlling for several possible confounders, they found that the presence of a living postreproductive mother and the length of her postreproductive life span had a significant positive effect, respectively, on the lifetime reproductive performance of her offspring and on the number of her grandchildren. These fitness benefits resulted from the effects of the postreproductive woman on life history traits of her offspring (e.g., earlier reproduction and reduced interbirth intervals) and on the survival probabilities of her grandchildren. On commenting these results, Hawkes (2004) noted, "The grandmother hypothesis attributes our slow ageing to the help that older females can give their descendants; females ageing more slowly in physiological systems other than their ovaries could help more." However, except for possible genetic effects related to having two X-chromosomes as opposed to one X- and one Y-chromosome (e.g., the heterogametic sex hypothesis for sex differences in longevity (Austad, 2006)), this should have implications for longevity in both sexes, because, as stated by Hawkes (2004), "Daughters and sons both inherit genes affecting levels of cellular maintenance and repair from their mothers."

Analogous to the distinction between proximate mechanisms and ultimate theories of aging in the beginning of this section, one can also distinguish between proximate mechanisms and evolutionary explanations of diseases (Nesse and Williams, 1998). Under this paradigm, aging and aging-related diseases may be seen as resulting from the same general evolutionary process, namely, the decline in the force of natural selection with age and the accumulation of deleterious mutations with late age-specific effects, but without necessarily sharing proximate mechanisms. As put forward by Rose and Archer (1996), "Some human diseases are distinguished by their late onset or their superficial resemblance to accelerated forms of normal aging; this ill-formed group of disorders are lumped together as diseases of aging. ...Despite the label, there is no reason to think that these diseases of aging are in fact disorders related to the aging process in normal humans. ...Nonetheless, these diseases of aging probably arise for the same reason as normal aging, the attenuation of natural selection at later ages."[11] This notion can already be found in Medawar (1952) with respect to cancer and cardiovascular diseases and has more recently been explored by others (Ackermann and Pletcher, 2008;

---

[11] Reproduced from *Current Opinion in Genetics & Development*, **6**, Rose, M. R. and Archer, M. A., Genetic analysis of mechanisms of aging, pages 366–370, Copyright 1996, with permission from Elsevier.

Kirkwood et al., 1999; Maynard Smith et al., 1999; Wick et al., 2003).[12] It is also important to recognize from this kinship of aging with aging-related diseases that from an evolutionary perspective, there is no such thing as "normal" or "healthy" aging, since it is inherent in the evolutionary explanation of aging that it results in nonadaptive phenotypes. Yet this does not go against the use of the term *normal aging* to signify aging in the absence of disease; the evolutionary perspective obviously says nothing about the very real difference for the individual between aging with and without a disabling disorder warranting a specific diagnosis.

In accordance with the view in the preceding text, some studies have pursued an evolutionary perspective on diseases in terms of the population genetic mechanisms of mutation accumulation and antagonistic pleiotropy. Albin (1993) gave criteria for considering four diseases (Huntington's disease, idiopathic hemochromatosis, myotonic dystrophy, and Alzheimer's disease) particularly good candidates for the ascertainment of antagonistic pleiotropy, while Cortopassi (2002) listed reasons why passive fixation of mutations with late deleterious effects (i.e., mutation accumulation) was likely to play a role in Alzheimer's disease and other late-onset neurodegenerative diseases. In a study assessing fitness (defined as the number of children surviving to 15 years of age) in patients with one of two trinucleotide repeat expansion diseases, Huntington's disease and spinocerebellar ataxia 1, the results supported the operation of antagonistic pleiotropy in the low/medium expansion range (Frontali et al., 1996). Another study examined the apolipoprotein E variation, a major risk factor for Alzheimer's disease, at the sequence haplotype level. Among other findings, the observed variation was a good fit to the expectations of selective neutrality, consistent with the operation of mutation accumulation, but the authors cautioned about the many limitations of this analysis (Fullerton et al., 2000).

With the advent of the evolutionary theory of aging, the Gompertz pattern of increase in mortality rates has been broadly explained in connection with the decline in the force of natural selection with adult age: "the 'Gompertz' form of mortality among iteroparous species [species that reproduce repeatedly, as opposed to species that reproduce only once or semelparous] may be due to a broad conformity of mortality to the intensity of natural selection acting on age-specific mortality rates" (Rose, 1991, p. 171). This is supported by theoretical studies using optimization and population genetics models, which have been able to produce results consistent with an approximately exponential increase in mortality rates with increasing age (Abrams and Ludwig, 1995; Mueller and Rose, 1996). However, the results of these studies do not go as far as warranting a conclusion that the exponential form of the increase in age-specific mortality rates is specifically accounted for by the evolutionary theory of aging (Partridge and Barton, 1996).

---

[12] This is how Medawar (1952) expressed the evolutionary underpinning of aging-related diseases in common with aging: "Susceptibility to both cancer and the cardiovascular diseases is in some degree influenced by heredity, and should therefore be subject to those forces, of 'natural selection,' that discriminate between the better and the genetically less well endowed. … But cancer and the cardiovascular diseases are affections of middle and later life. Most people will already have had their children before the onset of these diseases can influence their candidature for selection. In the post-reproductive period of life, the direct influence of natural selection has been reduced to zero, and the principal causes of death to-day lie just beyond its grasp."

Indeed, in the discussion of their findings, Mueller and Rose (1996) noted: "At this point in the development of the evolutionary theory of demography, we do not claim that the first 99% of all deaths [i.e., excluding deaths in 'late life,' which will be discussed in Section 2.2.2] might not be equally well described by one of the major competitors of the Gompertz model (e.g., the Weibull model). Whether there is a deeper connection between the Gompertz equation and the evolutionary theory than the phenomenological one we have pointed out must await further development of this theory."[13] Moreover, the relation between the intensity of natural selection and the pattern of age-specific mortality rates may be affected by pleiotropic effects between age classes, which motivated the following statement by Nusbaum et al. (1996): "We cannot really make strong statements connecting the force of natural selection to demographic patterns, except for the broadest qualitative assertions that are embodied in the evolutionary theory of aging in general." Or as asserted by Charlesworth and Partridge (1997), "The approximately exponential increase in death rates … is understandable qualitatively in terms of the conventional theory, but it would be nice to have deeper quantitative understanding."

2.2.1 The Argument for Gompertzian Mortality

For our reasoning in this section, we will build on the basic notions of the sufficient and component causes (SCC) model of causation in epidemiology (Rothman, 1976). The SCC model traces back to the work of the philosopher Mackie (1965), who defined an INUS condition as "an *insufficient* but *necessary* part of a condition which is itself *unnecessary* but *sufficient* for the result" (the acronym INUS derives from the first letters of the italicized words). An INUS condition corresponds to a necessary component cause in the SCC model (Rothman, 1976; Rothman and Greenland, 1998, chapter 2). Each component cause in the SCC model is part of one or more sufficient causes, while each sufficient cause includes one or more component causes and constitutes a minimal set of conditions that produce disease. This can be illustrated graphically with "causal pies," where a pie represents a sufficient cause and a slice represents a component cause. The SCC model provides a convenient way of conceptualizing biological interaction or joint effects, which makes it particularly useful for multifactorial diseases. Biological interaction between two or more factors is represented as a sufficient cause that includes all factors as component causes. The usefulness of the SCC model for conceptualizing gene–gene and gene–environment interactions is illustrated in Rothman and Greenland's (1998, pp. 11–14) and Khoury et al.'s (1993, pp. 63–64) epidemiology textbooks.

Although it is a popular way of thinking about causation in epidemiology, the SCC model has not been as useful in actual applications in terms of providing the basis for specific study designs or data analytical methods. Partly for this reason, the SCC model has recently received less attention in the health sciences and epidemiology literature than the potential outcomes (counterfactual) framework (Greenland, 2000; Little and Rubin, 2000). (A counterexample in this respect is the book by Aickin

---

[13] Reproduced from *Proceedings of the National Academy of Sciences of the United States of America*, **93**, Mueller, L. D. and Rose, M. R., Evolutionary theory predicts late-life mortality plateaus, pages 15249–15253, Copyright 1996, with permission from the National Academy of Sciences, USA.

(2002)). Greenland and Brumback (2002) identify the sufficient causes with "causal mechanisms" and consider that the basic units of analysis in the SCC model are the mechanisms (i.e., the sufficient causes) that determine the potential outcomes of individuals, rather than the individuals. Still, links between the potential outcomes framework and the SCC model have been established, and they may be seen as providing complementary perspectives (Flanders, 2006; Greenland and Brumback, 2002). According to VanderWeele and Hernán (2006), "Despite its seeming lack of utility in actual applications and data analysis, the sufficient-component cause model continues to be routinely taught in introductory epidemiology courses because it provides a useful framework in which to think about the actual causal mechanisms at work in bringing about a particular outcome."

For reasons that will become clear in the next section, we note that the causation model that we will develop here applies to intrinsic deaths (i.e., excluding deaths caused by extrinsic or accidental factors) occurring in a range of ages excluding neonatal and infant years as well as late life. In Section 3.2, we will extend our causation model to aging-related diseases of complex etiology, in addition to mortality. We initially build on the SCC model by defining the statistical nature of the sufficient causes. Rothman (1976) conceived of a sufficient cause in a deterministic way: "A cause which inevitably produces the effect is *sufficient*." That is, once all component causes of a sufficient cause express themselves, the sufficient cause is complete and death or disease follows. Rothman and Greenland (1998, p. 16) stated that the SCC model could accommodate chance but mostly by viewing chance as "deterministic events beyond the current limits of knowledge or observability." More recently, however, others have emphasized that the SCC model is not inherently deterministic, either because the component causes may be random and only the last component cause to occur determines the occurrence of disease (Poole, 2001) or because "the outcome affected by the completion of a sufficient cause may be a probability parameter rather than an observable event" (Greenland and Brumback, 2002).

We consider the occurrence of component causes as random events with a time-to-event distribution. The time to event is the age at which the component cause expresses its necessary causal role; more precisely, as will become clear in Section 3.2, we will be concerned with the residual lifetime after the earliest age at reproduction in the population. For environmental factors, the time-to-event distribution of the component cause is related to randomness in the timing and degree of exposure. For genetic factors, the time-to-event distribution of the component cause is related to the randomness inherent in the variability of biological phenomena. As reviewed earlier, a basic tenet of the evolutionary theory of aging is the existence of genes with age-specific effects. Here, the genetic component causes are understood to be "age-specific" in the sense that their age of expression is more common at a specific age, rather than being fixed in a deterministic way (i.e., they have a unimodal time-to-event distribution). Because a sufficient cause is only complete once all component causes occur, the time-to-event distribution of the sufficient causes is given by the distribution of the *maximum* time to event of the component causes. That is, we are treating the distributions of the component causes as the initial distributions, and, from the exact statistical theory of extreme values (Section 2.1), if the time-to-event distribution of each component cause in a sufficient cause is $F_i(x)$, the distribution of the sufficient cause is $\prod_{i=1}^{n} F_i(x)$.

We additionally consider that there are many sufficient causes of death in the population, each containing necessary component causes corresponding to genetic or environmental factors. Thus, death occurs at the time the first sufficient cause is complete in an individual, and if we now treat the distributions of the sufficient causes as the initial distributions, the time-to-event distribution in the population is the distribution of the *minimum* time to event of the sufficient causes. We must also take into account that each individual in the population may or may not inherit the genetic factors that constitute the sufficient causes of death. Similarly, an individual may or may not be exposed to (high enough doses of) the environmental factors that constitute the sufficient causes of death. If $F_i(x)$ is the time-to-event distribution of sufficient cause i given inheritance/exposure (i.e., given that an individual inherits all genetic component causes and is exposed to all environmental component causes of sufficient cause i), P_i is the probability of inheritance/exposure for sufficient cause i, and $Q_i = 1 - P_i$, $i = 1, 2, ..., n$, the survival function for sufficient cause i in the population is

$$P[X_i > x] = P[X_i > x | \text{ inheritance/exposure}]P_i + P[X_i > x | \text{ no inheritance/exposure}]Q_i$$

$$= P_i[1 - F_i(x)] + Q_i = P_i - P_i F_i(x) + Q_i = 1 - P_i F_i(x). \tag{2.77}$$

Note that this survival function (Eq. 2.77) is defective in that it never reaches 0 (the corresponding distribution function never reaches 1) as age goes to infinity. However, this does not affect the use that we will make of the following statement, as we will be concerned with the lower tail of the distributions of the sufficient causes: Because each individual in the population can die due to any of a large number of sufficient causes, the time-to-event distribution in the population is approximated by the limiting distribution of the *minimum* time to event of the sufficient causes, as the number of sufficient causes goes to infinity.

We will develop the SCC model further in the next chapter (Section 3.2); here we consider the simplifying scenario in which the sufficient causes of death in the population contain only genetic component causes or, more broadly, have time-to-event distribution determined only by genetic component causes. In this way, we will account for the emergence of the Gompertz distribution as a description of human mortality on exclusively biological grounds, in a sense that we will make more precise in Section 3.2. By referring to the original results in Section 2.1.2, if we assumed that the times to event of the sufficient causes under consideration were i.i.d. and their common time-to-event distribution were flat at the lower endpoint of the distribution, we would conclude that the limiting distribution of the minimum is the Gumbel distribution; hence, the time-to-event distribution in the population would approximately follow the Gompertz distribution. However, since the time-to-event distribution of each sufficient cause in our model is related to a different set of component causes, the times to event of the sufficient causes cannot be regarded as identically distributed. The results from Theorems 8 and 9 allow relaxing the requirement of identical initial distributions under certain assumptions. Still, these results presuppose that the observations are independent, and since the sufficient causes may share one or more component causes (i.e., the sets of component causes may intersect), the times to event of the sufficient causes cannot be regarded as independent either. However, as we discuss in the following text, it is reasonable to consider that the way in which the times to event of the sufficient causes of death fall short of being independent satisfies the assumptions in the definition of an E_n-sequence (Section 2.1.1). Then, Theorem 5, along with our results for the nonidentically distributed case, supports the claim that if the time-to-event distributions of the sufficient causes belong to a family of flat functions at the lower endpoint of the distribution, the limiting distribution of the minimum is the Gumbel distribution.

Potential applications for stochastic models that replace the assumption of independence by less restrictive assumptions, including the E_n-sequence, are given in Galambos (1981, 1987, pp. 224–232). The E_n-sequence was considered for the study of the strength of materials and for a reliability application, namely, the time to failure of a piece of equipment (a coherent system) with a large number of components. We briefly describe this reliability application here as it provides an analogy to our causation model. In system reliability theory, the definition of a coherent system of components simply excludes from consideration unusual situations, such as a system including components that do not play any direct role in the functioning of the system (irrelevant components) or a system that changes from a functioning to a failed state if a failed component is replaced by a functioning one (Barlow and Proschan, 1981, p. 6; Rausand and Høyland, 2004, pp. 125–126). A coherent system can be alternatively represented by a parallel structure of minimal path sets or a series structure of minimal cut sets. (In a parallel structure, the system fails when the last component fails, while in a series structure, the system fails when the first component fails.) A minimal path set is a minimal set of components whose functioning insures the functioning of the system. In other words, a minimal path set fails if one of its components fails and the system fails if all path sets fail. A minimal cut set is a minimal set of components whose failure causes the system to fail. That is, a minimal cut set fails if all its components fail and the system fails if one cut set fails (Barlow and Proschan, 1981, pp. 9–10; Rausand and Høyland, 2004, pp. 129–133).

In the case of the series structure of minimal cut sets, the time to failure of each minimal cut set is given by the maximum time to failure of its components, and the time to failure of the system is given by the minimum time to failure of the cut sets. This is analogous to our causation model, in which the time to event of each sufficient cause is given by the maximum time to event of the component causes, and the age at death is given by the minimum time to event of the sufficient causes. Thus, sufficient causes in the SCC model of causation correspond to minimal cut sets in systems reliability theory.[14] There is a distinction,

---

[14] The word *minimal* in "minimal cut set" is also used in a similar way in the definition of a sufficient cause by Rothman and Greenland (1998, p. 8): "A 'sufficient cause,' which means a complete causal mechanism, can be defined as a set of minimal conditions and events that inevitably produce disease; 'minimal' implies that all of the conditions or events are necessary." Aickin (2002, chapter 3) uses the term *minimal sufficient cause*.

however, between the reliability application and our causation model. In the reliability application, all pieces of equipment are produced such that they have the same components and the same minimal cut sets. In our causation model, as discussed earlier, each individual in the population may or may not inherit the genetic factors or be exposed to the environmental factors that constitute the sufficient causes. As in our causation model, if the number of minimal cut sets in the reliability application is large, asymptotic theory of extreme values can possibly be employed to approximate the time to failure distribution of the coherent system (the distribution of the minimum time to failure of the cut sets), but one clearly cannot assume independence of the time to failure of the cut sets, because different cut sets can share one or more components.

However, denoting the minimal cut sets $C_1, C_2, ..., C_n$, Galambos (1981, 1987, p. 232) notes that the construction of the set E_n is evident: if C_i and C_j have one or several components in common, then (i, j) belongs to E_n. Similarly, if we denote the sufficient causes in our causation model $S_1, S_2, ..., S_n$, we construct the set E_n by letting (i, j) belong to E_n if S_i and S_j have one or several component causes in common. We then assume that the pairs of sufficient causes that do not belong to the set E_n (i.e., pairs of sufficient causes that do not contain common component causes) are "almost independent," in the weak mathematical terms expressed in assumptions (i) and (ii) of the definition of the E_n-sequence in Section 2.1.1. Also, the requirement in assumption (iii) that the number of elements of the set E_n be of smaller order of magnitude than n^2 does not seem hard to satisfy from a biological point of view. For example, if we consider that there are 100 sufficient causes of death, the maximum possible number of pairs of sufficient causes is $\binom{100}{2} = 4950$. If we then imagine that we can divide these 100 sufficient causes into 10 groups of 10 sufficient causes, such that within a group each sufficient cause shares one or more component causes with each other, but no sufficient cause shares a component cause with a sufficient cause from another group, then the number of elements of the set E_n is $10\binom{10}{2} = 450$, which is of smaller order of magnitude than n^2.

It crucially remains to be argued why the time-to-event distributions of the sufficient causes under consideration would possibly belong to a family of functions that are flat at the lower endpoint of the distribution. We make that case on evolutionary grounds. As we noted at the end of the previous section, the Gompertz pattern of increase in mortality rates has been broadly explained in connection with the decline in the force of natural selection with adult age. Instead, we more specifically bring the evolutionary theory of aging into our causation model through the idea that since the time-to-event distributions of the sufficient causes under consideration are related to genetic component causes, they would have been "molded" over evolutionary history by the declining force of natural selection. A possible mechanism for such molding would be as follows. Consistent with the notion that the force of natural selection acting on a mutation that reduces survival decreases with age, the probability of fixation of a deleterious mutation, hence also its ultimate frequency in the population under mutation–selection balance, depends on its age of expression (Charlesworth, 1973;

Charlesworth and Williamson, 1975). For instance, a deleterious mutation that expresses its effect around age 40 years will be subject to stronger negative selection and be present at lower frequency in the population than a mutation that expresses its effect around age 60 years. This has been expressed in the context of describing mutation accumulation as follows: "If deleterious mutations are held in the population by a mutation-selection balance, if the strength of the selection declines with age, and if there are mutations with age-specific deleterious effects, they must increase in frequency as the age-class that they affect becomes older" (Stearns, 1992, p. 200). Or as stated by Partridge and Barton (1993), "Because the intensity of selection on later-acting mutants declines with age, alleles with deleterious effects will reach a higher frequency in a mutation-selection balance the later the age at which they reduce fitness."[15]

We follow this reasoning here but at the level of the sufficient causes, rather than at the level of a single mutation or component cause, because the phenotypic expression (i.e., death) for the action of natural selection only occurs in the context of our causation model once a sufficient cause is complete. However, the shaping of the frequencies of the sufficient causes by natural selection would be indirectly accomplished through the effects of the declining force of natural selection on the frequencies of the genetic component causes (since a sufficient cause is only present if all its component causes are present, the frequencies of the sufficient causes in the population depend on the frequencies of their component causes). In the case of the sufficient causes containing only genetic component causes or having time-to-event distribution determined only by genetic component causes, sufficient causes with time-to-event distributions shifted toward older ages of expression would be present at successively higher frequencies, while those with distributions shifted closer to the earliest age at reproduction in the population would be present at successively lower frequencies. At the extreme, sufficient causes with time-to-event distributions shifted heavily toward the earliest age at reproduction in the population and/or presenting a relatively heavy lower tail would tend to be eliminated from the population through the action of natural selection over evolutionary history.

We additionally postulate a second mechanism by which the declining force of natural selection could mold the time-to-event distribution of the sufficient causes, which involves genes whose effects are to modify the age of expression of the sufficient causes of death. These "modifier genes" would be subject to positive selection during evolutionary history if they delayed the age of expression of the sufficient causes and would have been more strongly selected for as they delayed the ages of expression of

---

[15] An analogous reasoning involving antagonistic pleiotropy is not as straightforward. For instance, it is easy to see that a mutation with both a deleterious effect on survival around age 40 years and a beneficial effect on survival (or reproduction) around age 20 years should be present at a higher frequency in the population than another mutation with solely a deleterious effect around age 40. Yet such mutation with beneficial and deleterious effects around ages 20 and 40, respectively, might be present at a higher frequency in the population than a mutation with solely a deleterious effect around age 60. That is, compared to the mutation with deleterious effect around age 60, the mutation with the antagonistic pleiotropic effect may end up with higher frequency in the population because of the early increased fitness, despite being subject to stronger negative selection later in life.

the sufficient causes closer to the earliest age at reproduction in the population. As such, this mechanism would have the effect of modifying the lower tail behavior of the time-to-event distribution of the sufficient causes. An analogous idea of postponement of the age of onset of genetic diseases had been proposed by Haldane (1942, pp. 191–194), and it was restated by Medawar (1952) as a mechanism for accounting for the evolution of aging separate from mutation accumulation and antagonistic pleiotropy: "If hereditary factors achieve their overt expression at some intermediate age of life; if the age of overt expression is variable; and if these variations are themselves inheritable; then natural selection will so act as to enforce the postponement of the age of the expression of those factors that are unfavourable, and, correspondingly, to expedite the effects of those that are favourable—a recession and a precession, respectively, of the variable age-effects of genes."[16] Wallace (1967) similarly considered the operation of modifier genes. However, this idea has been denied a major role as a population genetic mechanism of aging, because population genetics theory has shown that selection for modifier alleles is too weak to account substantially for the evolution of aging (Charlesworth, 1994, p. 200; Rose, 1991, pp. 70–71).

The two proposed mechanisms in the preceding text might not do enough to lead to time-to-event distributions of the sufficient causes that are flat at the earliest age at reproduction in the population, which we take as the lower endpoint of the distribution. However, we further consider that because of the extreme dependence of human offspring on parental care for a relatively long period of time, the force of natural selection acting on a mutation that reduces survival during reproductive years would be sustained at a high level for human populations, especially so during the earliest reproductive years. (As indicated in Section 2.2, this reasoning is generally consistent with Lee's (2003) formal theory incorporating selection due to intergenerational transfers.) That is to say that if a parent died soon after the earliest childbirth, the prospects of survival of any human offspring and propagation of the causal mutation would be greatly reduced. Previous authors have expressed this notion with respect to the death of human parents or the survival experience of the population, in contrast to our reasoning in terms of the time-to-event distribution of sufficient causes of death. For instance, Kirkwood and Austad (2000) stated: "human infants are born unusually early, relative to other species, with respect to the completion of brain growth and development. Infants remain highly dependent for extended periods and, in the ancestral environment, their survival will have been unlikely if their mother died in

---

[16] Both Haldane (1942, pp. 191–194) and Medawar (1952) proposed this idea based on the autosomal dominant neurological disorder Huntington's disease, with age of onset usually in the mid-30s to mid-40s. Haldane (1942, p. 193) wrote: "The present age of onset of that disease may merely mean that primitive men and women seldom lived much beyond forty, so postponement of onset beyond this age had no selective advantage." In considering the question of why a postponement of the age of onset of Huntington's disease to later ages had not already occurred, Medawar (1952) wrote: "My answer to this is based on an aside of Professor Haldane's. It is only in the last century or so that selection has had a real chance to get a grip on it, for it is only within this period that the average expectation of life at birth has come to equal the average age of onset of the disease." Although Haldane (1942) did not further develop this idea into a broader and more detailed evolutionary explanation of aging, Rose et al. (2008) attributed to him the initial publication of "the key insight into the evolution of ageing."

childbirth." Williams (1957) defined a reproductive probability function depending on both survival and fecundity and used this notion in the following reasoning: "In many primitive human societies the death of teen-age parents must have greatly reduced the survival prospects of any children they might have produced. The care of dependent offspring is as important to human reproduction as the production of gametes. So the rate of decline in reproductive probability in early adulthood must be very slight, and this factor should result in a very low rate of senescence during the first decade of man's reproductive life."[17]

Wallace (1967) explored in simple mathematical terms the consequences for fitness of a mutation that caused an increase in survival early in life and increased mortality later in life, according to whether or not the survival of a parent after reproduction had an effect increasing the survival of offspring. Under some simplistic and extreme assumptions for illustration purposes, the mutation caused an increase in fitness when the survival of the parent had no effect on the survival of the offspring but a decrease in fitness in the opposite scenario. For our purposes, we make a plausibility argument here. For the sufficient causes of death under consideration, if the age of expression of a sufficient cause were in a small right-neighborhood of the earliest age at reproduction in the population, denoted here by x_0, a "premium" in relation to the dependence of human offspring would be placed on the force of natural selection acting on this sufficient cause. The closer to x_0 the age of expression of the sufficient cause was, the higher the premium and the closer it would bring the force of natural selection to its maximum level at and before x_0. This would impact both proposed mechanisms, involving (i) negative selection against sufficient causes with time-to-event distributions shifted heavily toward x_0 and/or presenting a relatively heavy lower tail and (ii) positive selection for modifier genes delaying the ages of expression of the sufficient causes close to x_0. To the extent that the survival function for the sufficient causes under consideration reflected the force of natural selection, it would be more and more flat as age approached x_0. Thus, the molding by the declining force of natural selection of the lower tail behavior of the time-to-event distribution of the sufficient causes under consideration would plausibly lead to time-to-event distributions that are flat at the earliest age at reproduction in the population.

We conclude this section with three remarks. First, we have made our argument based on the underlying notion of mutation accumulation (i.e., the sufficient causes of death have time-to-event distributions determined by mutations with deleterious age-specific effects), apparently to the exclusion of antagonistic pleiotropy. However, the crux of the argument is not materially affected by the operation of antagonistic pleiotropy, for the following reason. Consider a mutation with a deleterious effect on survival at some age in a small right-neighborhood of x_0 and an earlier beneficial effect (on survival or reproduction). Given the extreme dependence of human offspring on parental care, the beneficial effect of the mutation for the purpose of natural selection would tend to be nullified by the deleterious effect occurring in a very short time frame after the earliest age at reproduction. Second, despite the fact that we have

[17] Reproduced from *Evolution*, **11**, Williams, G. C., Pleiotropy, natural selection, and the evolution of senescence, pages 398–411, Copyright 1957, with permission from Wiley.

argued in terms of an infinitely flat survival function, the survival and distribution functions for the group of sufficient causes under consideration could instead have a very large (say, in the hundreds) but finite number of derivatives at x_0 equal to 0. In this case, we need to assume that the results for an infinitely flat distribution function in Section 2.1.2 are valid to a satisfactory approximation for an initial distribution with such very large number of derivatives at x_0 equal to 0. Third, these asymptotic results involve only the lower endpoint of the initial distribution as they correspond to the mathematical scenario in which the number of sufficient causes goes to infinity. In the actual situation of a large but finite number of sufficient causes, the behavior of the initial distribution not only at the lower endpoint but supposedly in some right-neighborhood of the lower endpoint would have an effect on the distribution of the minimum.

2.2.2 Boundaries of the Argument

There are two sorts of boundaries on the extent to which the argument for Gompertzian mortality on evolutionary grounds is valid. The first boundary refers to the types of causes of death, and the second to the range of ages at death. These boundaries can be simply established based on the previous evolutionary reasoning. First, because the argument in Section 2.2.1 involves sufficient causes of death related to the accumulation of deleterious age-specific genetic effects over evolutionary history, the argument does not apply to those accidental causes of death striking haphazardly and affecting with approximately equal likelihood the young and the old. Second, since the force of natural selection acting on age-specific genetic effects starts to decline at the earliest age at reproduction and reaches 0 at the end of reproduction in the population (or at the end of the effective transfers of food and care in social species), the argument applies to the corresponding in-between range of ages at death. We address these boundaries in the following text based on empirical observations from the application of the Gompertz model to mortality data and further evolutionary reasoning.

With respect to the first boundary, another British actuary of the nineteenth century, William M. Makeham, observed in three mortality tables that the increase in the logarithm of the mortality rates between ages 40 and 60 years was higher than between ages 20 and 40 years (Makeham, 1860). Based on that, he proposed incorporating an additive parameter to the Gompertz equation, and this modification became known as the Gompertz–Makeham equation:

$$h_{GM}(x) = \omega + \lambda e^{\theta x}, \tag{2.78}$$

where $\lambda > 0$ and θ are the original parameters from the Gompertz equation and $\omega > 0$ is the age-independent additive Makeham parameter. Gavrilov and Gavrilova (1991, p. 58) called the Makeham parameter the background component of mortality and referred to the second term in Equation 2.78 as the age-dependent component of the Gompertz–Makeham equation. The increase in the slope of $\log h_{GM}(x)$ as age increases can be shown by taking the derivative of the log of the Gompertz–Makeham equation:

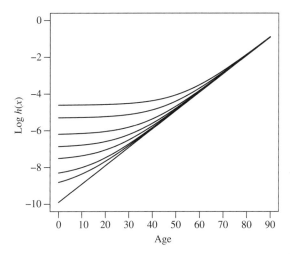

FIGURE 2.12 Semilog plots of the Gompertz–Makeham equation by age, for values of the Makeham parameter $\omega = 0, 0.0001, 0.0002, 0.0005, 0.001, 0.002, 0.005$, and 0.01, and keeping the other parameters fixed at $\lambda = 5e - 5$ and $\theta = 0.10$. The uppermost plot corresponds to the highest value of the Makeham parameter, and the straight line at the bottom corresponds to $\omega = 0$, in which case the Gompertz–Makeham equation reduces to the Gompertz equation.

$$\frac{d}{dx}\log\left(\omega + \lambda e^{\theta x}\right) = \frac{\theta \lambda e^{\theta x}}{\omega + \lambda e^{\theta x}} = \frac{\theta}{1 + (\omega/\lambda)e^{-\theta x}}, \tag{2.79}$$

which increases and approaches θ as x increases. This is illustrated in Figure 2.12 for different values of the Makeham parameter. The appropriateness of the Gompertz–Makeham equation in providing a good description of age-specific mortality rates over longer age ranges than the Gompertz equation, especially due to better fit in young adult ages, has been widely acknowledged (Beard, 1959; Greenwood, 1928; Perks, 1932; Sutter and Tabah, 1952).

In another article, Makeham (1867) additionally noted that a mortality schedule based only on "some diseases depending for their intensity solely upon the gradual diminution of the vital power" would be fitted by the Gompertz equation far more closely than a mortality schedule based on total mortality. This laid the ground for a partitioning of mortality into intrinsic mortality (including deaths that are "either caused or initiated by processes that originate within the body") and extrinsic mortality (including deaths that are "either caused or initiated by something that originates outside the body") (Carnes and Olshansky, 1997). Examples of causes of extrinsic mortality are accidents, homicides, suicides, predation, natural disasters, poisoning, starvation, and infectious diseases. Operationally, intrinsic causes of death are those that remain after the elimination of extrinsic causes of death (Carnes and Olshansky, 1997; Carnes et al., 2006).

Gompertz (1825) himself had thought along the lines of Makeham's (1867) reasoning: "It is possible that death may be the consequence of two generally co-existing causes; the one, chance, without previous disposition to death or deterioration; the other, a deterioration, or an increased inability to withstand destruction." He referred to the operation of each of these groups of causes using the following conditional statements: "If, for instance, there be a number of diseases to which the young and old were equally liable, and likewise which should be equally destructive whether the patient be young or old…"; "but if mankind be continually gaining seeds of indisposition, or in other words, an increased liability to death (which appears not to be an unlikely supposition with respect to a great part of life, though the contrary appears to take place at certain periods)…." He proceeded to point out the implications for the survival function and the force of mortality if each of these groups of causes occurred alone, yet this did not lead him to formulate Makeham's (1860) modification.

The following lines of evidence have supported the view that the age-independent additive parameter in Makeham's (1860) modification of the Gompertz equation is due to the contribution of extrinsic mortality to the mortality schedule. First, Jones (1956) analyzed life-table data from countries throughout the world and provided graphical evidence for widely different Makeham parameter estimates, supposedly reflecting varying impacts of infectious disease and malnutrition. Second, Gavrilov and Gavrilova (1991, pp. 77–85) fitted the Gompertz–Makeham equation to mortality data from the Swedish male population and reported a decrease in the Makeham parameter estimate from more than 5.5 in 1901–1910 to 0.5 in 1983, covering the relatively recent period corresponding to major advances in sanitation and public health. They obtained similar results using twentieth-century mortality data from males and females in other European countries, Japan, and the United States. Likewise, based on the analysis of mortality data from Swedish females, Jones (1959) provided graphical evidence for a substantial change in the Makeham parameter estimate during the period from 1751 through 1950. Data for four countries presented by Omran (1971) and Dutch data presented by Bonneux et al. (1998) are consistent with this pattern, as can be seen in Figure 2.13 and Figure 2.14, respectively. Third, by partitioning U.S. 1996 mortality data into intrinsic and extrinsic mortalities using the International Classification of Diseases (ICD) codes for the underlying cause of death, Carnes et al. (2006) observed a substantially better fit by the Gompertz model when extrinsic causes of death were excluded from total all-cause mortality data. The plots of the logarithm of age-specific mortality rates by age for all-cause, intrinsic, and extrinsic mortalities revealed that a "hump" in all-cause mortality between ages 15 and 40 years (peak at about 20 years) was related to mortality from extrinsic causes, and intrinsic mortality between ages 15 and 90 years conformed well to the Gompertz model. This is shown in Figure 2.15.

With respect to the second boundary—the range of ages at death for which the argument for Gompertzian mortality is valid—even as it was supposed to be related to inherent biological processes, the Gompertz equation was not originally intended to describe age-specific mortality rates over the entire human life span (Gompertz, 1825). For one clear inadequacy of the Gompertz equation, the observed mortality rates in the neonatal and infancy years tend to decrease with age and are substantially higher than those expected from fitting the Gompertz model to overall mortality data. This provides a justification for estimating the initial mortality rate (parameter λ of the

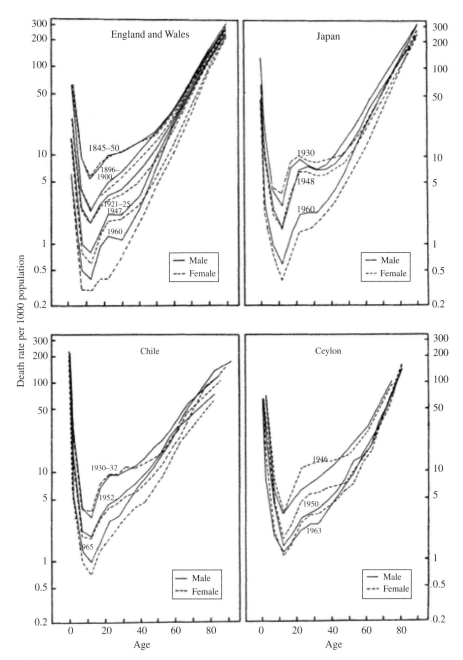

FIGURE 2.13 Semilog plots of mortality rates by age and sex in four countries at different time periods (reproduced from *The Milbank Memorial Fund Quarterly*, **49**, Omran, A. R., The epidemiologic transition: A theory of the epidemiology of population change, pages 509–538, Copyright 1971, with permission from Wiley); note the similarity of these plots to the Gompertz–Makeham equation plots in Figure 2.12.

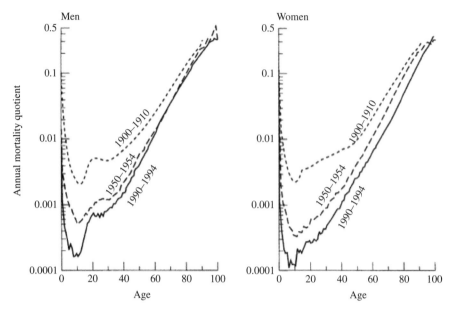

FIGURE 2.14 Semilog plots of mortality rates by age for the Dutch population at different time periods, separately for men and women (reproduced from *Journal of Epidemiology and Community Health*, **52**, Bonneux, L., Barendregt, J. J., and Van der Maas, P. J., The expiry date of man: A synthesis of evolutionary biology and public health, pages 619–623, Copyright 1998, with permission from BMJ Publishing Group Ltd.).

Gompertz equation) at the age of puberty or sexual maturity (Finch et al., 1990; Kirkwood, 1985). On the other extreme of the human life span, as survival to very old ages has become less of a rare event in human populations, a phenomenon of deceleration of mortality rates (i.e., less than exponential increase) has been observed, such that the fit of the Gompertz equation to human mortality data after approximately 90 years old is not satisfactory (Gavrilov and Gavrilova, 1991; Greenwood and Irwin, 1939; Olshansky and Carnes, 1997). Based on that, Gavrilov and Gavrilova (1991, p. 68) proposed that the dependence of human mortality on age consists of three periods: "a period of high child mortality, when the force of mortality decreases with age; a period of sexual maturity, when the force of mortality grows with age, usually following the Gompertz–Makeham law; and finally, a senile period, when the force of mortality is very high and grows comparatively slowly with age."

For the purposes of our argument for Gompertzian mortality, the lower bound of the relevant range of ages at death is given by the earliest age at reproduction in the population, and the germane earliest age at reproduction in the population is not the one in present human populations, but that which predominated during a continued period of time in human ancestors. From a statistical point of view, any population will have biological variation among its members in the age of first reproduction. The drawback of defining the earliest age at reproduction in the population by the minimum of the distribution of the ages of first reproduction over a period of time is that

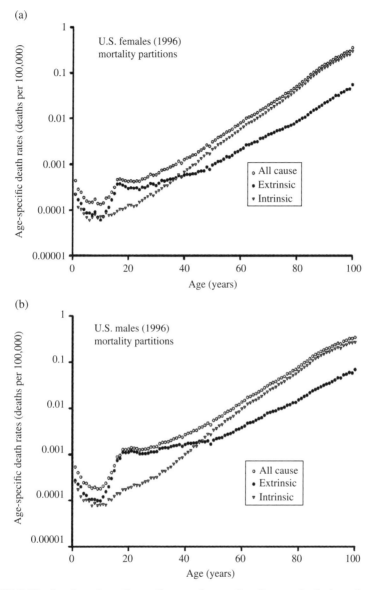

FIGURE 2.15 Semilog plots of mortality rates by age for all-cause, intrinsic, and extrinsic mortalities, separately for females and males (reproduced from *Biogerontology*, **7**, Carnes, B. A., Holden, L. R., Olshansky, S. J., Witten, M. T., and Siegel, J. S., Mortality partitions and their relevance to research on senescence, pages 183–198, Copyright 2006, with permission from Springer Science + Business Media).

this would not exclude outliers, occurring at one point in time or very sporadically during evolution. Thus, it seems more appropriate to think of the earliest age at reproduction in the population as a small percentile of the distribution, say, the first percentile. Based on estimates that menarche occurred in female human ancestors in Paleolithic and Neolithic times between the ages of 7 and 13 years and full reproductive competence in Neolithic females occurred between the ages of 9 and 14 years (Gluckman and Hanson, 2006), we take 10 years as an approximate earliest age at reproduction in the human population. This is admittedly a rough approximation based on limited evidence, but it is consistent with the observation in Figure 2.13, Figure 2.14, and Figure 2.15 that mortality rates in recent human populations reach a bottom and start to rise at approximately 10 years old.

The observation of a deceleration of mortality rates at very old ages in humans has been corroborated by experimental studies demonstrating late-life mortality plateaus, or even falling mortality rates, in very large laboratory cohorts of medfly and fruit fly (Carey et al., 1992; Curtsinger et al., 1992). These findings were initially met with skepticism and questions about possible artifactual explanations (Kowald and Kirkwood, 1993; Nusbaum et al., 1993; Robine and Ritchie, 1993), but they have been replicated in different species under diverse laboratory conditions (Carey, 2003, chapter 3; Rauser et al., 2006; Rose et al., 2005; Vaupel et al., 1998). While the previous observations of mortality deceleration in humans were attributed to reasons like inaccuracy of the data and older people having more careful behavior or receiving better health care (Horiuchi and Wilmoth, 1998; Rose et al., 2005, 2006) and thus did not prompt any major rethinking, the experimental observations on laboratory animals forced the question of whether very old individuals aged more slowly or showed "cessation of aging" (a nonincreasing hazard of death for individuals after a certain age).

The heterogeneity explanation put forward for late-life mortality plateaus would avoid that conclusion by considering that, within a population, there are different subpopulations defined by a general susceptibility of their members to death. Although each subpopulation would follow a pattern of ever-increasing mortality rates with increasing age, the overall mortality pattern in the population would eventually show a plateau due to the more susceptible individuals dying earlier, such that only the more robust individuals would live to late ages (Beard, 1959; Vaupel, 1988; Vaupel et al., 1979). As put by Vaupel and Carey (1993), "Death changes the composition of a cohort by differentially removing the frail," such that the mortality pattern of the population may be "an artifact of the evolving structure of the population" rather than reflecting changes in the hazard of death for individuals. Horiuchi and Wilmoth (1998) expressed it in terms of the deceleration in mortality rates at late ages being due to "a statistical effect of selection through the attrition of mortality" according to the "heterogeneity hypothesis," as opposed to a slowing down in the increase of mortality risk for individuals according to the "individual-risk hypothesis."

On initial examination, the heterogeneity explanation for late-life mortality plateaus has appealing characteristics. Under this explanation, one need not consider the implications for demography and the evolutionary theory of aging of a slowing down of individual aging at late ages. Also, heterogeneity in the broad sense of differences among individuals within a population is ubiquitous at all levels of bio-logical organization (Carnes and Olshansky, 2001). However, Rose et al. (2005, 2006) have emphasized that the heterogeneity explanation involves differences among individuals throughout the life span, rather than sporadic or intermittent het-erogeneity that pertains to some but not all age classes, hence their use of the term *lifelong heterogeneity*. Moreover, while mortality deceleration at late ages naturally arises whenever lifelong heterogeneity in susceptibility to death is present in a pop-ulation, the magnitude of lifelong heterogeneity must be large enough to explain observed mortality plateaus in experimental studies (Pletcher and Curtsinger, 1998; Rose et al., 2005). Mueller et al. (2003) compared predictions from models of lifelong heterogeneity to mortality observations in large laboratory populations of *D. melanogaster*; they found that the required levels of variation in demographic heterogeneity models far exceeded "what would be considered biologically plausi-ble." They further listed four predictions of the heterogeneity explanation that were refuted in their and others' (Drapeau et al., 2000; Khazaeli et al., 1998) exper-imental animal studies. Using human data, Horiuchi and Wilmoth (1998) tested three predictions of the heterogeneity hypothesis inferred through qualitative reasoning and illustrated quantitatively. Although the results were broadly consistent with the heterogeneity hypothesis, the authors noted that they were possibly also compatible with "specific versions of the individual-risk hypothesis." Overall, even if lifelong heterogeneity may have some impact on mortality rates at late life, experimental tests suggest that it is not a sufficient explanation of late-life mortality plateaus (Rauser et al., 2006; Rose et al., 2005, 2006).

Assuming that deceleration of mortality rates in the population actually reflects a slowing down of individual aging at late ages, it was not initially obvious how the evolutionary theory of aging could explain it, because the force of natural selection after the last age at reproduction (or the last age of transfer of food and care) in the population is 0, implying the absence of selection to maintain survival very late in life. Thus, it was claimed that the phenomenon of deceleration of mortality rates at very old ages called the evolutionary theory of aging into question (Charlesworth and Partridge, 1997; Gavrilov and Gavrilova, 2001).[18] The first indication that evo-lutionary theory might account for the observation of late-life mortality plateaus in experimental animal studies came from theoretical optimization and population genet-ics studies that produced results consistent with a deceleration of mortality rates at very old ages (Abrams and Ludwig, 1995; Mueller and Rose, 1996). However, criti-cisms have been made to some of the assumptions of the theoretical models in these studies (Charlesworth and Partridge, 1997; Pletcher and Curtsinger, 1998; Wachter,

[18] Given the long-standing notion among demographers of a Gompertzian pattern of ever-increasing mor-tality rates with age in the population taken as a whole, a deceleration of mortality rates at very old ages also challenged the field of demography. As stated by Mueller and Rose (1996), "late-life mortality plateaus pose a major problem for both demography and the evolutionary theory of aging, ostensibly challenging the foun-dations of two fields simultaneously." However, Carnes and Olshansky (2001) considered that "Although it is generally accepted that mortality over the entire age range of humans cannot be described by Gompertz's original equation, it is inappropriate to use this observation to declare that all Gompertz-based analyses are therefore flawed or that heterogeneity justifies the rejection of the Gompertz paradigm."

1999). Thus, although Mueller and Rose (1996) claimed that "evolutionary theory predicts late-life mortality plateaus" based on their study, this conclusion was challenged by Pletcher and Curtsinger (1998) and Wachter (1999). Importantly, Pletcher and Curtsinger (1998) argued that standard evolutionary models were not able to robustly account for the observation in experimental studies that mortality rates leveled off at values far below 100%, but both Charlesworth and Partridge (1997) and Pletcher and Curtsinger (1998) recognized that models incorporating positive pleiotropy at different ages held promise in addressing that. Indeed, Charlesworth (2001) showed with analytic and numerical results that by extending a standard model of mutation accumulation to include both age-specific and age-independent effects of mutations on mortality rates, maintenance of nonzero survival rates late in life was possible if there were enough alleles with age-independent beneficial effects, as these alleles would be favored by natural selection on the basis of their early beneficial effects and would have beneficial pleiotropic effects at later ages.

Within the context of Hamilton's (1966) work, as described in Section 2.2, the general evolutionary explanation for late-life mortality plateaus had simply been that it was a product of the plateau in the force of natural selection after the end of reproduction (Mueller and Rose, 1996). From that general explanation, Rose and Mueller (2000) derived the following prediction: "as the last age of reproduction should be relatively close to the age at which the force of natural selection reaches 0, experimental manipulation of that last age of reproduction should lead to the corresponding evolution of the age at which late-life mortality plateaus start." Thus, populations with later last age of reproduction should have later plateau onset. Rose et al. (2002) tested this prediction in computer simulations and experiments using *D. melanogaster* populations; their results showed that mortality plateaus shifted as predicted with the last age of reproduction in *D. melanogaster*, thus lending strong experimental support for the evolutionary explanation. In several articles, Rose et al. (2005, 2006, 2007, 2008) and Rauser et al. (2006) have elaborated on this explanation. In their account, the increase in age-specific mortality rates with increasing age arises from the decline in the force of natural selection, leading to a deterioration of the balance between selection and other evolutionary forces (e.g., mutation and genetic drift). Then, the late-life plateau in age-specific mortality rates would be due to the force of natural selection approaching a lower limit close to 0. This is not to say that age-specific genetic effects do not play a role in mortality after the force of natural selection reaches a plateau, but "natural selection will no longer discriminate among genetic effects that act at ages so late that they have had no impact on fitness during the evolutionary history of a population," because even in organisms that reproduce at all ages, the force of natural selection is overwhelmed by random genetic drift in late life (Rose et al., 2006).

However, a remaining puzzling aspect of this evolutionary account is that the force of natural selection in human populations reaches a plateau long before the observed onset of the deceleration of mortality rates (Charlesworth and Willliamson, 1975; see Fig. 2.11). Indeed, the force of natural selection drops to nearly 0 at 45–50 years in Figure 2.11, yet mortality deceleration in human populations starts at about 90 years (e.g., see Fig. 2.15). There are at least two potential explanations for that. First, similarly to how we argued in Section 2.2 that selection due to transfers of food and care in social species explained postreproductive survival (Lee, 2003) and implied that Hamilton's equation underestimated the force of natural selection at human adult ages, we can argue that intergenerational transfers, by substantially changing the "effective last age of reproduction," push the actual plateau in the force of natural selection to later ages. In this way, intergenerational transfers would contribute to the onset of the deceleration of mortality rates at a substantially later age than expected based on Hamilton's equation. Second, along the lines that positive pleiotropy was invoked to explain postreproductive survival in Section 2.2 and the leveling off of mortality rates below 100% in this section, positive pleiotropy may also contribute to a later onset of deceleration of mortality rates. That is, in parallel to their effect in enhancing postreproductive survival and maintaining nonzero survival rates late in life, alleles with early beneficial effects and pleiotropic beneficial effects at later ages would possibly also delay the onset of the deceleration of mortality rates (Rose et al., 2002).

Based on the evolutionary explanation for late-life mortality plateaus, Rose et al. (2005) claimed that "Late life is an evolutionarily distinct phase of life history, evolving according to strictures very different from those that mold both early life and aging." As such, they considered that late life represents a new frontier for physiology as well. In this and other reviews, these authors have argued that late life is as distinct in its fundamental evolutionary properties from aging as aging is from development (Rauser et al., 2006; Rose et al., 2005, 2006). Thus, they have proposed that, from an evolutionary perspective, there are three fundamentally distinct phases of life: development, aging, and late life. What separates aging from the two other phases of life are the two divides imposed by the decline in the force of natural selection, which starts at the earliest age at reproduction in the population and reaches a plateau late in life, in relation to the last age of reproduction or transfer in the population.

The limits for the evolutionarily defined aging phase of life in human populations also define the range of ages at death for which our argument for Gompertzian mortality is valid. By taking 10 years as the earliest age at reproduction (in human ancestors) and 90 years as the supposed onset of the deceleration of mortality rates in present human populations, the aging phase of human life and our argument for Gompertzian mortality would refer to the wide age range 10–90 years. This is to say that if life expectancy of human populations were 100 years, the aging phase of life would cover 80% of the human life span; at present values of life expectancy, this proportion is even larger. This similarly means that the scope of our argument for Gompertzian mortality (as well as the scope of the remainder of this work) is also that large as a proportion of the human life span. Clearly, and probably even shockingly, the evolutionarily defined aging phase of life is at odds on both ends with the customary, nontechnical understanding of the extent of the aging phase of human life. On one end, the technical evolutionary understanding includes in the aging phase of human life adolescence and early adult life, and on the other end, it excludes the late-life years that are most characteristically or extremely identified with aging in common language.

Regardless of the wide extent of the aging phase of life on evolutionary grounds, and in contrast with all-encompassing descriptive or mechanistic attempts to account for the total mortality experience of human populations (e.g., Gavrilov and Gavrilova, 2003; Witten, 1989), it may seem from this section that our account of Gompertzian mortality relies on a strategy of "divide and conquer" (i.e., divide the causes of death in intrinsic and extrinsic and divide the human life span in development, aging, and late life; then attack exclusively intrinsic mortality during the aging phase of life). However, as we made clear throughout this chapter, this was not a post hoc procedure adopted for convenience. Rather, as our account of Gompertzian mortality gradually emerged from statistical and evolutionary theories, so did the boundaries that we have described here. In the next chapter, we will argue that the Gompertz model does not even tell the whole story of the intrinsic mortality experience of human populations during the evolutionarily defined aging phase of life—as one might have guessed from the restriction in Section 2.2.1 of the sufficient causes of death under consideration to those that contain only genetic component causes or have time-to-event distribution determined only by genetic component causes.

3

THE ARGUMENT AGAINST GOMPERTZIAN MORTALITY

Even if we took into account the boundaries described in Section 2.2.2 by restricting mortality data to deaths due to intrinsic causes and occurring within an age range of 10–90 years, there would remain questions about how good the fit by the Gompertz model to the data is and whether another distribution can provide a similarly good or better fit. In this vein, Economos (1982) forcefully challenged the status of the Gompertz model as the most appropriate and widely applied description of human mortality data: "it cannot be overemphasized that the inverse-sigmoid form of the survivorship curve makes it amenable to curve-fitting by a great variety of possible mathematical functions, one of which is Gompertz's...the Gompertzian function is not a general 'law' of mortality, but rather one of the possible empirical models that are capable of fitting mortality kinetics. Once this is generally understood and accepted, the Gompertzian function will no longer be used as a Procrustean bed on which mortality kinetics are shortened or stretched until a straight line is magicked from the data!"[1] We briefly take this view in Section 3.1 as we lay out some arguments and evidence for it; we then offer an outline of a possible resolution for it. We fully develop this resolution in Section 3.2.

---

[1] Reproduced from *Archives of Gerontology and Geriatrics*, **1**, Economos, A. C., Rate of aging, rate of dying and the mechanism of mortality, pages 3–27, Copyright 1982, with permission from Elsevier.

3.1 DEPARTURES FROM THE GOMPERTZ MODEL

The long-standing notion of a good fit by the Gompertz model to human mortality data may have been overstated. Such overstatement could be related to the following: (i) the fit by the Gompertz model to mortality data has often been assessed based solely on visual inspection of semilog plots of mortality rates by age, and (ii) the Gompertz distribution has commonly been fitted to mortality data without concomitant consideration of other parametric models. As an example of a more formal assessment, Prentice and El Shaarawi (1973) devised a procedure for testing the fit by the Gompertz model to age-specific mortality rates involving weighted linear regression and marginal likelihood. This procedure was applied using mortality data from Ontario for the years 1964–1968. For the age range 30–70 years, the mortality data departed significantly from the Gompertz model in males (all causes of death), males dying of cardiovascular causes, and females dying of neoplasms (El Shaarawi et al., 1974). Other studies have compared the fits to human mortality data by the Gompertz, Weibull, and logistic distributions, assessing the goodness of fit of each model based on the mean squared deviations between the empirical and estimated survival probabilities. For instance, Juckett and Rosenberg (1993) observed a better fit (i.e., lower mean squared deviation) by the Gompertz than the Weibull distribution for all-cause mortality and a better fit by the Weibull than the Gompertz distribution for single causes of death, including ischemic heart disease. Wilson (1994) reported a better fit to human mortality data by the Gompertz distribution compared to the Weibull and the two-parameter logistic distributions but a similar fit by the Gompertz distribution and the three-parameter logistic distribution.

In quoting Beard (1959) in the beginning of Chapter 2 ("A satisfying basis for a law of mortality would be a formula that, starting from some fundamental concepts about the biological ageing process, led to a distribution of deaths by age which was comparable with observational data"), we omitted the subsequent sentence: "Such comparison would not be simple and straightforward because environmental and secular factors would introduce distortions as compared with the theoretical underlying distribution." A resolution for the challenge to the Gompertz model on the basis of its fit to mortality data might follow if we considered that the Gompertz equation reflects some underlying biological truth, but departures from the model emerge at least partly from the action of environmental factors. This was suggested by Greenwood (1928) long ago, as follows: "If it were true that the Gompertz 'law' expressed some important element of biological truth, would its distortion when adequate data, from a numerical point of view, are at command depend upon the fact, (a) that its functional expression is imperfect, or (b) upon the blurring effect of the 'environmental' factors which it cannot be supposed adequately to express? I surmise that both explanations are true."[2] As a matter of fact, both explanations would amount to the same phenomenon if we considered that the Gompertz distribution is but one component of a mixture of two or more

[2] Reproduced from *The Journal of Hygiene*, **28**, Greenwood, M., "Laws" of mortality from the biological point of view, pages 267–294, Copyright 1928, with permission from Cambridge University Press.

distributions describing the human mortality experience, with the other distribution(s) reflecting the action of environmental factors.

Greenwood (1928) preceded this proposition with an inquiry into "constitutional and environmental factors of mortality." He questioned the notion, formalized through the additive age-independent parameter in the Gompertz–Makeham equation, that environmental factors acted independently of constitution and age, where he uses the term *environmental* "in the man in the street's sense of preventable or removable without resort to eugenic action": "Were that separation credible, that is to say, if the Order of Dying-out of any animals, really depended upon two independent factors, one of which was wholly independent of the physiological constitution of the indivi- duals composing the population, the Makeham–Gompertz formula would be the ideal biometer—as Farr would have said—of the public health officer."[3] By also consid- ering it unlikely that the contribution of environmental factors to mortality would be covered by a term in the expression of the force of mortality that is independent of age, he concluded that "this easy separation of the environmental and constitutional is far too good to be true and that we must try to be a little clearer as to what we mean by these words." Bourgeois-Pichat (1952) in turn emphasized the difficulty of separ- ating "endogenous" and "exogenous" mortality due to the concurrence of endogenous and exogenous factors in causing death, especially at intermediate ages between early adult and late life. Presumably, accidental deaths occurring in earlier adult life would be more easily categorized as exogenous.

These authors' reservations seem largely to originate in the broad sense in which they use the terms *environmental* or *exogenous factors*, implying that we may begin to address them by distinguishing between the operation of accidental factors (i.e., extrinsic causes of death) and what we may call *environmental factors sensu stricto*. The following are proposed guidelines, which are intended only as first approxima- tions: (i) except for the fact that risk-taking behaviors are associated with age, accidental factors are roughly age-independent (i.e., they are equally likely to affect the young and the old), while environmental factors *sensu stricto* tend to show an increasing hazard of expression with increasing age; (ii) accidental factors usually strike suddenly or in a short period of time, while environmental factors *sensu stricto* usually take effect after reaching a certain threshold of cumulative exposure over longer periods of time; (iii) accidental factors generally operate by themselves, while environmental factors *sensu stricto* are component causes of sufficient causes containing other environmental or genetic component causes. Admittedly, accidental factors may not follow all these guidelines. For example, increasing susceptibility to infections due to immune system changes with increasing age implies that infections are not nearly age-independent, even though infections have traditionally been regarded as accidental factors. One may also claim that there is a propensity toward accidents, homicides, or suicides in relation to some predisposing genetic factors, in which case the accidental factor would not be operating by itself. More importantly, accidental factors may operate as actual environmental factors *sensu stricto* as they can be risk factors for

---

[3] Idem.

diseases associated with intrinsic mortality. For example, papillomavirus is a risk factor for cervical cancer, and traumatic brain injury has been shown to be a risk factor for Alzheimer's disease. Hence, infection and trauma are operating as environmental component causes in sufficient causes of diseases associated with intrinsic mortality and should be regarded in these instances as environmental factors *sensu stricto*.

If we restrict mortality data to intrinsic mortality, thus circumventing the need to add the age-independent Makeham parameter to the Gompertz equation, while keeping in mind the distinction between accidental factors and environmental factors *sensu stricto*, we can then address the challenge to the Gompertz model on the basis of its fit to mortality data by focusing on the operation of environmental factors *sensu stricto*, which are not claimed to act independently of age or, as Greenwood (1928) put it, constitution. In order to properly address how departures from the Gompertz model emerge from the action of these environmental factors (which henceforth we will refer to without the qualifying *sensu stricto*), we will further develop our model of causation based on evolutionary reasoning in the next section. The approach will take account of age-dependency of environmental effects and gene–environment interactions. Lest it be thought that this development is purely theoretical, we reiterate that this is a necessary step toward construction of the index of aging-relatedness in Chapter 4. Our goal is to progress in the direction charted by Perks (1932) in the following terms, with respect to mortality data: "most of us retain, consciously or unconsciously, a feeling that, underlying all the roughnesses in our data referable to errors of observation and an ever-changing environment, there may be an inherent mathematical system of law and order, which if it could but be discovered would give such insight into the meaning of the unadjusted figures that a considerable advance would be made in the practical application of our science."[4]

3.2   AN EVOLUTION-BASED MODEL OF CAUSATION

We further develop the SCC model by classifying the component causes based on evolutionary reasoning. Genetic effects are classified as "early onset" or "late onset" according to whether the expression of their causal role (as opposed to gene expression at the molecular level) occurs before or after the earliest age at reproduction in the population, respectively. This reflects the notion that the force of natural selection starts to decrease at the earliest age at reproduction in the population. The use of the term *genetic effect* as opposed to *genetic factor* serves the purpose of emphasizing the fundamental importance in our causation model of the age at which the genetic factor potentially affects the phenotype (*potentially* because that depends on the expression of other necessary component causes). Environmental factors are classified as "evolutionarily conserved" if they have been present through enough time during evolutionary history for adaptation to their effects to take place. Many of them are

---

[4] Reproduced from *Journal of the Institute of Actuaries*, **63**, Perks, W., On some experiments in the graduation of mortality statistics, pages 12–57, Copyright 1932, with permission from Cambridge University Press.

what we consider "part of nature" and tend to be ubiquitous, the implication being that virtually all members of the population are exposed to these environmental factors early in life. We thus make the simplifying assumption that enough exposure to evolutionarily conserved environmental factors for expression of their necessary causal role occurs before the earliest age at reproduction in the population. On the other hand, environmental factors are classified as "evolutionarily recent" if they are recent enough on an evolutionary scale so that adaptation to their effects has not occurred in most of the population. While this temporal characterization does not involve a precise boundary, the important practical implication is that environmental factors brought about by industrialization (e.g., exposure to chemicals and toxins) and modern life (e.g., cigarette smoking, sedentarism, changes in diet, and chronic stress) clearly fall under the category of evolutionarily recent environmental factors. Exposures brought about by industrialization involve mostly but not exclusively nonnaturally occurring substances; a naturally occurring substance may become present in the environment at higher doses than those that prevailed during evolutionary history and be regarded as evolutionarily recent.

We use the acronyms EOGE, LOGE, ECEF, and EREF as adjectival categories of necessary component causes, meaning, respectively, early-onset genetic effect(s), late-onset genetic effect(s), evolutionarily conserved environmental factor(s), and evolutionarily recent environmental factor(s). Sufficient causes contain any of 15 different combinations of from one to four categories (EOGE, LOGE, ECEF, EREF; EOGE + LOGE, EOGE + ECEF, …; EOGE + LOGE + ECEF, EOGE + LOGE + EREF, …; EOGE + LOGE + ECEF + EREF). The presence of any one of these categories in a sufficient cause means that *one or more* genetic effects or environmental factors of the given category are components of the sufficient cause. Since our causation model, like the evolutionary argument for Gompertzian mortality, applies to the evolutionarily defined aging phase of life (Section 2.2.2), we restrict the sufficient causes under consideration to those that are potentially related to death *after the earliest age at reproduction in the population.*

Thus, of the 15 possible combinations of categories, three will not be considered. First, a sufficient cause of death containing only EOGE would be either eliminated by natural selection or maintained through mutation–selection balance (e.g., in the case of a recessive mutation). In the latter case, a sufficient cause containing only EOGE would by definition cause death before the earliest age at reproduction in the population. Second, given our simplifying assumption that ECEF expresses its causal role before the earliest age at reproduction in the population, a sufficient cause containing EOGE and ECEF but not other categories of component causes would likewise cause death before the earliest age at reproduction in the population. Third, a sufficient cause containing only ECEF could not have been maintained during evolutionary history, because, by our definition of ECEF, a genetic variant that prevented its deleterious action would be adaptive and spread through the population by positive selection; otherwise, to the extent that the sufficient cause was ubiquitous, it could in principle extinguish the population. The remaining 12 combinations of categories of component causes into sufficient causes are listed in Table 3.1, classified according to whether they contain LOGE but not EREF, EREF but not LOGE, or both LOGE

TABLE 3.1   Combinations of categories of component causes into sufficient causes[a,b]

Containing LOGE but not EREF	Containing EREF but not LOGE	Containing both LOGE and EREF
LOGE	EREF	LOGE + EREF
LOGE + EOGE	EREF + EOGE	LOGE + EREF + EOGE
LOGE + ECEF	EREF + ECEF	LOGE + EREF + ECEF
LOGE + EOGE + ECEF	EREF + EOGE + ECEF	LOGE + EREF + EOGE + ECEF

[a] The presence of any category of component causes in a sufficient cause means that one or more genetic effects or environmental factors of the given category are part of the sufficient cause.
[b] ECEF, evolutionarily conserved environmental factor(s); EOGE, early-onset genetic effect(s); EREF, evolutionarily recent environmental factor(s); LOGE, late-onset genetic effect(s).

and EREF. We note that while LOGE component causes by definition express their causal role after the earliest age at reproduction in the population, this is not a requirement in the definition of EREF component causes. Hence, there is no guarantee that sufficient causes containing EREF but not LOGE (second column in Table 3.1) will only cause death after the earliest age at reproduction in the population. For the same evolutionary reasons that we are restricting the sufficient causes under consideration to those that are potentially related to death after the earliest age at reproduction in the population, we will consider that the time-to-event distribution of the sufficient causes containing EREF but not LOGE arises from the *conditional* time-to-event distribution of the EREF component causes given survival to the earliest age at reproduction in the population.

The combinations classified in Table 3.1 can be more broadly categorized according to whether or not the time-to-event distributions of the sufficient causes are molded by the declining force of natural selection. First, consider the sufficient causes of death containing LOGE but not EREF (first column in Table 3.1). Since we are only considering death after the earliest age at reproduction and the other possible component causes, ECEF and EOGE, either by definition or by assumption express their necessary causal role before the earliest age at reproduction, the last category to occur leading to completion of a sufficient cause in this group is LOGE. If only one LOGE participates in the sufficient cause, the age at death for the sufficient cause is given by the age of expression of the one LOGE, while if two or more LOGE participate in the sufficient cause, the age at death is given by the maximum age of expression of all LOGE. Thus, the time-to-event distribution of a sufficient cause in this group is the distribution of the maximum age of expression of the LOGE component causes. Because the age at death for these sufficient causes is given by the age of expression of heritable factors, their time-to-event distributions are molded by the declining force of natural selection.

For the sufficient causes containing EREF but not LOGE (second column in Table 3.1), the last category of component cause to occur leading to the completion of these sufficient causes is EREF. If only one EREF participates in the sufficient cause, the age at death is given by the age of expression of the one EREF, while if two or more EREF participate in the sufficient cause, the age at death is given by the maximum age of expression of all EREF. Thus, the time-to-event distribution of these sufficient causes is the distribution of the maximum age of expression of the EREF component causes. In this case, because the age at death for these sufficient causes is given by the age of expression of nonheritable factors, their time-to-event distributions are not molded by the declining force of natural selection.

For the sufficient causes containing both LOGE and EREF (third column in Table 3.1), the last category of component cause to occur leading to the completion of these sufficient causes is either LOGE or EREF. The age at death for the sufficient cause is given by the maximum age of expression of the two or more LOGE and EREF component causes, and the time-to-event distribution of these sufficient causes is the distribution of the maximum age of expression of the LOGE and EREF component causes. For these sufficient causes, unlike for the sufficient causes containing LOGE but not EREF, the inexistence (by definition) of EREF during most of evolutionary history would have prevented the action of natural selection except recently on an evolutionary scale—because sufficient causes containing both LOGE and EREF are only complete, so that phenotypic expression allows natural selection to act, in the presence of the EREF in the environment. Therefore, despite the presence of LOGE in these sufficient causes, the molding of the time-to-event distribution of the sufficient causes by the declining force of natural selection would not have occurred, since it requires that enough evolutionary time has elapsed such that natural selection may have acted over a large enough number of generations.

We have thus defined two groups of sufficient causes in our causation model on evolutionary grounds: a first group of sufficient causes whose time-to-event distributions are molded by the declining force of natural selection, including the sufficient causes containing LOGE in the absence of EREF (first column in Table 3.1), and a second group of sufficient causes whose time-to-event distributions are not molded by the declining force of natural selection, including the sufficient causes containing EREF with or without LOGE (second and third columns in Table 3.1). The argument in Section 2.2.1 applies to the group of sufficient causes whose time-to-event distributions are molded by the declining force of natural selection. That is, since the time-to-event distributions of these sufficient causes are related solely to genetic component causes, they would have been molded by natural selection over evolutionary history in such a way that they would tend to be flat at the lower endpoint of the distribution. Then, if we assume that the time-to-event distributions of the sufficient causes in this group belong to a given family of functions that are flat at the lower endpoint of the distribution, the limiting distribution of the minimum will have an exponential hazard function. In Section 2.2.1, we stated that by considering the simplifying scenario of sufficient causes containing only genetic component causes or having time-to-event distribution determined only by genetic component causes, we would be accounting for the Gompertz pattern of mortality on exclusively biological grounds. Here, we make the sense of "exclusively biological grounds" more precise by specifying that the sufficient causes under consideration are those containing LOGE in the absence of EREF, which corresponds to the evolutionary explanation of aging in its pure or essential form.

For the group of sufficient causes whose time-to-event distributions are not molded by the declining force of natural selection, such that there is no operation of the postulated mechanisms that flatten the distribution at the lower endpoint (Section 2.2.1), we argue that those distributions are regularly varying functions at the lower endpoint of the distribution with exponent $0 < \rho < \infty$. For sufficient causes whose time-to-event distributions are molded by the declining force of natural selection, it makes sense to reason at the level of sufficient causes, because phenotypic expression only occurs once the sufficient cause is complete and thus natural selection acts at that level. On the other hand, for sufficient causes whose time-to-event distributions are not molded by the declining force of natural selection, it makes more sense to reason at the level of the environmental and genetic component causes. To that end, we first show that if the component distributions are regularly varying at the lower endpoint of the distribution, so is the time-to-event distribution of the sufficient cause. From the exact statistical theory of extreme values, if $F_i(x)$ is the c.d.f. of each component cause, for $i = 1, 2, ..., j$, the c.d.f. of each sufficient cause is $F(x) = \prod_{i=1}^{j} F_i(x)$, that is, the distribution of the maximum age of expression of the component causes. Then, taking the lower endpoint of the distribution to be 0 without loss of generality, we show that if $X_1, X_2, ..., X_j$ are the independent times to event of the component causes with $X_i \sim F_i$, where F_i is regularly varying at 0 with exponent ρ_i for each i, the c.d.f. of $\max\{X_1, X_2, ..., X_j\}$ is also regularly varying at 0 with exponent given by the sum of the ρ_i's:

$$\lim_{t \downarrow 0} \frac{F(xt)}{F(t)} = \lim_{t \downarrow 0} \frac{\prod_{i=1}^{j} F_i(xt)}{\prod_{i=1}^{j} F_i(t)} = \lim_{t \downarrow 0} \prod_{i=1}^{j} \frac{F_i(xt)}{F_i(t)} = \prod_{i=1}^{j} \lim_{t \downarrow 0} \frac{F_i(xt)}{F_i(t)} = \prod_{i=1}^{j} x^{\rho_i} = x^{\sum_{i=1}^{j} \rho_i}.$$

(3.1)

For the group of sufficient causes under consideration here, whose time-to-event distributions are derived from EREF component causes only or both EREF and LOGE component causes, we next argue for the reasonableness of the assumption that the time-to-event distributions of the EREF and LOGE component causes are regularly varying at the lower endpoint of the distribution with exponent $0 < \rho < \infty$. Karamata (1933) showed that if the limit as t goes to 0 of $F(xt)/F(t)$ exists for all $x > 0$, then it must be of the form x^{ρ} for $\rho \in \Re$. The case $\rho < 0$ is ruled out for nondecreasing functions such as a c.d.f. F; $\rho = 0$ corresponds to F slowly varying at 0; and $\rho = \infty$ corresponds to F infinitely flat at 0. Thus, if a "well-behaved" c.d.f. with $F(0) = 0$ and $F(x) > 0$ for $x > 0$ is such that $\lim_{t \downarrow 0} F(xt)/F(t)$ exists, except for slowly varying functions, it is either flat at 0 or regularly varying at 0 with exponent $0 < \rho < \infty$. A value of ρ that is either zero or infinity corresponds to very special cases; absent some active process like the molding by natural selection, nature arguably will not produce such special cases, and a nonzero finite value of ρ should be expected as the norm. To illustrate that regularly varying functions at the lower endpoint of the distribution with exponent $0 < \rho < \infty$ correspond to a fairly wide class among "well-behaved" c.d.f.'s, the following are examples of such functions with $F(0) = 0$ and $F(x) > 0$ for $x > 0$: (i) power functions of the form x^{ρ}, (ii) polynomial functions where a power function x^{ρ} can be factored out, (iii) $-x^{\rho}/\log x$ (prototypical example (Eq. 2.61)), (iv) $\log (x^{\rho} + 1)$, and (v) $1 - \exp(-x^{\rho})$.

From Theorems 4 and 10 in Section 2.1.2, the limiting distribution of the minimum of these regularly varying event times, even in the case that they are not identically distributed, is the Weibull distribution. As we did in Section 2.2.1 for the group of sufficient causes whose time-to-event distributions are molded by the declining force of natural selection, we need to consider, for the results of Theorems 4 and 10 to be applicable, that the times to event of the sufficient causes in this second group, while not independent, satisfy the assumptions of an E_n-sequence. We also note that since we started by considering the behavior *at the lower endpoint* of the distributions of the component causes, we end up with the corresponding conclusion about the minimum times to event of the sufficient causes. That is, we are assuming that the distribution of the residual lifetime after the earliest age at reproduction in the population (i.e., after age 10 years) is approximately Weibull for this group of sufficient causes. Because truncating and changing the origin of a Weibull distribution changes the form of the distribution (see Equation C.18 in Appendix C), our assumption implies that the distribution over the entire age range is not Weibull. On the other hand, we note that most initial distributions starting from 0 would yield *conditional* distributions for the residual lifetime (given survival to the earliest age at reproduction) that are regularly varying, unless they were "molded" to be flat. For example, even if we begin with an unconditional distribution that is flat at age 0, say, our prototype flat distribution (Eq. 2.59), once we condition on survival to age 10, the *conditional residual* lifetime distribution is regularly varying at 10 years (with exponent 1).

Table 3.2 summarizes the characteristics of the two groups of sufficient causes in our causation model. Hypothetically, if all deaths in the population were caused by one of a large number of sufficient causes from group 1, the residual lifetime after age 10 years would follow an approximate Gompertz distribution, and if all deaths in the population were caused by one of a large number of sufficient causes from group 2, the residual lifetime after age 10 years would follow an approximate Weibull distribution. We now note that this evolution-based model of causation can be extended to *aging-related diseases of complex etiology*, in addition to intrinsic mortality, based on the notion put forward at the end of Section 2.2 that aging-related diseases result from the same general evolutionary process as aging, that is, the attenuation of natural selection at later ages. This can be accomplished by considering DS mortality, as in Figure 1.1, or incidence of specific aging-related diseases. For the latter case, we may simply replace "death" with "disease incidence" in many of the previous sentences in this section; likewise, we may replace "mortality rate" with "incidence rate," "sufficient cause of death" with "sufficient cause of a specific disease," and "age at death" with "age at disease onset." However, we must assume that the force of natural selection decreases with age for sufficient causes of a specific disease similarly to how it does for sufficient causes of death, such that our argument for Gompertzian mortality in Section 2.2.1 would similarly apply. This assumption is justified in terms of considering that these diseases are usually disabling and are themselves associated with intrinsic mortality. We must also assume that the number of sufficient causes of a specific disease is large enough for the asymptotic extreme value theory to be applicable, which we address at some length in the succeeding text. Figure 3.1 schematically illustrates our evolution-based

TABLE 3.2 Characteristics of two groups of sufficient causes

	Combinations of categories of component causes into sufficient causes[a]	Defining category of component causes	Time-to-event distributions of the sufficient causes	Time-to-event distribution for death or disease[b]
1. Time-to-event distributions molded by the declining force of natural selection	LOGE LOGE + EOGE LOGE + ECEF LOGE + EOGE + ECEF	LOGE in the absence of EREF	Family of flat functions at the lower endpoint of the distribution	Gompertz distribution
2. Time-to-event distributions *not* molded by the declining force of natural selection	EREF EREF + EOGE EREF + ECEF EREF + LOGE EREF + EOGE + ECEF EREF + EOGE + LOGE EREF + ECEF + LOGE EREF + EOGE + ECEF + LOGE	EREF	Family of regularly varying functions at the lower endpoint of the distribution	Weibull distribution

[a] ECEF, evolutionarily conserved environmental factor(s); EOGE, early-onset genetic effect(s); EREF, evolutionarily recent environmental factor(s); LOGE, late-onset genetic effect(s).
[b] Obtained from the limiting distribution of the minimum time to event of the sufficient causes, as the number of sufficient causes tends to infinity; time to event is the residual waiting time after age 10 years.

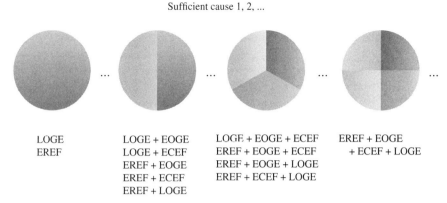

FIGURE 3.1   Schematic illustration of the evolution-based model of causation. ECEF, evolutionarily conserved environmental factor(s); EOGE, early-onset genetic effect(s); EREF, evolutionarily recent environmental factor(s); LOGE, late-onset genetic effect(s).

model of causation using the traditional causal pies and conveys the idea that the number of sufficient causes is "infinitely large."

In support of the assumption that the number of sufficient causes of aging-related diseases is "large enough" for the asymptotic theory to apply, we review the current thinking about the contribution of genetic variants to complex diseases. Most human diseases that have been genetically characterized are rare Mendelian disorders, caused by single (dominant or recessive) genes. In contrast, common aging-related diseases, whose etiology is largely unknown, are believed to be caused by multiple genetic and environmental factors. These diseases are usually described as multifactorial, polygenic, or complex, even though as stated by Risch (2000), "Often unwilling to cede to a notion of 'infinite' genetic complexity, geneticists refer to these cases as 'oligogenic' or 'multigenic', implicating a tractable degree of complexity." A popular hypothesis regarding the etiology of these complex diseases is the *common disease–common variant hypothesis*, which asserts that common diseases are caused by common genetic variants or polymorphisms that individually have little effect but in concert confer a high risk (Hardy and Singleton, 2009; Lander, 1996; Risch and Merikangas, 1996). Chakravarti (1999) described the common disease–common variant hypothesis in terms that are in keeping with our causation model: "If multiple genes are involved, then the central question is whether mutations at any one gene are necessary and sufficient to lead to the phenotype. The lack of Mendelian segregation of a complex phenotype in most families argues against the sufficiency of a mutation at any one gene: either there is a strong environmental effect and/or multiple genes are involved. A mutation may be necessary if strong epistacy were to prevail. Consequently, the nature of genetic variation for complex traits determined by many loci is likely to be common alleles (polymorphisms) at these loci."[5]

[5] Reproduced from *Nature Genetics*, **21**, Chakravarti, A., Population genetics — making sense out of sequence, pages 56–60, Copyright 1999, with permission from Macmillan Publishers Ltd.

The common disease–common variant hypothesis provided an important impetus for the International HapMap Project and subsequent genome-wide association studies (GWAS) (International HapMap Consortium, 2005; Pritchard and Cox, 2002). Based on the haplotype map of the human genome, GWAS have identified hundreds of genetic variants that contribute to more than 40 diseases and human phenotypes (Hirschhorn, 2009; Kraft and Hunter, 2009; Maher, 2008), such that, as stated by Hardy and Singleton (2009), "it is now routine to identify common, low-risk variants (i.e., those that are present in more than 5% of the population) that confer a small risk of disease, typically with odds ratios of 1.2 to 5.0." However, most common variants identified by GWAS are responsible for only a small fraction of the genetic contribution that is supposed to exist for these diseases, which has been referred to as "the case of the missing heritability" (Maher, 2008). Even when dozens of gene variants have been linked to a trait, the cumulative effects have been disappointingly small and far from accounting for earlier estimates of heritability (Goldstein, 2009; Kraft and Hunter, 2009). According to Goldstein (2009), "This observation is particularly troubling because the studies are largely comprehensive in terms of common single-nucleotide polymorphisms (SNPs), the genomic markers that are genotyped and with which disease associations are tested. We're finding the biggest effects that exist for this class of genetic variant, and common variation is packing much less of a phenotypic punch than expected."

Thus, finding the so-called missing heritability of complex diseases has become a preoccupation for researchers (Manolio et al., 2009). A basic question is whether the heritability estimates against which the results of GWAS studies have been reckoned actually represent a reliable measure of the genetic contribution to disease. In this respect, Vineis and Pearce (2011) considered that the premise of the issue of missing heritability "is based on two sources of misunderstanding: (i) confusion between variation and causation and (ii) confusion between heritability and genetic determination." We will discuss the limitations of the heritability index in Section 4.2. Apart from that, a possible explanation for unidentified genetic variants contributing to the cause of complex diseases is that a much larger number of variants of small effect size, acting independently or in gene–gene interactions, remain to be found (Gandhi and Wood, 2010; Manolio et al., 2009). This is related to the notion of genetic (or locus) heterogeneity, defined as the situation in which mutations in any one of several genes may result in identical phenotypes, such as when the genes are required for a common biochemical pathway or cellular structure (Lander and Schork, 1994). Galvan et al. (2010) listed reasons for what they called the "unidentified genetic 'dark matter' of cancer," many of which converged toward the underlying issue of genetic heterogeneity. Kraft and Hunter (2009) estimated the number of risk loci that would be needed to reach a level of risk equivalent to the sibling recurrence risks of complex diseases such as diabetes, heart disease, and cancer, assuming allele frequencies and relative risks similar to those of most markers that have been discovered through GWAS for these diseases. For a sibling relative risk of 2.0, the estimated number of risk alleles ranged from 347 to 867 assuming a relative risk per allele of 1.10 and from 87 to 231 assuming a relative risk per allele of 1.20. Hence, it has been proposed that GWAS conducted in larger samples and using genotyping platforms designed to test variants with population frequencies below 5%, as well as studies taking into account gene–gene and gene–environment interactions, will account for a larger proportion of the supposed heritability of specific diseases (Hirschhorn, 2009).

Some authors, however, believe that this strategy will not yield additional worthwhile findings given the likelihood that most genetic contribution to complex diseases is due to rare variants that have larger effects than common variants (the *common disease–rare variant hypothesis*) and cannot be detected by GWAS because of their very low population frequency (Goldstein, 2009; McClellan and King, 2010). The frequency in the population of genetic variants associated with complex diseases is in part related to allelic heterogeneity, in which there are multiple disease-causing mutations at a single gene (Lander and Schork, 1994). The higher the allelic heterogeneity at a particular locus, the lower the population frequency of any one variant at this locus tends to be. Based on a theoretical population genetics model for the evolution of complex disease loci, incorporating mutation, random genetic drift, and purifying selection, Pritchard (2001) concluded that "there is likely to be extensive allelic heterogeneity at many of these loci." Another theoretical study and empirical data have supported this conclusion (Pritchard and Cox, 2002; Reich and Lander, 2001). In evolutionary terms, the support for the common disease–rare variant hypothesis is broadly consistent with the rationale for our causation model. This can be seen in the following comment: "The apparently modest effect of common variation on most human diseases and related traits probably reflects the efficiency of natural selection in prohibiting increases in disease-associated variants in the population" (Goldstein, 2009). Or as put by McClellan and King (2010), "Genetic factors contributing to human disease are subject to the same evolutionary forces that dictate the architecture of the human genome. The overall magnitude of human genetic variation, the high rate of de novo mutation, the range of mutational mechanisms that disrupt gene function, and the complexity of biological processes underlying pathophysiology all predict a substantial role for rare severe mutations in complex human disease."[6]

It seems likely that both common and rare genetic variants play a role in the causation of most complex diseases (Bodmer and Bonilla, 2008). Under this scenario, extensive genetic and allelic heterogeneity for specific complex diseases would favor a large number of sufficient causes in our causation model by increasing the number of genetic component causes combining into sufficient causes. In the case of allelic heterogeneity, different susceptibility alleles in the same locus may have different magnitude of effects and require different causal partners (i.e., different complementary component causes within a sufficient cause), hence constituting different sufficient causes. Similarly, for the purpose of our causation model, if an allele has a higher deleterious effect when present in both homologous loci (i.e., an allelic dose effect), the double dose of the allele might constitute another sufficient cause with a different or more restricted set of causal partners than the set of causal partners for the single dose of the allele. Extensive genetic and allelic heterogeneity would contribute to the number of sufficient causes in both the group of sufficient causes containing LOGE in the absence of EREF and the group of sufficient causes containing EREF with or without LOGE, as both groups involve genetic component causes. For the group of sufficient causes containing EFEF, there would be the

---

[6] Reproduced from *Cell*, **141**, McClellan, J. and King, M., Genetic heterogeneity in human disease, pages 210–217, Copyright 2010, with permission from Elsevier.

additional contribution of the various environmental factors brought about by industrialization and recent changes in lifestyle. Analogous to the allelic dose effect, dose effects of environmental factors would be represented in different sufficient causes, since small doses would possibly require a larger set of causal partners than that required by large doses (Rothman, 1976).

Therefore, each of the two groups of sufficient causes in our causation model would conceivably involve hundreds of sufficient causes for specific complex diseases, making it plausible that the number of sufficient causes in each group is "large enough" for the asymptotic statistical theory of extreme values to be applicable. Consistent with that, Galvan et al. (2010) considered that "Regardless of frequency (i.e., common, rare, very rare) and type (i.e., SNP or CNV [copy-number variants]), it is likely that hundreds or even thousands of genetic variants are implicated in cancer risk." Although the normal distribution has traditionally been seen as a distribution whose minimum (or maximum) converges very slowly to the Gumbel-type distribution of the minimum (or maximum), Gumbel (1958, pp. 221–222) showed that the differences between the exact and asymptotic distributions are already barely visible in a plot for $n = 100$, except for the tails of the distributions. In our illustrative example in Section 2.1.2 (Fig. 2.9), the quality of the asymptotic approximation for the minimum of nonidentically distributed random variables whose parent distributions belong to a family of prototype flat functions is already reasonably good for $n = 100$. Overall, for the practical purposes of our application, the aforementioned suggests that the quality of the asymptotic approximations to the time-to-event distributions of the minimum for the two groups of sufficient causes of specific aging-related diseases is very good. Since the number of sufficient causes of death is higher than that for specific diseases, the quality of the approximations for intrinsic mortality is expected to be even better.

In the illustrative example for the i.i.d. case in Section 2.1.2 (Fig. 2.7), we fixed the approximating Gompertz distribution of the minimum and obtained the corresponding scale and shape parameters of the flat initial distribution $F(x) = e^{(-\sigma/x)^\rho}$ for different values of n, using estimates of the Gompertz parameters λ and θ from our data analysis of intrinsic mortality (first column in Table 4.5). We then plotted the exact and approximating distributions of the minimum. Here, we plot the flat initial distributions for $n = 100$, 200, 500, and 1000; the values of the scale and shape parameters are, respectively, $(\sigma, \rho) = (126.73, 3.25), (142.95, 2.82), (169.16, 2.41),$ and $(193.32, 2.17)$ (Fig. 3.2). We note from these graphs that, under this simplifying i.i.d. scenario, the initial distribution of the sufficient causes from group 1 (LOGE in the absence of EREF) is very close to 0 up to at least 70 years, which supports the notion that the force of natural selection is quite high until at least that age by virtue of humans being a social species—characterized, among other things, by the extreme dependence of human offspring and an apparently important role of grandparents during evolutionary history in the successful reproduction of their children and survival of their grandchildren. We can also visualize in these graphs that the time-to-event distribution of a sufficient cause of death is quite different from the age-at-death distribution for the human population, because the latter is the distribution of the minimum time to event of many sufficient causes. Only to make that point more striking, we note that if it were for a single sufficient cause from group 1 acting in isolation (i.e., to the exclusion of the other sufficient causes of death), the median

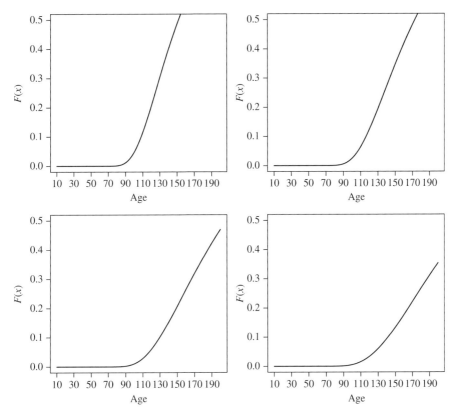

FIGURE 3.2   Plots of the time-to-event distribution of a sufficient cause of death from group 1, obtained under the simplifying i.i.d. scenario and using estimates of the Gompertz parameters λ and θ from our data analysis of intrinsic mortality, for $n = 100$, 200, 500, and 1000 (respectively, upper left, upper right, lower left, and lower right panel). See text for details.

age at death in the population would be close to 150 years in the scenario in which $n = 100$ and would substantially exceed that value for $n = 200$, 500, and 1000.

Our causation model also offers insights into some conundrums of complex diseases. For instance, Tanzi (1999) proposed that there exists a "genetic dichotomy" in Alzheimer's disease and other common aging-related diseases, such that rare early-onset forms of aging-related diseases are caused by rare and often fully penetrant autosomal dominant (or recessive) mutations and the more common late-onset forms of these diseases are associated with common polymorphisms. (For illustration, we draw in Figure 3.3 a hypothetical sufficient cause for Alzheimer's disease involving a genetic polymorphism and environmental factors; a fully penetrant mutation would be represented by a sufficient cause containing a single LOGE component cause.) This notion of a genetic dichotomy is supported by the existence of earlier-onset monogenic forms of complex diseases such as Alzheimer's disease, Parkinson's disease, and cancer (Bertram and Tanzi, 2005; Galvan et al., 2010). Consistent with this

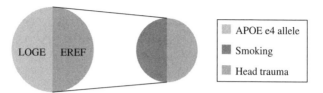

FIGURE 3.3 Hypothetical sufficient cause for Alzheimer's disease involving component causes that are risk factors for Alzheimer's disease. Each of the component causes would likely form several other sufficient causes for Alzheimer's disease with different causal partners. EREF, evolutionarily recent environmental factor(s); LOGE, late-onset genetic effect(s).

view, Pritchard (2001) parenthetically remarked: "For some complex traits, there are also rare Mendelian forms, but these can be considered separately from the more common, 'complex' forms of the diseases." With respect to neurodegeneration, Gandhi and Wood (2010) put it in a similar way but suggesting a spectrum rather than a clear-cut dichotomy: "The major neurodegenerative diseases share a common theme: they are mostly sporadic, late onset diseases that are caused by a complex etiology stemming from various genetic and environmental factors. When considering the genetic load in the etiology, Mendelian forms of the neurodegenerative disease have been noted in a minority of cases. These Mendelian (or familial) forms are clinically and pathologically similar to the sporadic forms (apart from an earlier age of onset)."[7]

In our causation model, rather than considering Mendelian forms of complex diseases separately, the monogenic causes and the sufficient causes involving several rare or common variants can be seen as part of a spectrum according to the number of component causes in each sufficient cause. The smaller the number of component causes, the higher the penetrance of each component cause (and vice versa), because the probability of expression of each component cause increases with fewer necessary conditions or causal partners. This is consistent with the notion that the penetrance function, given by the probability of disease for each genotype, depends on other genes and nongenetic factors (Lander and Schork, 1994). Moreover, the distinction between the common disease–common variant and the common disease–rare variant hypotheses is also expressed in terms of common variants being of low penetrance and rare variants being highly or moderately penetrant (Galvan et al., 2010; Maher, 2008). Under this scheme, it is easy to see that variants are common/rare because of their low/high penetrance, not the other way around. Since phenotypic expression is necessary for the action of natural selection, natural selection would have more of an opportunity to act on a highly penetrant variant over evolutionary history, so that it would become rare. Conversely, low-penetrance variants would become common as a result of their necessary causal partners "shielding" them

---

[7] Reproduced from *Nature Neuroscience*, **13**, Gandhi, S. and Wood, N. W., Genome-wide association studies: The key to unlocking neurodegeneration? pages 789–794, Copyright 2010, with permission from Macmillan Publishers Ltd.

from the action of natural selection, in a similar way that recessive genes causing early-onset disease are not subject to the action of natural selection in nonaffected carriers.

This scheme additionally provides a satisfactory explanation for the earlier onset of the monogenic forms of complex diseases. In contrasting Mendelian and complex diseases, Petronis (2001) asked: "If gene mutations underlie complex diseases, why is the age of onset delayed by a number of decades, whereas mutations in simple diseases express relatively early?" He offered a possible explanation in terms of the age-dependency of epigenetic changes leading to later onset of complex diseases. Bjornsson et al. (2004) elaborated on this explanation based on the "age-dependent degeneration of epigenetic patterns" (see review of epigenetics in the following text). Although not mutually exclusive with respect to this explanation, our causation model offers another explanation for the earlier/later age of onset in the setting of monogenic/multifactorial causation, applicable in contrasting separate Mendelian and complex diseases as well as Mendelian and complex forms of the same disease. It simply follows from the idea that as the time to event of each sufficient cause is given by the maximum time to event of the component causes, it tends to be smaller (earlier onset) for sufficient causes containing only one component cause, and it tends to become larger (later onset) as the number of component causes increases.

In the remainder of this section, we consider three relatively young and converging fields and their relevance to our evolution-based model of causation: life course epidemiology, the developmental origins of health and disease (DOHaD), and epigenetics. This will bring into focus the importance of environmental factors in the causation of complex diseases. A life course approach to chronic disease epidemiology is defined as "the study of long-term effects on chronic disease risk of physical and social exposures during gestation, childhood, adolescence, young adulthood and later adult life. It includes studies of the biological, behavioural and psychosocial pathways that operate across an individual's life course, as well as across generations, to influence the development of chronic diseases" (Ben-Shlomo and Kuh, 2002).[8] Despite the special interest devoted to early life exposures, the life course approach does not deny the importance of midlife lifestyle or other risk factors to chronic disease, and it goes beyond longitudinal study designs, as emphasized by Kuh et al. (2003): "Life course epidemiology implies more than a longitudinal study. The first is a theoretical model whereas the second is a study design. The purpose of life course epidemiology is to build and test theoretical models that postulate pathways linking exposures across the life course to later life health outcomes." Such pathways explicitly lay out the temporal ordering of exposures, their interrelationships, and connections, either directly or through intermediary variables, with the outcome measure (Ben-Shlomo and Kuh, 2002; Kuh et al., 2003). There does not seem to be any intrinsic incompatibility between our causation model and life course theoretical modeling. The life course approach to chronic disease "explicitly recognizes the importance of time and timing in understanding causal links between exposures and outcomes..." (Lynch and Davey Smith, 2005). The importance afforded

---

[8] Reproduced from *International Journal of Epidemiology*, **31**, Ben-Shlomo, Y. and Kuh, D., A life course approach to chronic disease epidemiology: Conceptual models, empirical challenges and interdisciplinary perspectives, pages 285–293, Copyright 2002, with permission from Oxford University Press.

to time and timing is reflected in our causation model, even if obliquely, in the time-to-event distribution of the component causes and the notion that the time-to-event distribution of the sufficient causes is given by the distribution of the maximum time to event of the component causes.

The broad idea behind the DOHaD—that adult disease is at least partly determined in early life—is more narrowly represented by the "fetal origins of coronary heart disease" hypothesis, which was suggested by studies showing an association between low birth weight and coronary heart disease later in life (Barker, 1993, 1995a). According to this hypothesis, fetal undernutrition in middle to late gestation leads to disproportionate fetal growth and "programmes" later coronary heart disease. The "programmed" changes would involve the fetuses' ability to respond to their mother's diet in utero through developmental plasticity, such that inadequate nutrition in intrauterine life might lead to lifelong alterations in the body's setting of metabolism and hormones or in the number of cells in key organs. The biological basis of the hypothesis further involves the notion that most organs and systems of the body go through periods of rapid cell division, or the so-called critical periods, during intrauterine development, in which they are plastic and sensitive to the environment (Barker, 2004). As a supposed benefit in evolutionary terms of developmental plasticity, the ability of the organism to take cues from the maternal environment enables the production of phenotypes that are better adapted to the future environment, but this can also be disadvantageous if there is a mismatch between the anticipated and actual future environments (Gluckman et al., 2010). In its current DOHaD form, the "fetal origins" hypothesis has been expanded in three ways. First, epidemiological and clinical studies have reported a relationship between undernutrition or low birth weight and other conditions, including hypertension, type 2 diabetes, osteoporosis, depression, schizophrenia, certain cancers, and obstructive lung disease. Second, there has also been an interest in the potential negative effects of nutrient excess. Third, long-term effects of inadequate or excess nutrition in infants and children have also been considered, despite constraints on the degree of plasticity as development proceeds (Barker, 1995b; Barker et al., 2002; Gluckman et al., 2010).

The life course approach to chronic disease epidemiology is more comprehensive than the DOHaD hypothesis in that an "accumulation of risk" conceptual model, in which factors that raise disease risk accumulate gradually over the life course, has its place next to the "critical period" conceptual model, in which an exposure acting during a specific period has lifelong structural or functional effects (Ben-Shlomo and Kuh, 2002). Moreover, the life course approach to chronic disease "emphasized from the start the importance of the postnatal social and physical environment, the psychological as well as physical developmental processes, and their interaction with later life social and biological factors in the development of disease risk" (Kuh and Davey Smith, 2004). However, attesting to the parallel development of life course epidemiology and the DOHaD hypothesis, both their origins can be traced back to studies conducted in the first half of the twentieth century suggesting a relation between early life experiences and mortality risk, such as the birth cohort study by Kermack et al. (1934), and the "fetal origins" work conducted by Barker (1993, 1995a, 2004) served as a catalyst for both (Davey Smith and Kuh, 2001; Kuh et al., 2003; Kuh and Davey Smith, 2004).

Recently, cellular epigenetic mechanisms have emerged as a potential mechanistic basis for the DOHaD hypothesis, and they are thus also relevant to the life course approach to chronic disease epidemiology (Gluckman et al., 2005, 2007, 2010). The term *epigenetics* is employed inconsistently and sometimes loosely (Bird, 2007; Goldberg et al., 2007; Jablonka and Raz, 2009). It is most often used in the sense of mitotically and meiotically heritable changes in gene expression that are not coded in the DNA sequence; yet the requirement of heritability has been questioned as a liability (Bird, 2007). In part, this is because of the dual facet of epigenetics as a response system involved in the regulation of gene expression and a memory and inheritance system. Jablonka and Raz (2009) defined epigenetics as "the study of the processes that underlie developmental plasticity and canalization [robustness or insensitivity of a phenotype to genetic and environmental variation] and that bring about persistent developmental effects in both prokaryotes and eukaryotes" and considered that epigenetic inheritance is a component of epigenetics: "It occurs when phenotypic variations that do not stem from variations in DNA base sequences are transmitted to subsequent generations of cells or organisms." In turn, these authors defined epigenetic inheritance in both a narrow and a broad sense. Epigenetic inheritance in a narrow sense, or cellular epigenetic inheritance, is "the transmission from mother cell to daughter cell of variations that are not the result of differences in DNA base sequence and/or the present environment." It occurs during mitotic cell division in the soma and sometimes in the meiotic division in the germline. Accordingly, cellular epigenetic mechanisms are those involved in cell-to-cell transmission of epigenetic variations. The most obvious manifestation of cellular epigenetic inheritance is the differentiation, during the development process of multicellular organisms, of cells with identical DNA content into organ- or tissue-specific types. Epigenetic inheritance in a broad sense further involves body-to-body information transference, which can take place through developmental interactions between mother and offspring, social learning, and symbolic communication.

To consider how epigenetics fits into our evolution-based model of causation, we focus here on cellular epigenetic mechanisms. Four types of cellular epigenetic mechanisms have been recognized: chromatin marking (e.g., DNA methylation and histone modifications), RNA-mediated, self-sustaining metabolic loops, and self-reconstructing three-dimensional structures. These four mechanisms, called epigenetic inheritance systems (EIS), interact in various ways, and the changes that they effect in the pattern of gene expression can be environmentally induced or stochastic events (Jablonka, 2004; Jablonka and Lamb, 2007). Referring to EIS, Jablonka and Lamb (2007) noted that "Like almost everything else in the biological world, these systems depend on DNA, but, by definition, epigenetic variations do not depend on DNA variations." While the transmission of induced changes in epigenetic states is crucial for normal development, Holliday (1987) was a pioneer in considering that epigenetic defects might contribute to the risk of disease and coined the term *epimutation* to designate "the heritable changes based on DNA modification," as distinguished from classical mutations that are changes in DNA sequence. The derivation of the term *epimutation* from *mutation* suggests a random process, which is supported by the occurrence of phenotypic and epigenetic differences in isogenic laboratory animals living in identical environmental conditions (Aguilera et al., 2010; Holliday, 2005). Yet, in the first place, we consider epigenetic modifications arising as repeatable and specific responses to environmental factors (Jablonka and Lamb, 1990). As such, epigenetic modifications provide a link between the environment and alterations in gene expression that might lead to disease phenotypes (Jirtle and Skinner, 2007). The potential relevance of epigenetics to human health has even led some to foresee a new branch of epidemiology (epigenetic epidemiology) that studies the effects of epigenetic changes on the occurrence and distribution of diseases (Feinberg, 2008; Jablonka, 2004).

For our causation model, epigenetic mechanisms mainly represent an alternative route for the action of environmental factors involving modification of patterns of gene expression, as opposed to a "direct" effect on pathogenetic pathways of disease causation. Such epigenetic mediation of environmental effects can involve mitotic inheritance of environmentally induced epigenetic changes within an individual's lifetime. In case the environmental induction occurs early in life and has lifelong effects on gene expression, this scenario might underlie the DOHaD hypothesis. Even if the environmental induction of an epigenetic state occurs in intrauterine or early postnatal life, our causation model takes such environmental effects into account as long as disease onset occurs after the earliest age at reproduction in the population. Epigenetic changes can also be inherited transgenerationally (i.e., meiotic transmission of epigenetic variants), in which case environmental effects induced in parents can be transmitted to one or more generations of descendents. This scenario has also been invoked with respect to the DOHaD hypothesis (Kaati et al., 2002; Pembrey, 2002). The importance of both the mitotic and meiotic transmission scenarios, especially the second one, may be limited by the following. The fidelity or replicative accuracy of transmission of epigenetic inheritance is not as great as with genetic inheritance (Bird, 2007; Jablonka, 2004). Studies have shown that the phenotypic stability for epigenetic inheritance, measured as the rate of change of the phenotype per generation in unicellular organisms, is orders of magnitude higher (less stable) than that for genetic inheritance (Rando and Verstrepen, 2007). More importantly, in sexually reproducing organisms, epigenetic variations often do not remain (i.e., they are reprogrammed) during the process of meiosis, and in multicellular organisms, they also have to survive gametogenesis and early embryogenesis in order to be transmitted to the next generation—"two developmental stages that involve significant restructuring of both cells and chromatin" (Jablonka and Raz, 2009).

In general, the potential role of epigenetics as a mediator of environmental effects on aging and aging-related diseases would involve three necessary conditions, for which the evidence is currently inconclusive. First, there must occur epigenetic changes with age. As recognized by Holliday (1987), it seems inevitable that there will be gradual loss of epigenetic marks with age: "If it is assumed there is a given low probability that a methyl group will be lost at each cell division and that de novo methylation either does not occur, or occurs at a lower rate, then it follows the level of methylation should progressively decline." Indeed, reviews of the evidence from *in vivo* and *in vitro* studies supported the idea that methyl groups were gradually lost during repeated cell division (Cooney, 1993; Lamb, 1994). However, more recent studies revealed, in addition to a global decrease in DNA methylation (hypomethylation) with age, a pattern of hypermethylation at specific loci with increasing age, especially in promoter regions (Bjornsson et al., 2008; Boks et al., 2009; Calvanese et al., 2009). These findings have been further refined as follows. Christensen et al. (2009) observed across several nonpathological human tissues an increase in methylation with age at loci in CpG islands[9] of promoter regions and a decrease at loci not in CpG islands. In the first genome-scale study of epigenomic dynamics during normal human aging, Rakyan et al. (2010) observed age-associated hypermethylated regions in precursor hematopoietic and buccal cells, "preferentially at a specific category of developmental gene promoters that bear a distinctive bivalent chromatin signature in precursor/stem cells, and are frequently hypermethylated in various cancers and cell culture." Using brain tissues from neurologically normal donors, Hernandez et al. (2011) reported that CpG loci showing a highly significant correlation between DNA methylation and chronological age were physically close to genes involved in DNA binding and regulation of transcription, suggesting that changes in DNA methylation with age may have a broad impact in gene expression. Changes in histone marks and histone-modifying enzymes with age were reviewed by Calvanese et al. (2009).

Second, epigenetic changes with age must have a functional outcome in terms of aging phenotypes or aging-related diseases. Bell et al. (2012) conducted epigenome-wide association scans to identify differentially methylated regions for 16 age-related phenotypes (previously defined "biomarkers of aging") in a healthy aging population. They identified 490 methylation variants significantly associated with age, of which 98% exhibited increased methylation with age. However, only one of these methylation variants was also associated with an age-related phenotype, suggesting that age-associated differentially methylated regions may be neutral with respect to surrogate measures of biological aging. Petronis (2001) argued that epigenetic dysregulation of genes is consistent with several features of complex diseases, such as discordance of monozygotic twins for disease phenotypes, age of onset, fluctuations in disease course, sex effects, and parent-of-origin effects. The prime example of complex disease in which epigenetic mechanisms have been implicated is cancer; other complex diseases associated with epigenetic alterations are type 2 diabetes, Alzheimer's disease, and other neurodegenerative diseases, but the evidence in these cases is not as strong as for cancer (Bjornsson et al., 2004; Calvanese et al., 2009; Egger et al., 2004; Feinberg, 2007, 2008; Qureshi and Mehler, 2011).

---

[9] CpG is shorthand for cytosine–phosphate–guanine, that is, cytosine and guanine linked in sequence and separated by a phosphate, as opposed to a cytosine–guanine base pair. In mammals, DNA methylation mostly consists of the addition of a methyl group to the 5-carbon of the cytosine ring of a CpG dinucleotide. In normal human tissues, 5-methylcytosine accounts for 3–6% of the total cytosine. DNA methylation is a means of suppressing (or silencing) gene expression. CpG islands are CpG-rich regions of DNA found in the promoter of approximately half of all genes; they are at least 200 bases long, of which more than half are cytosine or guanine. CpG islands are usually unmethylated in normal cells, while sporadic CpG sites in the rest of the genome are generally methylated (Aguilera et al., 2010; Callinan and Feinberg, 2006; Calvanese et al., 2009).

Third, specific environmental factors must be implicated in the generation of epi-genetic changes. Epigenetic mechanisms such as DNA methylation, methylation of histones, and acetylation of chromatin proteins may respond to levels of dietary and metabolic precursors and cofactors for methylation and acetylation (Cooney, 1993, 2007), and this likely accounts for diet and nutritional supplements effecting epigenetic changes. The list of environmental factors that can result in epigenetic changes also includes drugs, xenobiotic chemicals, smoking, endocrine disruptors, heavy metal toxins, low-dose radiation, and behavioral cues (Aguilera et al., 2010; Belinsky et al., 2002; Calvanese et al., 2009; Cooney, 2007; Feinberg, 2007; Jirtle and Skinner, 2007; Sutherland and Costa, 2003). Aguilera et al. (2010) cautioned that it is not known whether all substances that can effect epigenetic changes are "authentic epigenetic modifiers," because it has not been determined whether the epigenetic modifications that they induce are stable over time. One study that investigated meth-ylation changes in relation to environmental factors in specific tissues found that exposures were not strongly associated with methylation profiles, but locus-specific analysis revealed hypermethylation at 24 CpG loci in pleural tissue related to asbestos, altered methylation at 30 CpG loci in blood related to drinking status, and altered methylation at 138 CpG loci in lung tissue related to smoking status (Christensen et al., 2009). Barrès et al. (2012) showed a decrease in whole genome methylation in skeletal muscle biopsies from healthy sedentary men and women after acute exer-cise and provided evidence that exercise alters promoter methylation of exercise-responsive genes in a dose-dependent manner. In a study of the genome-wide meth-ylation pattern of human adipose tissue before and after a 6-month exercise interven-tion, global DNA methylation changed and 17,975 individual CpG sites in 7663 genes showed altered levels of methylation in response to exercise; also, there was differ-ential methylation of 39 candidate genes for obesity and type 2 diabetes (Rönn et al., 2013).

Although preliminary, the evidence in the preceding text suggests that the potential role of epigenetics as a mediator of environmental effects on chronic diseases goes beyond the DOHaD hypothesis, and in our causation model, it is particularly relevant to the operation of EREF. As stated by Cooney (2007), "Epigenetics appears to have evolved in part to allow for an adaptation to last for one or a few generations while preserving the potential for other epigenetic phenotypes should conditions change. How do epigenetic systems evolved over millions of years respond when encounter-ing new environmental variables such as refined foods, drugs, xenobiotics, etc.? Do once adaptive epigenetic responses within a natural range of nutrient balances become maladaptive when responding to extreme nutrient imbalances in refined foods and lead to diabetes and other chronic diseases?"[10] Indeed, the very responsiveness and flexibility that give epigenetics a fundamental role in development may make it a conduit for environmental effects on disease causation, especially if they are evolutionarily recent.

---

[10] Reproduced from *Disease Markers*, **23**, Cooney, C. A., Epigenetics — DNA-based mirror of our environment?, pages 121–137, Copyright 2007, with permission from Wiley.

We must also consider the possibility that epigenetic changes may contribute to aging and aging-related diseases as stochastic events rather than in response to environmental factors, as clearly proposed by Holliday (2005) with respect to cancer: "Nowadays it is commonly stated that disease is either genetic or environmental, when in reality stochastic events are equally important. In the absence of strong predisposing factors, such as asbestos-related mesothelioma, the cumulative changes that characterize many carcinomas are the result of chance. It is simply bad luck if a mutation occurs in an oncogene or tumor suppressor gene, and the same can be said of epigenetic defects in these or other genes."[11] This would imply that aside from the sufficient causes contemplated in our causation model, involving genetic effects and environmental factors, random or unsystematic sources of epigenetic changes would contribute to death or disease in the guise of EREF component causes. The current picture of epigenetic changes with age, as reviewed earlier, shows a combination of loss of epigenetic control (e.g., global loss of DNA methylation) and aberrant epigenetics (e.g., hypermethylation of specific genes) (Cooney, 2010). Aguilera et al. (2010) proposed that global loss of DNA methylation could be the result of a passive process due to the failure of a maintenance methyltransferase, while hypermethylation of specific genes could be due to the overexpression of a de novo methyltransferase. This supports a conjecture that loss of epigenetic control may be random or due to the so-called epigenetic drift, but aberrant epigenetics would more likely arise from environmental induction. In this scenario, we may further conjecture that, to the extent that specific rather than global epigenetic changes are more important for aging and aging-related diseases, the relative contribution of stochastic events might be limited.

Also relevant to this discussion, an influential paper in behavioral genetics by Plomin and Daniels (1987) raised the question of why children in the same family were as different from each other as pairs of children randomly selected from the population, in terms of personality, cognitive function, and psychopathology. Plomin and Daniels (1987) proposed that the reason was the importance of aspects of the environments of children that are not shared with siblings (nonshared environment). They also considered a "gloomy prospect" that the nonshared environment might be unsystematic ("It is possible that nonshared environmental influences could be unsystematic in the sense of stochastic events that, when compounded over time, make children in the same family different in unpredictable ways"), but they put it aside because such stochastic events "are likely to prove a dead end for research." As a consequence, an extensive research effort focused on the assessment of the effects of measured environmental differences among siblings on behavioral outcomes. A review by Turkheimer and Waldron (2000) of 43 studies measuring specific environmental variables relevant to Plomin and Daniels' (1987) proposal showed that although the variance component due to the nonshared environment accounted for upwards of 50% of the phenotypic variation in most outcomes, specific environmental variables accounted for a median of about 3% of the observed variation

---

[11] Reproduced from *Biochemistry*, **70**, Holliday, R., DNA methylation and epigenotypes, pages 500–504, Copyright 2005, with permission from Springer Science + Business Media.

in behavioral outcomes. This led Turkheimer (2000) to plainly state, "The gloomy prospect is true." More recently, Davey Smith (2011) brought together the "gloomy prospect," with respect to the causation of chronic diseases, and epigenetics, as an underlying mechanism of chance events. While he suggested that epidemiologists should embrace randomness in population health research and practice, he also noted that what seemed random at one level might be predictable at a different level. Chance events are also one of the reasons that made Buchanan et al. (2006) liken the search for the causes of complex diseases to the quest for the Philosopher's Stone: "Because of the vagaries of biology and timing of exposures and so forth, chance plays a much larger role in disease, beyond simple measurement 'noise', than generally acknowledged, and may not be quantifiable in any sense that we currently understand."

We summarize the main points about the relevance of life course epidemiology, DOHaD, and epigenetics to our causation model: (i) the importance given by the life course approach to time and timing in understanding the links between exposures and disease is translated in our causation model into the time-to-event distributions of the component and sufficient causes; (ii) epigenetics refers to changes in gene expression that can be environmentally induced or stochastic events; (iii) epigenetic mechanisms may underlie the "accumulation of risk" and "critical period" conceptual models of life course epidemiology and the DOHaD hypothesis that adult disease is at least partly determined in early life; (iv) for our causation model, epigenetic mechanisms represent an additional route for the action of environmental factors, aside from direct effects on pathogenetic pathways of disease causation; (v) in case environmental induction of epigenetic changes occurs in intrauterine or early postnatal life and has long-term effects into adult life, consistent with the DOHaD hypothesis, our causation model takes such environmental effects into account; (vi) in our causation model, the potential role of epigenetics as a mediator of environmental effects is particularly relevant to EREF; (vii) nevertheless, epigenetic changes may also contribute to aging and aging-related diseases as stochastic events.

The evolution-based model of causation developed here plays an essential role in creating a framework and providing a motivation for a survival mixture model of the Gompertz and Weibull distributions for the description of intrinsic mortality and disease incidence, which is presented in the next chapter, and from which an evolutionarily grounded index of aging-relatedness—thus far lacking in the literature—naturally emerges. Thus, it is possible that our causation model and mixture statistical model provide for a level and type of analysis in which most of the effect of chance is integrated, and the "gloomy prospect" is not so gloomy after all.

4

THE INDEX OF AGING-RELATEDNESS

In previous chapters, we laid out an extensive theoretical foundation for the index of aging-relatedness proposed here, which we briefly recapitulate. The Gompertz distribution was developed based on empirical human mortality observations and has played a central role in demography for describing the survival time of human populations. The Gumbel-type distribution is one of just two possible limiting distributions of the minimum of i.i.d. time-to-event random variables and becomes the Gompertz distribution when restricted to the positive half line. The other limiting distribution of the minimum of i.i.d. time-to-event random variables is the Weibull-type distribution, which plays a prominent role in reliability theory for describing the time to failure of mechanical devices. In the context of offering an account of the Gompertz pattern of mortality through the statistical theory of extreme values and biological evolution, we extended the applicability of some classical theorems on the asymptotic behavior of the minimum of time-to-event random variables. These results showed that if the initial distributions belong to a certain family of functions that are infinitely flat at the lower endpoint of the distribution (i.e., all derivatives evaluated at the lower endpoint of the distribution equal 0), the limiting distribution of the minimum is the Gumbel-type distribution; and if the initial distributions belong to a family of functions that are regularly varying at the lower endpoint of the distribution with exponent $0 < \rho < \infty$, the limiting distribution of the minimum is the Weibull-type distribution.

Further, in addressing the challenge to the Gompertz model on the basis of its fit to mortality data, we considered that departures from the model emerge from the action

The Biostatistics of Aging: From Gompertzian Mortality to an Index of Aging-Relatedness,
First Edition. Gilberto Levy and Bruce Levin.
© 2014 John Wiley & Sons, Inc. Published 2014 by John Wiley & Sons, Inc.

of environmental factors. This in turn led us to develop an evolution-based model of causation, which builds on the SCC model of causation in epidemiology and motivates a mixture statistical model presented in this chapter for describing intrinsic mortality and the incidence of aging-related diseases of complex etiology. We present the survival mixture model of the Gompertz and Weibull distributions in Section 4.1 and discuss the interpretation of one parameter of this model as an index of aging-relatedness in Section 4.2. In Section 4.3, we justify our survival mixture model in the context of the theory of competing risks (CR), and in Section 4.4, we cover the statistical procedures necessary for obtaining a point and an interval estimate of the index of aging-relatedness and the other parameters of the mixture model using maximum likelihood estimation. As an illustration of the application of the proposed method, we obtain the index of aging-relatedness for intrinsic mortality in Section 4.5 using data from a 43-year long prospective study. Finally, we discuss the precision of the parameter estimates in Section 4.6.

4.1   A SURVIVAL MIXTURE MODEL OF THE GOMPERTZ AND WEIBULL DISTRIBUTIONS

We defined two groups of sufficient causes in our evolution-based model of causation. In group 1, the time-to-event distributions of the sufficient causes are shaped or "molded" by the declining force of natural selection, and the sufficient causes are characterized by the presence of LOGE in the absence of EREF. In group 2, in which the time-to-event distributions of the sufficient causes are not molded by the declining force of natural selection, the sufficient causes are characterized by the presence of EREF component causes. We argued on statistical and evolutionary grounds that the time-to-event distributions of the sufficient causes in group 1 meet conditions to be in the minimum domain of attraction of the Gumbel-type distribution, and the time-to-event distributions of the sufficient causes in group 2 meet conditions to be in the minimum domain of attraction of the Weibull-type distribution. Thus, if all deaths or cases of a specific disease in a population were caused by one of a large number of sufficient causes from group 1, the residual time to event after age 10 years would follow an approximate Gompertz distribution, while if all deaths or cases of a specific disease in a population were caused by one of a large number of sufficient causes from group 2, the residual time to event after age 10 years would follow an approximate Weibull distribution.

A mixture of the Gompertz and Weibull survival distributions represents a theoretically motivated model for the situation in which deaths or cases of a specific disease in an actual population can be due to sufficient causes from group 1 or group 2. A justification of this statement in the context of CR theory will be discussed in Section 4.3. Here we emphasize that we consider the mixture of Gompertz and Weibull distributions *not* from an arbitrary or phenomenological attempt at model fitting. As a matter of fact, there are more flexible families of statistical models from which one could choose to fit mortality or disease incidence data. Rather, the preceding theoretical development *requires* us to consider this model. A mixture of the Gompertz and

Weibull distributions as a representation of a real-world phenomenon has not, to our knowledge, been previously considered. The evolutionary, causal, and statistical considerations leading us to the mixture model are multilayered, which goes in step with the represented real-world phenomenon being nonobvious. Indeed, if the phenomenon were obvious, the mixture model would arguably have been considered long ago.

Our consideration of the mixture model can also be said to have the "weakness of its strength." To the extent that it is theory-driven, skepticism directed toward the theory simultaneously puts into question the descriptive use of the model as well as the definition and interpretation of the index of aging-relatedness (Section 4.2). In other words, if the theory does not stand on its feet, neither does the application. However, this is a general limitation of any practical application deeply grounded in theoretical work, and that's why we have gone to great lengths to make our theory explicit and open to evaluation. Moreover, as we illustrated in Section 2.1.2, the Gompertz and Weibull components of the mixture model are approximations to the "true" exact distributions, and in this sense, the mixture model can strictly be regarded as misspecified. Yet, as we argued in Section 3.2, the approximations are supposed to be very good. Aside from these foundational caveats, one can anticipate that this theoretically motivated model represents a major statistical challenge to estimate. The estimation of the model parameters can be seen as an effort to discriminate between the Gompertz and Weibull models. Given how closely both the Gompertz and Weibull models each fit mortality data, we can take for granted neither the identifiability nor estimability of the mixture model parameters, let alone having enough information to obtain reasonably narrow confidence intervals (CIs) with usual sample sizes in prospective studies. We will return to this point in Section 4.6.

We now make the mixture model mathematically explicit. The Gompertz hazard function, $h_G(x) = \lambda e^{\theta x}$, describes an exponential relation between mortality or incidence rates and age, where, as in Chapter 2, $\lambda > 0$ and θ are parameters. The Gompertz survival function and p.d.f. are, respectively, $S_G(x) = \exp[-(\lambda/\theta)(e^{\theta x} - 1)]$ and $f_G(x) = \lambda e^{\theta x} \exp[-(\lambda/\theta)(e^{\theta x} - 1)]$. In turn, the Weibull hazard function, $h_W(x) = \alpha \gamma x^{\gamma - 1}$, describes a power relation between mortality or incidence rates and age, where $\alpha > 0$ and γ are parameters. The Weibull survival function and p.d.f. are, respectively, $S_W(x) = \exp(-\alpha x^\gamma)$ and $f_W(x) = \alpha \gamma x^{\gamma - 1} \exp(-\alpha x^\gamma)$. We state these and other relevant properties of the Gompertz and Weibull distributions in Appendix C. We shall denote the mixing parameter by π, so that the density function of the mixture is

$$f(x) = \pi f_G(x) + (1 - \pi) f_W(x). \tag{4.1}$$

Similarly, the mixture survival function is

$$S(x) = \pi S_G(x) + (1 - \pi) S_W(x). \tag{4.2}$$

It follows that the life expectancy or mean survival time of the mixture distribution, from Equations C.11 and C.13, is

$$E[X] = \pi E_G[X] + (1 - \pi) E_W[X] = \pi \frac{e^{\lambda/\theta}}{\theta} \int_{\lambda/\theta}^{\infty} y^{-1} e^{-y} dy + (1 - \pi) \alpha^{-1/\gamma} \Gamma(\gamma^{-1} + 1), \tag{4.3}$$

where $\Gamma(x) = \int_0^\infty y^{x-1}e^{-y}dy$ is the gamma function, and the median survival time of the mixture distribution is obtained by solving the following equation for x_{50}:

$$\pi \exp\left[-\frac{\lambda}{\theta}\left(e^{\theta x_{50}} - 1\right)\right] + (1-\pi)\exp\left(-\alpha x_{50}^{\gamma}\right) = \frac{1}{2}. \tag{4.4}$$

In contrast, the hazard function of the mixture distribution is

$$h(x) = \frac{f(x)}{S(x)} = \frac{\pi f_G(x) + (1-\pi)f_W(x)}{\pi S_G(x) + (1-\pi)S_W(x)} = \frac{\pi S_G(x)h_G(x) + (1-\pi)S_W(x)h_W(x)}{\pi S_G(x) + (1-\pi)S_W(x)}$$

$$= \frac{\pi S_G(x)}{\pi S_G(x) + (1-\pi)S_W(x)}h_G(x) + \frac{(1-\pi)S_W(x)}{\pi S_G(x) + (1-\pi)S_W(x)}h_W(x). \tag{4.5}$$

Thus, unlike the mixture density and survival functions, the mixture hazard function is an average of the Gompertz and Weibull hazard functions weighted by the age-dependent terms $\pi S_G(x)/S(x)$ and $(1-\pi)S_W(x)/S(x)$, rather than being the average of the Gompertz and Weibull hazard functions weighted by the constant terms π and $(1-\pi)$, respectively. Let the weights of the Gompertz and Weibull hazard functions in the mixture hazard function be denoted by $w(x)$ and $1 - w(x)$, respectively, and write Equation 4.5 as $h(x) = w(x)h_G(x) + [1 - w(x)]h_W(x)$. Then, the derivative of the mixture hazard function is

$$h'(x) = w(x)h_G'(x) + [1-w(x)]h_W'(x) + w'(x)[h_G(x) - h_W(x)], \tag{4.6}$$

where the derivative of $w(x)$ is

$$w'(x) = \frac{\pi(1-\pi)\left[S_G'(x)S_W(x) - S_G(x)S_W'(x)\right]}{S(x)^2}$$

$$= \frac{\pi(1-\pi)S_G(x)S_W(x)\left[S_G'(x)/S_G(x) - S_W'(x)/S_W(x)\right]}{S(x)^2}$$

$$= \frac{\pi(1-\pi)S_G(x)S_W(x)[(d/dx)\log S_G(x) - (d/dx)\log S_W(x)]}{S(x)^2}$$

$$= \frac{-\pi(1-\pi)S_G(x)S_W(x)[h_G(x) - h_W(x)]}{S(x)^2}. \tag{4.7}$$

Hence, Equation 4.6 becomes

$$h'(x) = w(x)h_G'(x) + [1-w(x)]h_W'(x) - \frac{\pi(1-\pi)S_G(x)S_W(x)[h_G(x) - h_W(x)]^2}{S(x)^2}. \tag{4.8}$$

Because we restrict the application of our model to the relevant situation in which the Gompertz and Weibull components of the mixture distribution have monotonically increasing hazard functions (i.e., $\theta > 0$ for the Gompertz component and $\gamma > 1$ for the Weibull component), the first and second terms in Equation 4.8 are positive. The third term, however, is always negative and may dominate the sum of the first two, especially when the difference between the hazard rates of the Gompertz and Weibull components is large. Thus, even if the hazard functions of the Gompertz and Weibull components are monotonically increasing, the hazard function of the mixture distribution is not necessarily monotonic.

4.2 DEFINITION AND INTERPRETATION OF THE INDEX OF AGING-RELATEDNESS

We take our index of aging-relatedness to be the mixture parameter π, and it thus represents the proportion of the intrinsic mortality or disease incidence experience of the population that follows a Gompertz as opposed to a Weibull distribution. The interpretation of the mixture parameter in terms of genetic and environmental contributions to mortality or disease incidence in a population follows from the definition of the two groups of sufficient causes as described in Sections 3.2 and 4.1, specifically the defining categories of component causes in each group (i.e., LOGE in the absence of EREF in group 1 and EREF in group 2). Thus, the mixture parameter indicates the proportion of deaths or cases of a specific disease in the population due to sufficient causes from group 1. That is to say, the index of aging-relatedness measures the relative retrospective contribution of sufficient causes containing LOGE in the absence of EREF to intrinsic mortality or disease incidence in a population.

It will also be helpful to introduce two age-dependent proportions. Let Y denote a latent random group indicator taking the value $Y = 1$ for an observation arising from the Gompertz distribution and $Y = 0$ for an observation arising from the Weibull distribution. Then, we define

$$\pi_f(x) = P[Y = 1 | X = x] = \frac{\pi f_G(x)}{\pi f_G(x) + (1-\pi)f_W(x)}, \tag{4.9}$$

$$\pi_S(x) = P[Y = 1 | X > x] = \frac{\pi S_G(x)}{\pi S_G(x) + (1-\pi)S_W(x)}. \tag{4.10}$$

In words, based on the fitted mixture model, $\pi_f(x)$ represents the probability that the death or disease of a population member occurring at age x is aging-related (i.e., due to a sufficient cause containing LOGE in the absence of EREF), while $\pi_S(x)$ represents the probability that the death or disease of a population member occurring after age x is aging-related. Both $\pi_f(x)$ and $\pi_S(x)$ have been previously recognized as relevant quantities in analogous contexts (Cox, 1959; Mendenhall and Hader, 1958). For instance, Mendenhall and Hader (1958) described a quantity equivalent to $\pi_S(x)$, which they denoted $p(t)$ in a reliability application: "If the entire population were put on test (or into service) the proportion of items belonging to each subpopulation would, in general, change with time. This is because the items from one subpopulation would die off more rapidly than those from the other. At time t, the subpopulations would be mixed in the proportions $p(t) : 1 - p(t)$. The quantities $p(t)$ and $1 - p(t)$ will be called the conditional mixture proportions."[1] Note that $\pi_S(x)$ is equivalent to $w(x)$ in Section 4.1, that is, the weight of the Gompertz hazard function in the mixture hazard function; note also that $\pi_S(0) = \pi$. We will graph $\pi_f(x)$ and $\pi_S(x)$ by age in the data analysis in Section 4.5.

The definition and interpretation of the index of aging-relatedness must be contrasted with that of the heritability index, which was developed in the context of quantitative genetics and applies primarily to continuous traits such as height and intelligence quotient (IQ). The concept of heritability originated in Fisher's (1918) article, "The correlation between relatives on the supposition of Mendelian inheritance," in connection with the idea of polygenic inheritance. Heritability has been defined as "the proportion of variation [in a trait] directly attributable to genetic differences among individuals relative to the total variation in a population (which includes variation due to both genetic and nongenetic factors)" (Khoury et al., 1993, p. 200). The concept of heritability has also been applied to qualitative traits or diseases by considering the variation in risk of disease, rather than in the measurement of a continuous trait, that can be attributed to genetic differences among individuals. In this case, one assumes an underlying continuous "liability" to the disease, such that individuals are affected by disease when their liability crosses a particular threshold, and "incidence" of the disease is conceived as the proportion of individuals with liabilities exceeding the threshold (Falconer, 1965). The analysis-of-variance approach of the heritability index involves partitioning the observed phenotypic variance into components reflecting differences in unobserved genetic and environmental factors. The heritability index is then obtained as a ratio of the genetic variance (i.e., the phenotypic variance attributable to genotypic or allelic differences among individuals) to the total phenotypic variance in the population.

For the estimation of heritability, two kinds of genetic variance are distinguished. The "additive variance" is attributable to the average effects of genes considered singly, as transmitted in the gametes. The "nonadditive variance" is attributable to the additional effects of these genes when combined in diploid genotypes; it arises from dominance ("dominance variance") and interaction between genes at nonhomologous loci ("epistatic variance") (Falconer, 1965). This distinction leads to the definition of two types of heritability: heritability in the broad sense, which is the ratio of variance attributed to all genetic differences among individuals to the total phenotypic variance, and heritability in the narrow sense, which is the ratio of variance contributed by the additive effects of alleles at one or more loci (i.e., additive variance) to the total phenotypic variance. Since both these measures of heritability are ratios of a genetic

---

[1] Reproduced from *Biometrika*, **45**, Mendenhall, W. and Hader, R. J., Estimation of parameters of mixed exponentially distributed failure time distributions from censored life test data, pages 504–520, Copyright 1958, with permission from Oxford University Press.

component of variance to the total variance, they lie between 0 and 1. The estimation of the heritability index in human studies relies on family-based data and takes advantage of the theoretical genotypic correlation among relatives in naturally occurring families (Khoury et al., 1993, pp. 206–209; Weiss, 1993, p. 106). Additive genetic variance represents variation in the phenotype that is transmissible from parents to offspring. The dominance effect cannot be transmitted to an offspring, which receives only one allele from each parent, but it contributes to the covariance between full siblings. The formulation of the model in terms of which parameters can be estimated depends on the study design and the types of relatives and involves specific assumptions. Commonly used study designs include nuclear families (parents and their biological offspring), extended pedigrees with pairs of relatives of different degrees, twin studies, and the full adoption design (Rice and Borecki, 2001; Vitzthum, 2003).

In relation to Fisher's (1958, pp. 22–51) fundamental theorem of natural selection implying that the speed of achieving desirable phenotypes through artificial selection is determined by the magnitude of narrow-sense heritability, several authors have emphasized the utility of heritability in predicting the effectiveness of artificial breeding programs in domesticated animals and crops (Kempthorne, 1997; Stoltenberg, 1997; Surbey, 1994; Vitzthum, 2003). However, the use of the heritability index in human studies, most commonly with respect to quantitative traits in behavioral genetics but also with respect to qualitative traits or diseases, involves observational rather than controlled experimental data. In this context, three fundamental shortcomings of the heritability index have been emphasized (Falconer, 1965; Khoury et al., 1993, chapter 7; Rice and Borecki, 2001; Susser and Susser, 1987). First, the heritability index assumes independence between genotype and environment (i.e., no gene–environment covariance), but this is not warranted in observational human studies, as noted by Wahlsten (1994a): "Genuine absence of gene-environment covariance is most unlikely in research with humans." This is also reflected in Kempthorne's (1997) commentary: "The theory of correlation between relatives has been of vast importance in plant and animal breeding because it is possible to design and carry out experiments to estimate variance components in expressions for covariances between relatives. However, data on humans is observational and individuals are not randomly assigned to environments, so that estimation of heritability from such data is not on the same firm foundation as it is in plant and animal breeding contexts."[2]

Second, expected genetic variation but not environmental variation can be well specified from the known degrees of relatedness among individuals. The variation in the phenotype shared by individuals is assigned to the genotype according to their different degrees of relatedness, and the residue is assigned to the environment. However, this "genotypic variance" includes any shared environmental variance that has not been removed by design or analysis. Third, estimates of the heritability index depend on the extent of variation of environmental and genetic factors in the population. In principle, irrespective of the genetic contribution to a phenotypic trait, the heritability index could be equal to 0 if there were no genetic variation in the

---

[2] Reproduced from *Genetica*, **99**, Kempthorne, O., Heritability: Uses and abuses, pages 109–112, Copyright 1997, with permission from Springer Science + Business Media.

population under study, or it could approach 1 if there were very little variation in the population for the environmental factors influencing the trait. Turkheimer (2011) considered that this issue—in his words, "that biometric components are not invariant across the genetic, environmental and phenotypic variances of uncontrolled traits in their naturally occurring populations"—lies at the heart of the problem with the endeavor of partitioning phenotypic variance. Hence, his verdict: "Practitioners of the art wanted it to be about cause, in the sense that the relative magnitudes of the various components were supposed to tell us something about the importance of genetic and environmental causes underlying a trait, but they do not." That conclusion was previously reached based on the notion of *norm of reaction* by Lewontin (1974), who additionally emphasized the distinction between this issue and that of obtaining different results merely from sampling from a population: "the relation of sample to universe in statistical procedures is not the same as the relation of variation in spatiotemporally defined populations to causal and functional variation summed up in the norm of reaction."

The heritability index has been the subject of an intense debate and controversy originating in its use in behavioral genetics, especially for the study of IQ. Table 4.1 lists articles that presented a thorough and comprehensive criticism of the use of the heritability index, starting with Lewontin's (1974) now classic article, titled "The analysis of variance and the analysis of causes," which was reprinted by the *International Journal of Epidemiology* in 2006 along with several commentaries (Freese, 2006; Lewontin, 2006; Rose, 2006; Taylor, 2006; Vreeke, 2006). The methodological issues raised, including but not restricted to the three described previously, go beyond the IQ controversy and certainly apply to the use of the heritability index to ascertain the genetic contribution to complex diseases. Adding to the methodological discussion initiated by Lewontin's (1974) article, Stoltenberg (1997) focused on the difference between the common and technical meanings of heritability and the

TABLE 4.1 Articles presenting a thorough and comprehensive criticism of the use of the heritability index in human studies

Article title	Author (year)
The analysis of variance and the analysis of causes	Lewontin (1974)
Logical, epistemological and statistical aspects of nature-nurture data interpretation	Kempthorne (1978)
Heritability: One word, three concepts	Jacquard (1983)
Is the nature-nurture debate on the verge of extinction?	Bors (1994)
The intelligence of heritability	Wahlsten (1994a)[a]
On models and muddles of heritability	Schönemann (1997)
Hereditarian scientific fallacies	Bailey (1997)
A number no greater than the sum of its parts: The use and abuse of heritability	Vitzthum (2003)

[a] A rebuttal of this article is given in Surbey (1994), with a response in Wahlsten (1994b).

resulting confusion. In the epidemiology literature, Pearce (2011) further considered the distinction between the analysis of variance and the analysis of causes with respect to nongenetic factors, particularly environmental risk factors that become ubiquitous over time.

Several authors have expressed forceful opinions against the abuse of heritability in human studies, which seems justified in the face of widespread uncritical research practice. For instance, Lewontin (1974) stated, "In view of the terrible mischief that has been done by confusing the spatiotemporally local analysis of variance with the global analysis of causes, I suggest that we stop the endless search for better methods of estimating useless quantities." In the introduction of her critique of heritability's use, especially in the fields of evolutionary anthropology and genetic epidemiology, Vitzthum (2003) noted, "The difficulty is that heritability, a worthy instrument when used for the purposes for which it was designed, cannot provide a meaningful answer to the nature-nurture debate for either behavioral or biological phenotypes." With respect to the estimation of heritability for multifactorial diseases, in particular cardiovascular diseases, van Asselt et al. (2006) concluded: "To accept a quantitative heritability estimate from any study as a fact of nature is but an illusion." Yet, as recently as in 2011, Turkheimer (2011) lamented, "not a month goes by without another outbreak of credulous surprise that one trait or another has turned out to be 50% heritable." On the methodological front, Visscher et al. (2008), while acknowledging the limitations of heritability, reaffirmed its importance in the genomics era and described new ways in which it can be useful. The persistence of the estimation of heritability in human studies despite the methodological shortcomings seems to be at least in part due to a hunger for easy answers in the nature–nurture debate, both in the scientific community and the public at large. It also attests to the fact that the path to finding an alternative to the heritability index is far from obvious.

Given this contested but enduring history of the concept of heritability as applied to human studies, our index gains additional significance. The index of aging-relatedness is similarly claimed to be interpretable in terms of genetic and environmental contributions to mortality and disease incidence in a population, but there are fundamental distinguishing characteristics of our index compared to the heritability index. The index of aging-relatedness emerges, on one hand, from the notion of aging-relatedness rather than the concept of heritability and, on the other hand, from evolutionary biology and population genetics rather than Mendelian genetics. The index of aging-relatedness is based on the analysis of population-based data, as opposed to family-based data. The survival-mixture-model approach of the index of aging-relatedness naturally applies to yes/no traits such as death or disease, which contrasts with the analysis-of-variance approach of the heritability index more naturally applying to quantitative traits. Importantly, assumptions of the linear model underlying the heritability index often involve no gene–gene interaction and no gene–environment interaction; while a term can be added for gene–environment interactions, they are difficult to detect and the term is often dropped in practice (Rice and Borecki, 2001; Vitzthum, 2003; Wahlsten, 1994a). The index of aging-relatedness does not assume the absence of biological interaction. Instead, our evolution-based model of causation makes biological interaction explicit, and the interpretation of the index prominently takes gene–environment interaction into account, especially in that sufficient causes containing both LOGE and EREF are subsumed under the group of sufficient causes containing EREF with or without LOGE (group 2).

In discussing how estimates of the heritability index in twin studies attribute unmeasured gene–environment interactions to the genetic component of variance and contribute to systematically underestimating the influence of environmental factors, Schwartz and Susser (2006) reasoned: "In one sense, this is correct because without the genetic component the outcome would not have happened. Thus, the heritability estimate is not invalid. What is incorrect, however, is the conclusion that the shared environmental component had little influence, and therefore that intervention on the environmental component would have little effect." They proceeded to consider the epidemiological measure of attributable proportion or attributable fraction: "In epidemiology, the measure of 'attributable proportion' is most analogous to heritability measures. It simply means the proportion of the cases that would be removed from the population if this particular risk factor were eliminated." The index of aging-relatedness is consistent with attributable proportion in a way that has important implications from a public health point of view. The index of aging-relatedness measures the attributable proportion of genetic factors in the sense of sufficient causes containing LOGE in the absence of EREF. Then, the complement of the index of aging-relatedness, that is, $1 - \pi$, represents the proportion of deaths or cases of an aging-related disease that would be removed from the population (or postponed) if all EREF were eliminated.

From a practical standpoint, the argument in the preceding text suggests that when analyzing a dataset containing information on exposure to an EREF supposedly playing an important role in causing death or disease incidence in the population, stratification by exposure to the EREF would have a predictable effect on the index of aging-relatedness relative to the overall analysis. In the stratum of those not exposed to the EREF, all those dying or being affected by a specific disease from sufficient causes containing the particular EREF would be excluded, and the index of aging-relatedness would tend to be larger than in the overall analysis. On the other hand, all those dying or being affected by a specific disease from sufficient causes containing the particular EREF would be included in the stratum of those exposed to the EREF, and the index of aging-relatedness would tend to be smaller than in the overall analysis. We will be able to test this prediction using information on smoking in the data analysis presented in Section 4.5.

We must lastly consider that, as described in Section 3.2, epigenetic changes may arise not only in response to environmental factors but also as stochastic events. This would imply that even in the hypothetical situation in which all EREF contributing to death or disease in a population were eliminated, the theoretical value of the index of aging-relatedness would not be equal to 1. That is, because of random or unsystematic sources of epigenetic changes contributing to death or disease, acting as if EREF component causes in sufficient causes from group 2, there would be a ceiling to the index of aging-relatedness below 1, representing how high the index could possibly go through intervention on environmental factors. Assuming that the effect of stochastic epigenetic changes is nonnegligible, the actual value of the ceiling for death or specific diseases would depend on the relative importance of stochastic vis-à-vis environmentally induced epigenetic changes, which is currently unsettled.

4.3 THE SURVIVAL MIXTURE MODEL AND COMPETING RISKS

In this section, we clarify how our survival mixture model reflects what we call a cause-specific (CS) approach rather than a CR approach to analyzing population mortality or disease incidence and offer arguments to justify the CS approach. The traditional approach in CR analysis involves hypothetical "latent failure times," corresponding to the failure times of each cause of failure in the absence of the others (Prentice et al., 1978). An essential feature of the CR problem is that independent individuals are exposed to two or more causes of failure, and on failure, an individual is withdrawn from risk. Except for censored observations, the cause of failure is observed; thus, the failure observation can be assigned to a given cause (Cox, 1959). This distinguishes the typical CR problem from our application, in which we cannot observe from which of two groups of sufficient causes in our evolution-based model of causation an individual died or suffered disease.

The formulation of the CR problem in terms of latent failure times usually defines X_j to be the time of failure from cause j that would be observed if the possibility of failure from causes other than j were removed (Prentice et al., 1978). If we consider two causes of death and let X_j be the latent failure time due to cause j ($j = 1, 2$) in the absence of the other cause, the following is observed for each individual: $X = \min(X_1, X_2)$, the cause of death, and the event/censoring indicator; for censored observations, the time and cause of death are unknown. Moreover, it is assumed that the CR are independent (David and Moeschberger, 1978, chapter 1; Lawless, 2003, chapter 9). Under this assumption, letting $S_j^{(l)}(x)$ and $h_j^{(l)}(x)$ be the survival and hazard functions, respectively, for the latent failure time X_j, we obtain

$$P[\min(X_1, X_2) > x] = \exp\left[-\int_0^x h_1^{(l)}(u) + h_2^{(l)}(u)du\right], \qquad (4.11)$$

which shows that the hazard function for $X = \min(X_1, X_2)$ is the sum of the hazard functions for the latent failure times X_1 and X_2, that is, $h(x) = h_1^{(l)}(x) + h_2^{(l)}(x)$.

McLachlan and McGiffin (1994) advocated that "finite mixture distributions provide a way of modeling time to failure in the case of competing risks or failures." McLachlan and Peel (2000, pp. 269–271) elaborated on the relation between the traditional latent failure-time approach of CR analysis and the use of mixtures of survival functions as an alternative approach. In the case of a two-component mixture model like ours, in which the survival function is modeled as $S(x) = \pi_1 S_1(x) + \pi_2 S_2(x)$, where $\pi_1 + \pi_2 = 1$, the jth component survival function is viewed as the conditional survival function given that failure is due to cause j and π_j is the probability of failure from cause j ($j = 1, 2$). They also noted that by writing the survival function $S(x)$ for $X = \min(X_1, X_2)$ in the latent failure-time approach as, from the independence of CR and Equation 4.11,

$$S(x) = \int_x^\infty f_1^{(l)}(u) S_2^{(l)}(u)\,du + \int_x^\infty f_2^{(l)}(u) S_1^{(l)}(u)\,du, \qquad (4.12)$$

where $f_1^{(l)}(x), f_2^{(l)}(x)$, and $f(x)$ are the density functions of X_1, X_2, and $X = \min(X_1, X_2)$, respectively, Equation 4.12 can be expressed as a two-component mixture model if one takes $\pi_1 = 1 - \pi_2 = \int_0^\infty f_1^{(l)}(u) S_2^{(l)}(u)\,du, \quad S_1(x) = \left[\int_x^\infty f_1^{(l)}(u) S_2^{(l)}(u)\,du\right] \Big/ \pi_1,$

and $S_2(x) = \left[\int_x^\infty f_2^{(l)}(u) S_1^{(l)}(u)\,du\right] \Big/ \pi_2.$

To clarify the distinction between these two approaches, we contrast here the two respective probability models, which we call the CR model and the CS model. In the two-cause CR model, two latent event times X_1 and X_2 are assumed to exist with survival functions $S_j^{(l)}(x) = P[X_j > x]$ ($j = 1, 2$) and X_1 independent of X_2 (assumption CR). We define the indicator function $Y = I[X_1 < X_2]$ and let

$$\pi = P[Y = 1] = P[X_1 < X_2]. \qquad (4.13)$$

We observe $X = \min(X_1, X_2) = YX_1 + (1 - Y)X_2$. Note that Y is not independent of X_1 or X_2; for example, $P[Y = 1 | X_1 = x] = P[X_1 < X_2 | X_1 = x] = P[X_2 > x] = S_2^{(l)}(x)$. The conditional survival functions $S_1(x) = P[X > x | Y = 1]$ and $S_2(x) = P[X > x | Y = 0]$ are not equal to $S_1^{(l)}(x)$ and $S_2^{(l)}(x)$. For example,

$$S_1(x) = \frac{\int_x^\infty f_1^{(l)}(u) S_2^{(l)}(u)\,du}{\int_0^\infty f_1^{(l)}(u) S_2^{(l)}(u)\,du}. \qquad (4.14)$$

This is to say that, within the CR framework, the conditional survival functions S_1 and S_2 would not be Gompertz and Weibull for the purpose of our application.

In the CS model, two latent event times X_1 and X_2 are assumed to exist with survival functions $S_j(x) = P[X_j > x]$ ($j = 1, 2$), which we can write without the latency superscript l as will become clear in the succeeding text. Now we define the indicator function differently from the CR model, $Y = I[\text{event occurs due to cause 1}]$, and let

$$\pi = P[Y = 1] = P[\text{event occurs due to cause 1}]. \qquad (4.15)$$

Note that, relative to Equation 4.13, since the definition of Y has changed, so has the meaning of π. We make the key assumption that the vector random variable (X_1, X_2) is independent of Y (assumption CS). That is, the mechanism that determines Y

TABLE 4.2   Distinction between the CR and CS models[a]

	CR model	CS model
Assumption	X_1 independent of X_2	(X_1, X_2) independent of Y
Indicator function	$Y = I[X_1 < X_2]$	$Y = I$ [event occurs due to cause 1]
Meaning of π	$\pi = P[X_1 < X_2]$	$\pi = P$ [event occurs due to cause 1]
$P[X > x \mid Y = 1]$	$\displaystyle \int_x^\infty f_1^{(l)}(u)S_2^{(l)}(u)\,du \bigg/ \int_0^\infty f_1^{(l)}(u)S_2^{(l)}(u)\,du$	$S_1(x)$

[a] CR, competing risks; CS, cause-specific.

is independent of the two CS event times. This assumption differentiates the CS model from the CR model, since in the CR model $Y = I[X_1 < X_2]$ is not independent of (X_1, X_2). If we define the observable event time as $X = YX_1 + (1 - Y)X_2$, then the conditional survival function of X given $Y = 1$ is

$$P[X > x \mid Y = 1] = P[X_1 > x \mid Y = 1] = P[X_1 > x] = S_1(x), \qquad (4.16)$$

and similarly, $P[X > x \mid Y = 0] = P[X_2 > x] = S_2(x)$, which justifies omitting the latency superscript on $S_j(x) = P[X_j > x]$. Lastly, note that the survival function of the observable event time is $S(x) = P[X > x] = E_Y P[X > x \mid Y]$, which gives $S(x) = \pi S_1(x) + (1 - \pi) S_2(x)$. Table 4.2 summarizes the distinction between the CR and CS models.

We mention in passing that $Y = I[X_1 < X_2]$ in the CR model is clearly a retrospective variable, and it might appear that $Y = I$[event occurs due to cause 1] in the CS model is similarly retrospective insofar as whether the cause of death or disease pertains to group 1 or group 2 is not known in advance for any individual. Indeed, we interpret π as the proportion of individuals having died or suffered a disease from a sufficient cause in group 1. This does distinguish our mixture model from other mixture models wherein two a priori identifiable subpopulations mingle. Yet we ask, is it not possible in our mixture model to infer two identifiable subpopulations independently of the actual time and specific cause of death or disease for an individual? We might tentatively justify assumption CS for our application by considering that the primary mechanism that determines Y in an individual is the pattern of inheritance/exposure of the component causes in the sufficient causes from each of the two groups (i.e., whether or not an individual inherits all genetic component causes and is exposed to all environmental component causes of each sufficient cause from each group). Hypothetically, if the pattern of inheritance/exposure were completely determinative of the type of cause, this would lead to (X_1, X_2) being independent of Y. Although this justification in itself within the CS framework is not completely tenable, we use it in the subsequent text to provide a heuristic argument for the assertion that (reasoning now within the CR framework) the asymptotic distribution of the minimum time to event for one set of many causes of one type, given that it is smaller than the minimum time to event for a large set of causes of another type, does not depend on that conditioning event, that is, the conditional survival functions S_1 and S_2 are still approximately Gompertz and Weibull.

We use special notation to formalize our assertion. Let $W_{1m} = \min\{X_{11}, X_{12}, ...,$ $X_{1m}\}$ and $W_{2n} = \min\{X_{21}, X_{22}, ..., X_{2n}\}$. Suppose there exist normalizing coefficients $a_m > 0$ and b_m $(m = 1, 2, ...)$ such that $P[W_{1m} > a_m x + b_m] \rightarrow \exp(-e^x)$ as $m \rightarrow \infty$ and normalizing coefficients $c_n > 0$ and d_n $(n = 1, 2, ...)$ such that $P[W_{2n} > c_n x + d_n] \rightarrow \exp$ $(-x^\rho)$ as $n \rightarrow \infty$, where $\rho > 0$ is a shape parameter. That is, the limiting distribution of the shifted and scaled minimum $W_{1m}^* = (W_{1m} - b_m)/a_m$ is the Gumbel-type distribution, and the limiting distribution of the shifted and scaled minimum $W_{2n}^* = (W_{2n} - d_n)/c_n$ is the Weibull-type distribution. Then, we assert that, for each individual in the population, either Equation 4.17 or Equation 4.18 will pertain:

$$P\left[W_{1m}^* > x \,\middle|\, W_{1m} < W_{2n}\right] \rightarrow \exp(-e^x) \quad \text{as } m, n \rightarrow \infty, \tag{4.17}$$

$$P\left[W_{2n}^* > x \,\middle|\, W_{2n} < W_{1m}\right] \rightarrow \exp(-x^\rho) \quad \text{as } m, n \rightarrow \infty. \tag{4.18}$$

Expressing the conditioning events $W_{1m} < W_{2n}$ and $W_{2n} < W_{1m}$ in terms of the variables W_{1m}^* and W_{2n}^*, the assertion is equivalently that, for each individual, either Equation 4.19 or Equation 4.20 will pertain:

$$P\left[W_{1m}^* > x \,\middle|\, W_{1m}^* < W_{2n}^* \frac{c_n}{a_m} + \frac{d_n - b_m}{a_m}\right] \rightarrow \exp(-e^x) \quad \text{as } m, n \rightarrow \infty, \tag{4.19}$$

$$P\left[W_{2n}^* > x \,\middle|\, W_{2n}^* < W_{1m}^* \frac{a_m}{c_n} + \frac{b_m - d_n}{c_n}\right] \rightarrow \exp(-x^\rho) \quad \text{as } m, n \rightarrow \infty. \tag{4.20}$$

The heuristic argument for the assertion, incorporating our tentative justification of assumption CS, is as follows. For any given individual, the particular pattern of inheritance/exposure of the component causes in the sufficient causes from each of the two groups will result, *with exceedingly high probability* as the number of sufficient causes increases, in the realization of the minimum time to event *from only one of the two sets* of sufficient causes. Even as we are not assuming a deterministic or actual future time to event for a given person, unless there were an amazingly coincidental balancing of normalization factors, the probability would approach 1 that the minimum over all possible sufficient causes would be from either one or the other set of sufficient causes, because eventually the normalization factors cause one minimum to strongly dominate the other in distribution. That is to say that the conditioning events have limiting probability approaching 0 or 1. Thus, for a given person, conditioning on the fact that the minimum time to event from one set of sufficient causes is smaller than the minimum time to event from the other set of sufficient causes is really no conditioning in the limit. Hence, we would expect a Gumbel/Gompertz or Weibull time-to-event limiting distribution after normalization, assuming only the typical situation wherein two normalization schemes for differently distributed minima result in asymptotic dominance of one over the other.

Based on this heuristic argument, we then justify our statement in Section 4.1 that a survival mixture model of the Gompertz and Weibull distributions represents a theoretically motivated model for the situation in which deaths or cases of a specific disease in a population can be due to sufficient causes from group 1 or group 2. We do that by additionally arguing that, on a population basis, the patterns of inheritance/exposure of the component causes are mixed, with mixing proportions π and $1 - \pi$, respectively, for the patterns leading to the realization of the minimum time to event from the set of sufficient causes from group 1 or group 2. It is precisely that population-level mixture that produces (and justifies) the mixture model of the Gompertz and Weibull distributions based on the CS framework.

4.4   ESTIMATION OF THE MODEL PARAMETERS

We next describe the procedures necessary for obtaining a point and an interval estimate of the index of aging-relatedness and the other parameters of the mixture model from prospective data using maximum likelihood estimation. In addition to taking right-censoring into account, we shall also take the age at entry into the study into account for each subject, so as to accommodate the fact that in prospective studies (such as the one whose mortality data we will analyze in the next section) subjects are entered into the study at a certain age and followed from that point on but only conditional on survival up to age at entry. Using the parametrization for the Gompertz and Weibull models introduced in Chapter 2, the five-parameter mixture p.d.f. is

$$f(x) = \pi\lambda e^{\theta x}\exp\left[-\frac{\lambda}{\theta}\left(e^{\theta x}-1\right)\right] + (1-\pi)\alpha\gamma x^{\gamma-1}\exp(-\alpha x^{\gamma}), \qquad (4.21)$$

and the mixture survival function is

$$S(x) = \pi\exp\left[-\frac{\lambda}{\theta}\left(e^{\theta x}-1\right)\right] + (1-\pi)\exp(-\alpha x^{\gamma}). \qquad (4.22)$$

Note, however, that the estimates of λ and θ for the Gompertz component and α and γ for the Weibull component of the mixture model will generally differ from the estimates that either pair of parameters would have in separate single Gompertz or single Weibull models.

The likelihood function we shall use for estimating the model parameters is

$$L(\lambda,\theta,\alpha,\gamma,\pi) = \prod_{i=1}^{n}\left[\frac{f(x_i)}{S(a_i)}\right]^{\delta_i}\left[\frac{S(x_i)}{S(a_i)}\right]^{1-\delta_i} = \prod_{i=1}^{n}\frac{f(x_i)^{\delta_i}S(x_i)^{1-\delta_i}}{S(a_i)}$$

$$= \prod_{i=1}^{n}\frac{\begin{aligned}&\left\{\pi\lambda e^{\theta x_i}\exp\left[-(\lambda/\theta)\left(e^{\theta x_i}-1\right)\right] + (1-\pi)\alpha\gamma x_i^{\gamma-1}\exp(-\alpha x_i^{\gamma})\right\}^{\delta_i}\times\\&\left\{\pi\exp\left[-(\lambda/\theta)\left(e^{\theta x_i}-1\right)\right] + (1-\pi)\exp(-\alpha x_i^{\gamma})\right\}^{1-\delta_i}\end{aligned}}{\pi\exp\left[-(\lambda/\theta)(e^{\theta a_i}-1)\right] + (1-\pi)\exp(-\alpha a_i^{\gamma})},$$

$$(4.23)$$

where δ_i is the event/censoring indicator, taking the values 1 for event and 0 for censoring, and a_i denotes the age at entry into the study for the ith subject ($i = 1, \ldots, n$). Each factor in the likelihood function is divided by the mixture survival probability $S(a_i)$ to account for the fact that subject i had to survive to age a_i in order to be included in the study. Thus, the likelihood function comprises conditional mixture probabilities given survival to age at entry into the study.

In order to constrain the point estimate and endpoints of the interval estimate of the mixture parameter π to be between 0 and 1, we reexpress the likelihood function using a logit parametrization of the mixture parameter. That is, we define $\Lambda = \log[\pi/(1 - \pi)]$ and replace in the likelihood function π with $e^{\Lambda}/(1 + e^{\Lambda})$ and $1 - \pi$ with $1/(1 + e^{\Lambda})$. Moreover, we constrain the estimates of λ and α to be positive by defining $\mu = \log(\lambda) \Rightarrow \lambda = e^{\mu}$ and $\beta = \log(\alpha) \Rightarrow \alpha = e^{\beta}$. Then, the log-likelihood function becomes

$$\log L(\mu,\theta,\beta,\gamma,\Lambda) = \sum_{i=1}^{n} \left\{ \delta_i \log \left\{ \frac{e^{\Lambda}}{1+e^{\Lambda}} e^{\theta x_i} \exp\left[\mu - \frac{e^{\mu}}{\theta}\left(e^{\theta x_i}-1\right) \right] + \frac{1}{1+e^{\Lambda}}\gamma x_i^{\gamma-1}\exp\left(\beta - e^{\beta}x_i^{\gamma}\right) \right\} \right.$$

$$+ (1-\delta_i)\log\left\{ \frac{e^{\Lambda}}{1+e^{\Lambda}}\exp\left[-\frac{e^{\mu}}{\theta}\left(e^{\theta x_i}-1\right) \right] + \frac{1}{1+e^{\Lambda}}\exp\left(-e^{\beta}x_i^{\gamma}\right) \right\}$$

$$\left. - \log\left\{ \frac{e^{\Lambda}}{1+e^{\Lambda}}\exp\left[-\frac{e^{\mu}}{\theta}\left(e^{\theta a_i}-1\right) \right] + \frac{1}{1+e^{\Lambda}}\exp\left(-e^{\beta}a_i^{\gamma}\right) \right\} \right\}. \qquad (4.24)$$

We provide formulas for the first and second partial derivatives of the log-likelihood function (Eq. 4.24) with respect to these five parameters for use in the Newton–Raphson (NR) iterative algorithm in Appendix D. Because obtaining an appropriate initial value of the parameter estimates for the NR algorithm can be challenging in any mixture model, we specify in Appendix E an expectation–conditional maximization (ECM) algorithm (Meng and Rubin, 1993). This ECM algorithm, while slow to converge, provides suitable initial estimates in the NR domain of attraction. Given this restricted purpose of the ECM algorithm, it uses the original parameters λ, θ, α, γ, and π. To construct large-sample CIs, we use the usual observed Fisher information matrix for parameters μ, θ, β, γ, and Λ. Confidence intervals for λ, α, and π are obtained by back-transformation.

Concerning the expected Fisher information per observation, $I(p)$, for the proportion $p = 1 - q$ in a simple mixture of two densities, $f(x) = p f_1(x) + q f_2(x)$, with no censoring or conditioning on age at entry, Hill (1963) found that

$$I(p) = \frac{1}{pq}\left[1 - \int_{-\infty}^{\infty} \frac{f_1(x)f_2(x)}{pf_1(x)+qf_2(x)}dx \right]. \qquad (4.25)$$

Since $(pq)^{-1}$ is the information per observation for p in a pure Bernoulli model and $0 \le \int_{-\infty}^{\infty} \frac{f_1(x)f_2(x)}{f(x)}dx \le 1$, the additional uncertainty as to which component of the mixture an observation comes from is reflected in the factor $\left[1 - \int_{-\infty}^{\infty} \frac{f_1(x)f_2(x)}{f(x)} dx\right]$.

From this expression, one can see that if the two component densities do not overlap, the integral is equal to 0 and the expected information for the mixture parameter is the same as for the parameter p from a pure Bernoulli model, while if the densities are identical, the integral is equal to 1 and the expected information for the mixture parameter is equal to 0. Thus, if the two densities overlap to a large extent, the expected information for the mixture parameter may be quite small. Based on approximations for the cases of mixtures of two normal and two exponential distributions, Hill (1963) concluded that "extremely large, and often impractical, sample sizes are required to obtain even moderate precision in estimating p unless the mixed distributions are very well separated." This is a cautionary note germane to our application, since the Gompertz and Weibull component densities can have substantial overlap. Adding to this challenge, for our application, one needs to take right-censoring and age at study entry into account. Moreover, Hill's formula also ignores the information penalty for having to estimate the component parameters λ, θ, α, and γ, which can be substantial in our application.

We implement three modifications of the observed data for the estimation procedures, based on previous arguments. First, given that only intrinsic causes of death are contemplated in our evolution-based model of causation, extrinsic causes of death (e.g., accidents, homicides, suicides, intoxications, and infectious diseases) are excluded from the analysis of mortality data. This is accomplished by replacing an event due to an extrinsic cause of death with a right-censoring at that age of death, since we know that the subject did not die from an intrinsic cause of death up to that age. We assume the censoring time is independent of the residual time to death from any intrinsic cause of death; for example, suicides completed due to an illness might be a violation of this assumption. Second, as discussed in Section 2.2.2, given the evolutionary basis for considering late life a distinct phase of life, we wish to administratively right-censor all observations at the supposed onset of the late-life mortality plateau in human populations, which we take to be 90 years based on empirical observations. Third, an approximate earliest age at reproduction in the population is subtracted from both the age at event/censoring and the age at entry into the study of each subject for the estimation procedures. For our purposes, as discussed in Section 2.2.2, the relevant earliest age at reproduction in the population is that which predominated among human ancestors during a continued period of time over evolutionary history, which we take to be 10 years.

A program for implementing the estimation procedures, given in Appendix F, was written in the R language and environment for statistical computing (R Development Core Team, 2010) and was used for the data analysis presented in the next section.

4.5 ILLUSTRATIVE APPLICATION: THE ISRAELI ISCHEMIC HEART DISEASE STUDY

We apply the method for obtaining the index of aging-relatedness using mortality data from the Israeli Ischemic Heart Disease (IIHD) study, a prospective study of 10,059 Israeli male civil servants and municipal employees at least 40 years old (Goldbourt et al., 1993; Groen et al., 1968; Medalie et al., 1973a, b; Weitzman and Goldbourt, 2006). The dataset we analyzed contained no identifying information. The study obtained almost complete mortality information over a 43-year follow-up period (1963–2006), resulting in the ascertainment of 8472 (84.2%) deaths in 10,059 subjects. The mortality information includes International Classification of Disease (ICD) codes for the underlying cause of death, allowing the partitioning of mortality into intrinsic and extrinsic. In addition, the study collected information on smoking.

We describe the design and methods of the IIHD study here, focusing on those aspects most relevant to our analysis. The IIHD study was designed as a prospective epidemiological study of ischemic heart disease. The study population was limited to men at least 40 years old working for the government of Israel or the three largest municipalities. Many types of occupations corresponding to different educational and socioeconomic levels were represented in the study population, ranging from those in high-level administrative posts to professional and clerical positions and unskilled labor. Pension and other social benefits tended to keep these workers from leaving government employment, thereby facilitating the task of long-term follow-up. Another advantage of a cohort of government and municipal employees was that the records of disability with medical certification and reports of retirement were available. Because of an interest in investigating differences among diverse cultural/geographical groups, stratified random sampling was used to provide roughly equal representation from six areas of birth: Eastern Europe, Central Europe, Southeastern Europe, Israel (born in the pre-1948 British Mandate of Palestine), the Middle East, and North Africa. Initially, 11,876 subjects were invited to participate in the study, with a response rate of 86.2% (10,232 subjects). Comparison of respondents and nonrespondents showed that nonrespondents were slightly older, reported slightly more heart attacks and associated diseases, and had more unpleasant previous contacts with medical personnel and institutions. Of the 10,232 responders, 173 were found not to meet the inclusion criteria and were excluded from the study, leaving 10,059 subjects for follow-up (Groen et al., 1968; Medalie et al., 1973a).

The design of the study involved standardized procedures to determine the incidence of ischemic heart disease during a 5-year follow-up. A baseline evaluation was conducted in 1963, and two follow-up evaluations were conducted in 1965 and 1968. At baseline, the evaluation included a brief physical examination, electrocardiogram, dietary and psychosocial questionnaires, and selected laboratory tests. In 1965, some information collected at the baseline evaluation was reassessed, and additional information was obtained. All subjects were accounted for in 1968, and 98% of the living subjects were reexamined. Mortality information for the period between 1963 and 1968 was ascertained by several means, such as obtaining information from the central Government Bureau of Statistics for all males (aged 40 and over) who died during the follow-up period, investigating all subjects reported by their employers as having died, checking all those who changed their workplace, writing to those subjects who had gone overseas, and following up all nonrespondents to the 1965 and 1968 exams. Copies of death certificates, hospital summaries, and autopsy reports were obtained on notified deaths. When death occurred at home, the subject's personal physician was contacted (Medalie et al., 1973a).

Further mortality information was obtained for an extended period, at first through 1986, with 3473 deaths being recorded over 23 years. Mortality information was obtained for another period through 2006, totaling 43 years of mortality information on the IIHD study cohort, with 8472 deaths being recorded. Since all subjects were at least 40 years old at baseline, all reached age 83 years or died prior to that by 2006. Information on mortality after 1970 was derived from the Israeli Mortality Registry, which is virtually complete in terms of death reports. The likelihood of migration among Israeli men holding a tenured civil servant position during the 1960s and 1970s was extremely low, because of a state-budgeted pension and given the socio-political environment, their family ties, and their advancing ages. Thus, it is safe to assume that loss to mortality follow-up was negligible. The underlying cause of death was recorded in different ways during the 43-year follow-up period. A review panel determined the underlying cause of death until 1970; thereafter, the underlying cause of death was classified according to the ICD, 9th or 10th revisions (Goldbourt et al., 1993; Weitzman and Goldbourt, 2006).

The IIHD study dataset contained year of birth information, but not complete date of birth. For the calculation of age at baseline and age at death or censoring, we used June 30th as the approximate day and month of birth for all subjects. Information on smoking was obtained at both the 1963 and the 1965 study visits, and the combined information was used to define smoking status. We considered a subject an "ever smoker" if he reported current or past smoking in either the 1963 or the 1965 visit and a "current smoker" if he reported currently smoking in either visit. Thus, those classified as "past smokers" stopped smoking before 1963 and were not smoking again at the 1965 visit. "Never smokers" were those who did not report ever smoking. Only two subjects had missing information on smoking. For the purpose of restricting the mortality analysis to intrinsic mortality, we used a list of ICD codes to identify extrinsic causes of death (see Table 4.3). Among 8472 deaths that occurred during the 43-year follow-up period, 560 (6.6%) were due to extrinsic causes, of which 214 (38.2%) were due to injuries and poisoning and 124 (22.1%) to infectious diseases of the respiratory system. Therefore, there remained 7912 deaths due to intrinsic causes. The mean age at baseline of the 10,059 subjects in the IIHD study was 49.3 years (standard deviation, 6.9; median, 48.7; minimum, 39.5; maximum, 74.5). Of 10,057 subjects with information on smoking, 2877 (28.6%) were never smokers, 1619 (16.1%) were past smokers, and 5561 (55.3%) were current smokers. Summary intrinsic mortality statistics by 5-year age intervals are given in Table 4.4. There were 431 subjects who died after age 90 years. These subjects were administratively right-censored at age 90 years; the intrinsic mortality analysis thus involved 7481 events occurring before age 90 years.

The ECM algorithm for the estimation of the parameters of the mixture model took 27,578 iterations to converge, with relative change less than $1e-5$ for all five parameter estimates as the convergence criterion. Figure 4.1 shows plots of the log-likelihood function and the estimate of π versus iteration of the ECM algorithm; the plot of the log-likelihood function versus iteration shows that the ECM algorithm monotonically increases the likelihood function, as expected, and that the increase is initially fast but then, after approximately the first 1000 iterations, becomes extremely slow.

TABLE 4.3   List of the ICD codes used to identify extrinsic causes of death (adapted from Carnes et al., 2006)[a]

ICD 9 code	ICD 10 code	Extrinsic causes of death
E800–E999	S00–T98	Injuries and poisoning
001–139	A00–B99	Infectious and parasitic diseases
291		Alcoholic psychosis
303	F10–F19	Alcohol dependence syndrome
304		Drug dependence
320–326	G00–G09	Inflammatory diseases of the central nervous system
390–398	I00–I02, I05–I09	Rheumatic fever and rheumatic heart disease
460–487	J00–J39	Infectious diseases of the respiratory system
571.0–571.3		Chronic liver diseases and cirrhosis, alcohol-related
	K70–K77	deaths
571.4–571.7		Chronic hepatitis and biliary cirrhosis
590	N39	Infections of the kidney
595	N30	Cystitis
597	N34	Urethritis, not sexually transmitted
601	N70–N77	Inflammatory diseases of the female genitourinary system
630–676	O00–O99	Complications of pregnancy, childbirth, and the puerperium
730	M86, M90	Osteomyelitis, periostitis, and other infections involving bone

[a] As an example of how our list differs from that of Carnes et al. (2006), these authors listed lung cancer as an extrinsic cause of death, supposedly because of the important etiologic contribution of smoking. From our perspective, we did not consider a disease to be an extrinsic cause of death if it could be thought of as aging-related or if the question of genetic versus environmental contributions was relevant. Different forms of cancer are often qualified in the medical literature as "aging-related," and they are an appropriate target for the application of our method, including those types of cancer for which the environmental contribution may be extremely important. This is also consistent with our proposed guidelines (see Section 3.1) for distinguishing between the operation of accidental factors (i.e., extrinsic causes of death) and environmental factors *sensu stricto*, which would prominently include smoking.

TABLE 4.4   Intrinsic mortality by 5-year age intervals

Age group	At risk	Events	Person-years	Event rate	Log event rate
40–45	3564	17	10,175.9747	0.001670602	−6.394571
45–50	5646	71	22,495.3806	0.003156204	−5.758385
50–55	7699	181	32,951.4812	0.005492925	−5.204294
55–60	8939	384	40,445.7112	0.009494208	−4.657073
60–65	9286	693	42,988.4894	0.016120594	−4.127658
65–70	8602	964	40,476.3196	0.023816395	−3.737381
70–75	7563	1254	34,496.6543	0.036351351	−3.314524
75–80	6214	1486	27,166.1342	0.054700459	−2.905883
80–85	4618	1486	17 956.8145	0.082754099	−2.491882
85–90	2310	945	7,074.6092	0.133576283	−2.013083
90–95	711	350	1,932.4374	0.181118418	−1.708604
>95	155	81	390.8029	0.207265620	−1.573754

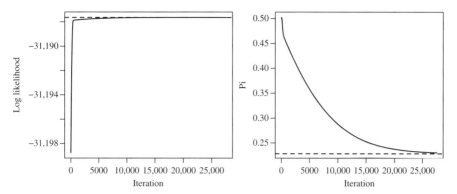

FIGURE 4.1   Plots of the log-likelihood function (left) and the estimate of π (right) versus iteration of the ECM algorithm for the analysis of intrinsic mortality. Dashed lines correspond to the final values of the maximized log-likelihood function and the estimate of π, after running the NR algorithm.

With initial values of the parameter estimates provided by the ECM algorithm, the NR algorithm converged in four steps (convergence criterion: relative change less than $1e-10$ for all five parameter estimates). Table 4.5 shows the results of fitting the mixture model to the intrinsic mortality data. We give point and interval estimates for parameters μ, θ, β, γ, and Λ and those obtained by back-transformation for λ, α, and π. The estimate of π and the 95% CI are 0.23 (0.018, 0.83). Putting aside for the moment the width of the CI, which we will address in the next section, the interpretation of the estimate of π is that 23% of the intrinsic deaths in the population are due to sufficient causes containing LOGE in the absence of EREF (77% of the intrinsic deaths are due to sufficient causes containing EREF). We might also say that 23% of the intrinsic deaths in the population are due to "aging-related causes of death." Table 4.5 additionally shows the results of the analysis of intrinsic mortality stratified by smoking status. As predicted toward the end of Section 4.2, the estimates of π are, respectively, higher and lower in never and ever smokers than the estimate of π in the overall analysis; and the estimates of π are, respectively, higher and lower in past and current smokers than the estimate of π in ever smokers.

Figure 4.2 shows four graphs relative to the overall analyses. The curves in the first graph correspond to data fitting by separate Gompertz and Weibull models. The curve in the second graph shows the result of fitting the mixture model to the data. In the third graph, the same curve is shown again with dashed lines that represent the Gompertz and Weibull components. That is, we use the estimates of λ, θ, α, and γ from the mixture model but fix π at 1 and 0 to visualize the Gompertz and Weibull components of the mixture, respectively. These dashed lines can be interpreted as what the intrinsic mortality experience of the population would be if all intrinsic deaths were due to only sufficient causes containing LOGE in the absence of EREF (Gompertz component) or only sufficient causes containing EREF (Weibull component). The former case can also be understood as the hypothetical (or counterfactual) situation in which exposure

TABLE 4.5 Results of fitting the mixture model to intrinsic mortality data, overall and stratified by smoking status. The estimated index of aging-relatedness corresponds to $\hat{\pi}$. Parameter estimates are followed by 95% CIs in parenthesis[a]

	Overall	Never smokers	Ever smokers	Past smokers	Current smokers
n	10,059	2877	7180	1619	5561
Events	7481 (74.4%)	1958 (68.1%)	5521 (76.9%)	1221 (75.4%)	4300 (77.3%)
$\hat{\mu}$	-16.6 (-29.5, -3.7)	-14.4 (-28.5, -0.4)	-17.6 (-39.8, 4.6)	-13.6 (-25.0, -2.2)	-99.0 (-220.2, 22.2)
$\hat{\lambda}$	$6.0e{-}8$ ($1.5e{-}13$, $2.5e{-}2$)	$5.5e{-}7$ ($4.4e{-}13$, $6.8e{-}1$)	$2.3e{-}8$ ($5.3e{-}18$, $9.6e{+}1$)	$1.2e{-}6$ ($1.4e{-}11$, $1.1e{-}1$)	$1.0e{-}43$ ($2.4e{-}96$, $4.4e{+}9$)
$\hat{\theta}$	0.19 (0.015, 0.36)	0.16 (-0.018, 0.34)	0.20 (-0.098, 0.50)	0.15 (0.0012, 0.30)	1.3 (-0.30, 2.8)
$\hat{\beta}$	-25.8 (-27.2, -24.3)	-26.4 (-30.6, -22.3)	-25.7 (-27.3, -24.2)	-26.0 (-31.2, -20.9)	-25.9 (-26.7, -25.1)
$\hat{\alpha}$	$6.4e{-}12$ ($1.5e{-}12$, $2.7e{-}11$)	$3.3e{-}12$ ($5.3e{-}14$, $2.1e{-}10$)	$6.6e{-}12$ ($1.4e{-}12$, $3.0e{-}11$)	$5.0e{-}12$ ($3.0e{-}14$, $8.4e{-}10$)	$5.6e{-}12$ ($2.4e{-}12$, $1.3e{-}11$)
$\hat{\gamma}$	6.1 (5.7, 6.4)	6.3 (4.8, 7.8)	6.1 (5.7, 6.4)	6.2 (5.0, 7.4)	6.1 (5.9, 6.3)
$\hat{\Lambda}$	-1.2 (-4.0, 1.6)	0.3 (-5.5, 6.1)	-1.7 (-5.5, 2.0)	-0.2 (-5.0, 4.6)	-3.8 (-4.7, -3.0)
$\hat{\pi}$	0.23 (0.018, 0.83)	0.58 (0.0043, 1.0)	0.15 (0.0040, 0.88)	0.45 (0.0069, 0.99)	0.021 (0.0091, 0.049)
Log likelihood	$-31,187.635919$	-8343.133168	$-22,748.004651$	-5014.358325	$-17,710.836313$

[a] Sample sizes in the analyses of never and ever smokers do not add up to the sample size in the overall analysis because two patients had missing information on smoking.

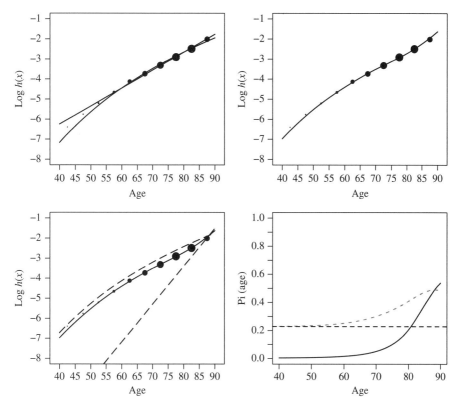

FIGURE 4.2   Intrinsic mortality ($n = 10{,}059$, events: 7481). Upper left panel: data fitting by separate Gompertz (straight line) and Weibull (curved line) models. Upper right panel: data fitting by mixture model. Lower left panel: data fitting by mixture model with dashed lines representing the Gompertz (straight dashed line) and Weibull (curved dashed line) components of the mixture. These three graphs are semilog plots of the hazard function by age in years; the points are the observed log hazard rates for each 5-year age interval, and dot diameters are proportional to the number of events in the age intervals. Lower right panel: $\pi_f(x)$ (solid line) and $\pi_S(x)$ (dashed gray line) by age in years; dashed black line marks the estimate of π.

to EREF is completely removed from the population. The final graph gives the two versions of $\pi(x)$ described in Section 4.2 (Eqs. 4.9 and 4.10) by age. We make the following observations based on these four graphs: (i) The separate Gompertz and Weibull models apparently provide similarly good fits to the data. The Gompertz and Weibull fitted lines cross at two points and are close together, such that it is difficult to discern by visual inspection which one is providing a better fit. (ii) The five-parameter mixture model provides a very good fit to the data, which is clearly better than the fits by the separate Gompertz and Weibull models. (iii) The graph in the lower left panel suggests that the intrinsic mortality experience of the population would be appreciably different, especially by showing reduced log mortality rates in midadult

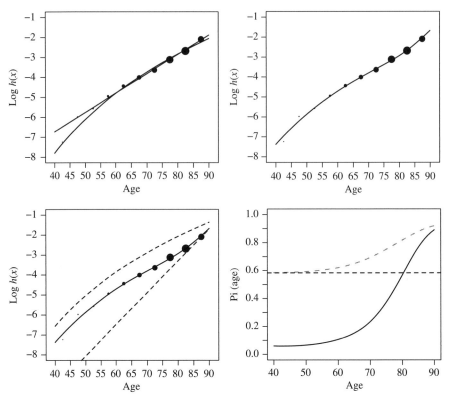

FIGURE 4.3 Intrinsic mortality in never smokers ($n = 2877$, events: 1958). Upper left panel: data fitting by separate Gompertz (straight line) and Weibull (curved line) models. Upper right panel: data fitting by mixture model. Lower left panel: data fitting by mixture model with dashed lines representing the Gompertz (straight dashed line) and Weibull (curved dashed line) components of the mixture. These three graphs are semilog plots of the hazard function by age in years; the points are the observed log hazard rates for each 5-year age interval, and dot diameters are proportional to the number of events in the age intervals. Lower right panel: $\pi_f(x)$ (solid line) and $\pi_S(x)$ (dashed gray line) by age in years; dashed black line marks the estimate of π.

ages, if all intrinsic deaths were due to sufficient causes containing LOGE in the absence of EREF (i.e., if exposure to EREF were to be completely eliminated). (iv) Consistent with that, the graph in the lower right panel shows that the probability that the death of a population member at a given age is aging-related increases with age.

In Figure 4.3, Figure 4.4, Figure 4.5, and Figure 4.6, we present the same graphs as in Figure 4.2 for the analysis of intrinsic mortality in never, ever, past, and current smokers. As can be seen in the lower left panels of these figures, the lower estimates of π in the analysis of ever and, especially, current smokers are reflected in the prox- imity of the fit by the mixture model to the curved dashed line (Weibull component of

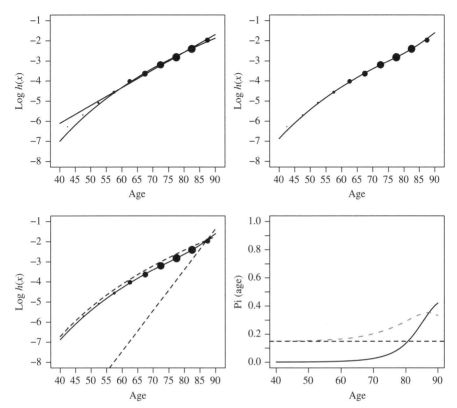

FIGURE 4.4 Intrinsic mortality in ever smokers ($n = 7180$, events: 5521). Upper left panel: data fitting by separate Gompertz (straight line) and Weibull (curved line) models. Upper right panel: data fitting by mixture model. Lower left panel: data fitting by mixture model with dashed lines representing the Gompertz (straight dashed line) and Weibull (curved dashed line) components of the mixture. These three graphs are semilog plots of the hazard function by age in years; the points are the observed log hazard rates for each 5-year age interval, and dot diameters are proportional to the number of events in the age intervals. Lower right panel: $\pi_f(x)$ (solid line) and $\pi_S(x)$ (dashed gray line) by age in years; dashed black line marks the estimate of π.

the mixture). In the analysis of current smokers (Fig. 4.6), one notes a peculiar bump in the fitted curve for the mixture model at about age 90 years, as well as a rather steep straight dashed line reflecting a large estimate of θ. This suggests the possibility of "statistical instability," which might occur under two scenarios. When π gets relatively close to 0 (i.e., the contribution of the Gompertz component to the mixture model becomes virtually null), the statistical instability is characterized by a very small estimate of λ and large estimate of θ (see Table 4.5, fifth column). On the other hand, when π gets relatively close to 1 (i.e., the contribution of the Weibull component to the mixture model becomes virtually null), the statistical instability would be characterized by a very small estimate of α and large estimate of γ. In both these cases,

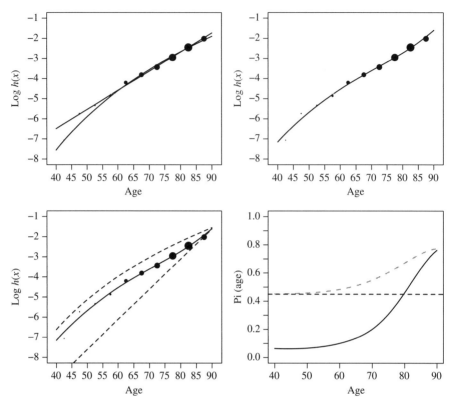

FIGURE 4.5 Intrinsic mortality in past smokers ($n = 1619$, events: 1221). Upper left panel: data fitting by separate Gompertz (straight line) and Weibull (curved line) models. Upper right panel: data fitting by mixture model. Lower left panel: data fitting by mixture model with dashed lines representing the Gompertz (straight dashed line) and Weibull (curved dashed line) components of the mixture. These three graphs are semilog plots of the hazard function by age in years; the points are the observed log hazard rates for each 5-year age interval, and dot diameters are proportional to the number of events in the age intervals. Lower right panel: $\pi_f(x)$ (solid line) and $\pi_S(x)$ (dashed gray line) by age in years; dashed black line marks the estimate of π.

the instability would emerge as an attempt by the model to "overfit" observations at an extreme of the age range. In Figure 4.7, we present semilog plots of the hazard function by age and smoking group (superposed in the same graph) with the respective fits by the mixture model. These plots show that, aside from smoking being associated with lower estimates of π (Table 4.5), the mortality rates were as expected higher at all ages for ever smokers than for never smokers, and among ever smokers, the mortality rates were as expected higher at all ages for current smokers than for past smokers.

Finally, we assessed the goodness of fit of the mixture as well as the separate Gompertz and Weibull models to the overall intrinsic mortality data. To that end,

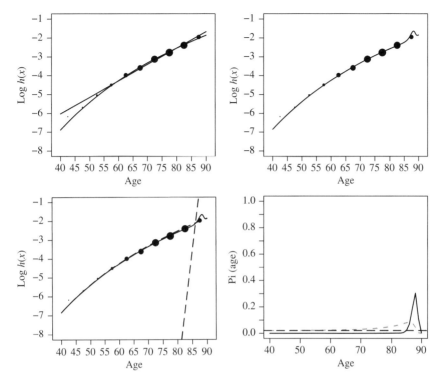

FIGURE 4.6 Intrinsic mortality in current smokers ($n = 5561$, events: 4300). Upper left panel: data fitting by separate Gompertz (straight line) and Weibull (curved line) models. Upper right panel: data fitting by mixture model. Lower left panel: data fitting by mixture model with dashed lines representing the Gompertz (straight dashed line) and Weibull (curved dashed line) components of the mixture. These three graphs are semilog plots of the hazard function by age in years; the points are the observed log hazard rates for each 5-year age interval, and dot diameters are proportional to the number of events in the age intervals. Lower right panel: $\pi_f(x)$ (solid line) and $\pi_S(x)$ (dashed gray line) by age in years; dashed black line marks the estimate of π.

we first plotted the Nelson–Aalen estimate of the cumulative hazard function along with the parametric estimate for each model (Andersen et al., 1993, pp. 445–450). For comparison purposes, we were interested in the "net" parametric cumulative hazard function beginning at the lower limit in the sample of age 40 years at baseline. Thus, for the parametric cumulative hazard rates, we subtracted the cumulative hazard predicted by the models at age 40 years. Second, we conducted a formal chi-squared test based on grouped data and the comparison of the Nelson–Aalen and parametric estimates of the cumulative hazard function (Andersen et al., 1993, pp. 462–464; Hjort, 1990). In particular, we used the "very simple but slightly conservative test procedure" described by Hjort (1990, p. 1235), in which the chi-squared statistic, analogously to the classical Pearson chi-squared statistic, is given by $\sum_{i=1}^{m} (N_i - E_i)^2 / E_i$,

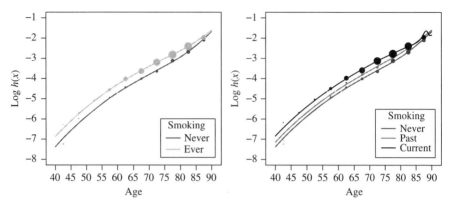

FIGURE 4.7   Semilog plots of the hazard function by age in years and smoking group for intrinsic mortality. Data fitting by mixture model showing smoking groups superposed in the same graph. The points are the observed log hazard rates for each 5-year age interval, and dot diameters are proportional to the number of events in the age intervals.

where m is the number of age intervals and N_i is the observed number of events in interval I_i; $E_i = \int_{I_i} Y(x)h(x)dx$ is the expected number of events or a model-based estimate of N_i, where $Y(x)$ gives the observed number at risk just before age x and $h(x)$ is the model hazard function using the maximum likelihood parameter estimates. In our application, $Y(x)$ differs from the usual nonincreasing number-at-risk process because subjects enter into the cohort at different ages at baseline, but this also satisfies the regularity conditions used in Hjort's (1990, section 2) theoretical results. Third, given that the separate Gompertz and Weibull models are embedded in the mixture model, we conducted a generalized log-likelihood ratio test comparing each to the mixture model. Unlike the chi-squared goodness-of-fit test, which is an absolute measure in the sense that it considers only the observed events and a given model-based expectation, the generalized log-likelihood ratio test gives a relative measure of goodness of fit, speaking to the significance of the improvement in fit by the mixture model over the Gompertz or Weibull model.

Figure 4.8 (upper panel) shows the graph with the Nelson–Aalen and mixture model estimates of the cumulative hazard function. The fit is strikingly good by visual inspection; the superposition of the empirical and parametric estimates makes them virtually undistinguishable. Consistent with that, the chi-squared goodness-of-fit test assessing the fit by the mixture model to the intrinsic mortality data produced a P-value close to 1 (chi-squared statistic, 0.58; d.f., 5; P-value = 0.99). On the other hand, the chi-squared test rejected the hypothesis of a good fit by the separate Gompertz (chi-squared statistic, 13.50; d.f., 5; P-value = 0.019) and Weibull (chi-squared statistic, 17.24; d.f., 5, P-value = 0.0041) models, despite the fact that the fits by these models also seemed very good by visual inspection (Fig. 4.8, lower panels). Moreover, the generalized log-likelihood ratio test showed a significant improvement of fit by the mixture model over the Gompertz (likelihood ratio statistic,

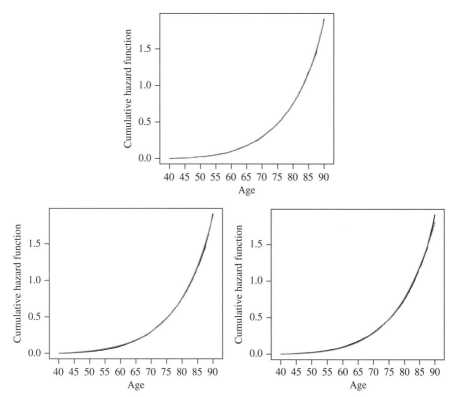

FIGURE 4.8 Goodness-of-fit cumulative hazard plots for intrinsic mortality. Upper panel: Nelson–Aalen (black line) and mixture model (gray line) estimates of the cumulative hazard function (the black line is concealed underneath the gray line). Lower left panel: Nelson–Aalen (black line) and Gompertz model (gray line) estimates of the cumulative hazard function. Lower right panel: Nelson–Aalen (black line) and Weibull model (gray line) estimates of the cumulative hazard function. For the model cumulative hazard rates, we subtracted the cumulative hazard predicted by the model at age 40 years, such that the accumulation of hazard starts at 0 at age 40 years.

25.38; d.f., 3; P-value $= 1.29e - 5$) and Weibull (likelihood ratio statistic, 47.87; d.f., 3; P-value $= 2.27e - 10$) models.

We summarize the results of the data analysis by making three broad points: (i) In the overall analysis of intrinsic mortality, 23% of the intrinsic deaths in the population under study were due to aging-related causes of death (reflecting the contribution of the Gompertz component of the mixture distribution), notwithstanding the long-standing view that the Gompertz model alone provides a good description of human mortality data. (ii) In the intrinsic mortality analysis stratified by smoking status, we confirmed a prediction that in those not exposed to a causally important environmental factor, the index of aging-relatedness would be larger than in the overall analysis, while in those exposed, the index of aging-relatedness would be smaller than in the overall analysis. (iii) The results of the goodness-of-fit analysis strongly supported the appropriateness of the mixture model for the description of intrinsic mortality. The outstanding graphical fit and highly nonsignificant result for the mixture model, in the face of the significant rejection of the Gompertz and Weibull models, which themselves also showed very good graphical fits, should allay concerns about lack of statistical power.

4.6   PRECISION OF ESTIMATION

Overall, despite the plausible results presented in Section 4.5, the CIs for the index of aging-relatedness, as well as for the other parameters of the mixture model, were very wide. In Section 4.1, we considered that the estimation of the mixture model parameters might be seen as an effort to discriminate between the Gompertz and Weibull models. Since the Gompertz and Weibull models each fit mortality data closely (suggesting that they are also close to each other), one might anticipate that the estimation of the mixture parameters would represent a challenge. Indeed, Figure 4.2 (upper left panel) shows that the separate Gompertz and Weibull models provide a good fit by visual inspection to the intrinsic mortality data. Figure 4.9 presents the plots of the Gompertz and Weibull densities corresponding to the semilog hazard plots in Figure 4.2 (upper left panel); it shows that the densities overlap almost completely, thus making discrimination between the two extremely challenging. A related but different consideration introduced in Section 4.4 is Hill's (1963) result (Eq. 4.25), showing that if the two component densities of a mixture distribution overlapped to a large extent, the expected information per observation for the mixture parameter could be quite small. This overlap, represented by the second multiplicative factor in Equation 4.25, is illustrated in Figure 4.10 for the components of our mixture model, based on the analysis of intrinsic mortality overall and in never and ever smokers.

We can also account for the width of the CIs for π in terms of the penalty for having to estimate the parameters λ, θ, α, and γ, which is not included in Hill's (1963) result, as mentioned in Section 4.4. For example, in the analysis of intrinsic mortality overall, the information matrix component that we would use for the standard error of the estimate of the logit mixture parameter Λ, namely, $\hat{I}_{\Lambda\Lambda}^{-1/2}$, was 0.055, while the standard error of $\hat{\Lambda}$ reflecting the estimation of the other parameters, namely, $\hat{I}_{\Lambda\Lambda.\Psi}^{-1/2} = \left(\hat{I}_{\Lambda\Lambda} - \hat{I}_{\Lambda\Psi}\hat{I}_{\Psi\Psi}^{-1}\hat{I}_{\Psi\Lambda}\right)^{-1/2}$, was 1.43, where we have written $\Psi = (\mu, \theta, \beta, \gamma)$. The 95% CI for π ignoring the penalty for estimating the other parameters (i.e., assuming the other parameters were known) would be (0.21, 0.25), as contrasted with the actual 95% CI: (0.018, 0.83). Therefore, the penalty was quite substantial.

We explored the impact of larger sample sizes on the width of the CIs for the index of aging-relatedness by sampling with replacement from the original intrinsic mortality data, so as to obtain "bootstrapped samples" 4, 9, and 25 times larger than the original sample. The results of fitting the mixture model to these bootstrapped samples are presented in Table 4.6. The standard error of the logit parameter estimate for the original and increasingly larger bootstrapped samples was, respectively, 1.43, 0.73, 0.59, and 0.26. Thus, it was closely reduced by the anticipated factor of $\sqrt{4} = 2$ for the first bootstrapped sample, less than the anticipated factor of $\sqrt{9} = 3$

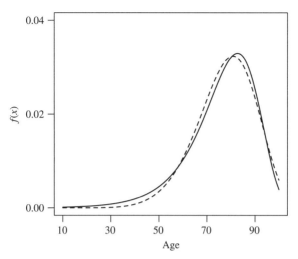

FIGURE 4.9 Plots of the densities of the Gompertz (solid line) and Weibull (dashed line) models fitted separately to the overall intrinsic mortality data.

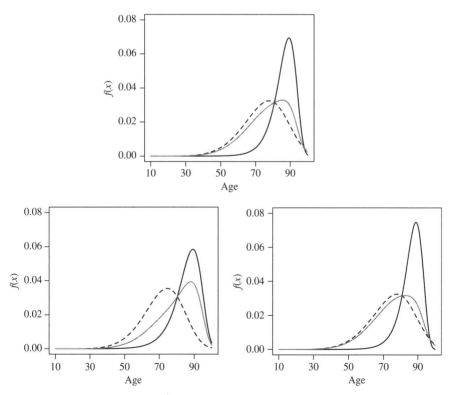

FIGURE 4.10 Plots of the densities of the Gompertz (solid black line) and Weibull (dashed black line) components of the mixture distribution and the density of the mixture distribution (gray line), for the analysis of intrinsic mortality overall (upper panel) and in never (lower left panel) and ever (lower right panel) smokers.

TABLE 4.6 Results of fitting the mixture model to intrinsic mortality data, using the original data and bootstrapped samples 4, 9, and 25 times larger than the original sample size. Parameter estimates are followed by 95% CIs in parenthesis

	Original data	Bootstrapped sample (×4)	Bootstrapped sample (×9)	Bootstrapped sample (×25)
n	10,059	40,236	90,531	251,475
Events	7481 (74.4%)	29,901 (74.3%)	67,351 (74.4%)	186,763 (74.3%)
$\hat{\mu}$	−16.6 (−29.5, −3.7)	−16.1 (−22.0, −10.2)	−18.9 (−25.9, −11.8)	−17.6 (−20.3, −14.8)
$\hat{\lambda}$	6.0e−8 (1.5e−13, 2.5e−2)	1.0e−7 (2.8e−10, 3.8e−5)	6.4e−9 (5.6e−12, 7.4e−6)	2.3e−8 (1.5e−9, 3.6e−7)
$\hat{\theta}$	0.19 (0.015, 0.36)	0.18 (0.10, 0.26)	0.22 (0.12, 0.31)	0.20 (0.16, 0.24)
$\hat{\beta}$	−25.8 (−27.2, −24.3)	−25.8 (−26.5, −25.1)	−26.3 (−26.7, −25.9)	−25.7 (−26.0, −25.4)
$\hat{\alpha}$	6.4e−12 (1.5e−12, 2.7e−11)	6.1e−12 (3.0e−12, 1.3e−11)	3.7e−12 (2.5e−12, 5.6e−12)	6.8e−12 (5.2e−12, 8.9e−12)
$\hat{\gamma}$	6.1 (5.7, 6.4)	6.1 (5.9, 6.3)	6.2 (6.1, 6.3)	6.1 (6.0, 6.1)
$\hat{\Lambda}$	−1.2 (−4.0, 1.6)	−1.1 (−2.5, 0.3)	−1.6 (−2.7, −0.4)	−1.4 (−1.9, −0.8)
$\hat{\pi}^a$	0.23 (0.018, 0.83)	0.25 (0.074, 0.58)	0.18 (0.062, 0.40)	0.20 (0.13, 0.30)
Log likelihood	−31,187.635919	−124,576.901718	−280,564.226684	−779,250.873919

[a] GLRT-based 95% CIs for π, in the analysis of the original data and bootstrapped samples 4, 9, and 25 times larger than the original sample size, are, respectively, (0.051, 0.92), (0.10, 0.65), (0.079, 0.42), and (0.14, 0.31); see also Figure 4.12.

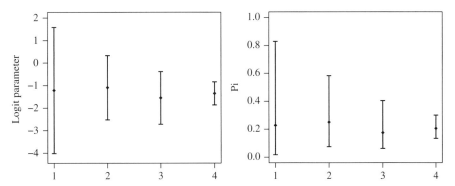

FIGURE 4.11 Plots of the point and 95% interval estimates for the logit mixture parameter Λ (left) and for π (right) obtained from fitting the mixture model to intrinsic mortality data, using the original data and bootstrapped samples 4, 9, and 25 times larger than the original sample size (labeled 1, 2, 3, and 4 in the x-axis, respectively).

for the second bootstrapped sample, and more than the anticipated factor of $\sqrt{25} = 5$ for the third bootstrapped sample. With sample size 25 times larger than the original sample size, we obtained a point estimate of the index of aging-relatedness close to the original result and a reasonably narrow 95% CI, namely, $\hat{\pi} = 0.20$ (0.13, 0.30). Figure 4.11 shows plots of the point and interval estimates for the logit parameter and for π in this analysis.

For the original data and bootstrapped samples, we additionally obtained the profile log-likelihood function of π. That is, for each given value of π or the logit parameter Λ, we obtained the maximum likelihood estimates of $\Psi = (\mu, \theta, \beta, \gamma)$ and calculated the value of the maximized log-likelihood function. This is shown in Figure 4.12. These graphs show that the profile log-likelihood function is very flat at the overall maximum for the original data but becomes more peaked as the sample size increases. The profile log-likelihood function of π also allowed us to obtain generalized likelihood ratio test (GLRT)-based CIs for π (Fig. 4.12 and footnote in Table 4.6). Compared to the Wald-based CIs, the GLRT-based CIs are wider and shifted to the right, but the two intervals get closer to each other with increasing sample size.

The previous analysis implies that population registry data are necessary for more informative results, with event counts in the hundreds of thousands. While this is certainly a limitation of the proposed index of aging-relatedness, we regard it not as a shortcoming of the method per se but as an indication of the general and inherent difficulty in discerning two close mathematical models. What makes the effort and resources worthwhile is that, despite the closeness of the Gompertz and Weibull models, they reflect meaningfully different causal explanations for mortality and disease incidence, conferring biomedical and public health relevance upon the index of aging-relatedness. Furthermore, needing large event counts is arguably not impractical in today's age of "big data." Indeed, moving forward, appropriate sources of data for estimating the index of aging-relatedness include national vital statistics (e.g., vital

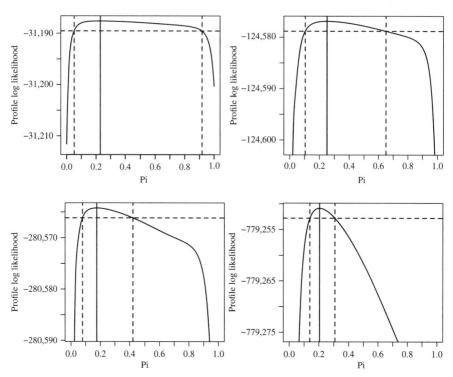

FIGURE 4.12   Profile log-likelihood function of π for original data (upper left panel) and bootstrapped samples 4 (upper right panel), 9 (lower left panel), and 25 (lower right panel) times larger than the original sample size. The vertical solid line marks the maximum likelihood estimate of π. The horizontal dashed line marks the overall maximum of the log-likelihood function minus 1.92 (the chi-squared 5% critical value of 3.84 on 1 d.f. divided by 2) and defines the limits of the GLRT-based 95% CIs for π (vertical dashed lines).

statistics collected by the U.S. National Center for Health Statistics), death registries for whole countries (e.g., the U.K. General Register Office), and countrywide or state-wide morbidity registries (e.g., the Danish National Hospital Register). Contingent on a large enough number of events, potential outcomes of interest include, in addition to intrinsic mortality, DS mortality, disability, and incidence of common aging-related diseases of complex etiology.

Estimating the index of aging-relatedness for a whole population within a geographical area and within a period of time is informative in itself, but estimating the index of aging-relatedness across geographical areas or across time in the same area may provide more useful or interesting information. If one is to analyze a mortality dataset with men and women, given the longer survival of women compared to men (Austad, 2006; Kirkwood, 1999, chapter 13), it is advisable to also estimate the index of aging-relatedness separately by sex. For the application of the index of aging-relatedness to complex diseases, incidence data would be preferable to DS mortality data, because the latter is to some extent "distorted" by progress in tertiary medical care improving survival after disease onset (e.g., interventional cardiology or surgical procedures for ischemic heart disease). Moreover, two recent reports indicate that there is reason for concern about the accuracy of cause-of-death information in death certificates in the United States (Al-Samarrai et al., 2013; Wexelman et al., 2013). However, one would expect that large enough incidence datasets are at the present time scant, even for common aging-related diseases such as ischemic heart disease and Alzheimer's disease.

5

DISCUSSION: IMPLICATIONS

The causation framework and the method proposed here have widespread potential implications. In this chapter, we discuss the following topics from the perspective of our causation model and the index of aging-relatedness: the meaning of the Gompertz parameter (Section 5.1), age as a risk factor for disease (Section 5.2), the question of whether aging-related diseases are an integral part of aging (Section 5.3), biological versus chronological aging (Section 5.4), and the public health notions of compression of morbidity and mortality (Section 5.5). Finally, in Section 5.6, we draw a current picture of aging that emerges from this work.

5.1 THE MEANING OF THE GOMPERTZ PARAMETER

Our work provides a theoretical basis based on evolutionary biology and statistical theory for a Gompertz pattern of mortality in human populations, but it does so by eventually considering the Gompertz distribution as one of two components of a mixture distribution. That the already very good fit by the Gompertz (or the Weibull) model to the mortality data analyzed in Section 4.5, as judged by visual inspection, was substantially improved by the mixture model suggests it provides a more fundamental description of human mortality. This is arguably so even though some improvement over the Gompertz fit would follow merely from the increased flexibility afforded by the greater number of parameters in the mixture model. We note that, given the role

The Biostatistics of Aging: From Gompertzian Mortality to an Index of Aging-Relatedness, First Edition. Gilberto Levy and Bruce Levin.
© 2014 John Wiley & Sons, Inc. Published 2014 by John Wiley & Sons, Inc.

played by the extreme dependence of human offspring in our evolutionary reasoning, the theoretical basis for the Gompertz pattern of mortality applies to humans and similarly social species, but not to species that do not exhibit such dependence. We also note that the Gompertz exponential rate parameter in the mixture model is not the same as the Gompertz parameter under the assumption of a purely Gompertz model. So not only does the mixture model provide a better description of intrinsic mortality data, it also permits the estimation of the Gompertz parameter in the presence of a Weibull component under the assumption that the mixture model is true. The difference is quantitatively nontrivial, as the estimate of the Gompertz parameter in our mixture model analysis was about 0.20, while the estimate of the Gompertz parameter in most analyses of human mortality data using the pure Gompertz model is about 0.10. As reviewed in the following text, several analyses of human mortality data using the pure Gompertz model have demonstrated a relative stability of the Gompertz exponential rate parameter estimate. Based on such stability, we offer an interpretation for the biological meaning of the Gompertz parameter, but this presupposes a similar stability of the Gompertz parameter estimate under the mixture model.

The analysis by Gavrilov and Gavrilova (1991, pp. 77–85), first mentioned in Section 2.2.2, revealed a striking stability of the age-dependent component of the Gompertz–Makeham equation (comprising parameters λ and θ) during the period covered by the study and for most countries included in the analysis. Such stability, which the authors referred to as "the historical stability of the age-dependent component of mortality," was particularly noticeable for the estimates of the Gompertz parameter θ, which ranged from 0.101 to 0.112 in the Swedish male population during the period 1901 through 1983, as contrasted with a 2.4-fold difference between the minimum and maximum values of the λ parameter estimate. Based on a graphical analysis of mortality data from Swedish females, Jones (1959) also provided evidence for relative stability of the Gompertz parameter during an even longer period from 1751 through 1950. Other studies have reported similar stability of the Gompertz parameter estimate for human mortality data across geographical areas. Jones (1956) analyzed life-table data from countries throughout the world over the period 1900–1951 and evidenced a mortality rate doubling time (MRDT) (MRDT = (log 2)/θ, see Appendix C) between 7 and 8.5 years, corresponding to a Gompertz parameter estimate between 0.082 and 0.099. Carnes et al. (1996) analyzed mortality data from the second half of the twentieth century drawn from vital registration systems in Australia, Japan, the Netherlands, Sweden, and the United States, restricting the analysis to intrinsic mortality. The MRDT across gender, countries, and calendar year (1960 through 1990) ranged from 6.5 to 8.2 years (Gompertz parameter estimate: 0.085–0.107), and the parameter λ estimate showed roughly a sevenfold difference between minimum and maximum values.

Relative stability of Gompertz parameter estimates has also been demonstrated in populations experiencing severe adverse conditions over a limited period of time. Based on data reported by Bergman (1948), Jones (1959) plotted the age-specific mortality rates of Australian internees in World War II Japanese prison camps in Java in the years 1944 and 1945, together with age-specific mortality rates of the male civilian

Australian population in 1944–1945. The semilog plots of age-specific mortality rates by age revealed that the three groups had different intercepts (the intercept for prisoners of war in 1945 was greater than the intercept for prisoners of war in 1944, which was greater than the intercept for civilians in 1944–1945), but the slopes estimating the Gompertz parameters were indistinguishable. Finch et al. (1990) further expanded this comparison with data from the U.S. 1980 female population; again, the slope of the Gompertz fit was virtually indistinguishable from the other groups, while the intercept for the U.S. 1980 female population was the lowest. Similar results with respect to the stability of the Gompertz parameter were obtained when Jones (1959) examined the effect of the starvation and duress that afflicted the entire population of the Netherlands in 1945, by comparing age-specific mortality rates of Netherlands males in the years 1945 and 1946.

Such apparent stability of the Gompertz parameter has suggested that it may have an underlying biological meaning with respect to the aging process. Jones (1956) stated, "the fact that all of the human populations have essentially the same slope [Gompertz parameter] in the latter half of adult life means that the doubling time of q_x [age-specific death rate] is the same for all populations, as though physiologic deterioration, in an average sense, is progressing on a very accurate time schedule." Gavrilov and Gavrilova (1991, p. 80) argued based on their empirical observations that "the age-dependent component of mortality is determined not by social conditions, but by significantly more stable biological characteristics of human populations." These authors also stated, "The historical stability of this component of mortality shows that it is determined by the fundamental (genetic and ecological) characteristics of human populations, which evolve significantly more slowly than socioeconomic living conditions" (Gavrilov and Gavrilova, 1991, p. 87). This is generally consistent with the conclusions of Carnes et al. (1996), who referred to the age pattern of intrinsic mortality in a population as the "intrinsic mortality signature" and argued that it should remain invariant given stability in the "genetic composition of a population."

The field of biodemography, whose central themes are the biology of the life table and the search for a law of mortality (Olshansky and Carnes, 1997), has offered an explanation for a relatively stable Gompertz parameter in evolutionary terms. In addition to the evolutionary theory of aging, it involves the evolutionary notion that growth and development have been molded by the forces of extrinsic mortality, such that organisms would attain the age of sexual maturity before the likelihood of dying from an extrinsic cause of death was too high (Carnes and Olshansky, 1997). That is, given a hostile environment and the strong contribution of extrinsic causes of death to mortality during most of evolutionary history, natural selection has favored organisms that can reproduce sooner rather than later. The general reasoning then follows: "We contend that the logic used to link natural selection and reproduction, and reproduction and senescence for individuals has a direct bearing on when intrinsic mortality should occur in a population. The timing of genetically determined processes such as growth and development is driven by a reproductive biology molded by the necessity for early reproduction. If individual senescence is an inadvertent consequence of these developmental processes, then age patterns of intrinsic mortality in a population should also be calibrated to some element(s) of the species' reproductive biology" (Carnes et al., 1996).[1]

We offer a more precise interpretation for the biological meaning of the Gompertz parameter θ in the context of our causation model and using an interesting result in Gumbel's (1958, p. 246) classical book with respect to the Gompertz distribution. Starting from the definition of the hazard function, $h(x) = f(x)/[1 - F(x)] \Rightarrow h(x)[1 - F(x)] = f(x)$, where $f(x)$ and $F(x)$ are a general p.d.f. and c.d.f., respectively, Gumbel (1958, p. 21) takes the derivative of both sides of this equation to obtain

$$h'(x) = h(x)^2 \left[1 + \frac{f'(x)}{f(x)h(x)} \right] \quad \text{for } f(x) \neq 0. \tag{5.1}$$

If $f(x)$ has a modal value, say, $\tilde{x}$, then $f'(\tilde{x}) = 0$ and we obtain

$$h'(\tilde{x}) = h(\tilde{x})^2. \tag{5.2}$$

For the Gompertz distribution, $h'_G(x) = \theta \lambda e^{\theta x} = \theta h_G(x)$. Thus, we obtain

$$h'_G(\tilde{x}) = h_G(\tilde{x})^2 \Rightarrow \theta h_G(\tilde{x}) = h_G(\tilde{x})^2 \Rightarrow \theta = h_G(\tilde{x}). \tag{5.3}$$

This shows that θ is the hazard rate at the modal age of the distribution, which gives a tangible meaning to the Gompertz parameter, like the one for λ, which represents the hazard rate at age 0 or another arbitrary age taken as the lower endpoint of the distribution. Moreover, implicit in Gumbel (1958, pp. 118–123) is the fact that the ratio of the mode of the Gumbel-type distribution of the minimum to $F^{-1}(1/n)$ converges to 1 as n tends to infinity, where here F is an initial distribution in the minimum domain of attraction of the Gumbel-type distribution. That is, the mode of the Gumbel-type distribution of the minimum converges in ratio toward the $(1/n)$th quantile of the initial distribution. To obtain this result, it suffices to assume that (i) $f(x)$ increases in a right-neighborhood of 0 (taken without loss of generality as the lower endpoint of the distribution) and (ii) $\lim_{x \downarrow 0} [xf(x)/F(x)] > 0$ (i.e., that the limit exists and is not equal to 0, where the limit is allowed to be $+\infty$) (proof omitted).

In our application, to the extent that natural selection molds the distributions of the sufficient causes containing LOGE in the absence of EREF, it influences $F^{-1}(1/n)$ for each sufficient cause and indirectly the mode of the distribution of the minimum. Then, as θ is a parameter of the approximately Gompertz distribution of the minimum time to event of these sufficient causes and the hazard rate at the mode of the distribution, it ultimately reflects the molding of the initial distributions of the group of sufficient causes containing LOGE in the absence of EREF by the declining force of natural selection. This is consistent with the aforementioned idea by Carnes et al. (1996) of a "calibration" of the schedule of intrinsic mortality in a population to elements of the species' reproductive biology. In general, for a survival function $S(x)$, from $S(x) = 1 - F(x)$, we obtain $S'(x) = -f(x)$ and $S''(x) = -f'(x)$. It follows that

$$f'(\tilde{x}) = 0 \Rightarrow S''(\tilde{x}) = 0; \qquad (5.4)$$

that is, the mode of the distribution corresponds to the point of inflection of the survival function, indicating more concretely how such calibration may operate. (See also Appendix C for further details on the point of inflection of the Gompertz survival function.) Overall, according to this argument, since the evolutionary processes underlying the Gompertz parameter are relatively stable within a shorter nonevolutionary time scale, the Gompertz parameter could take the meaning of a species-specific "biological constant" with respect to aging.

5.2   AGE AS A RISK FACTOR FOR DISEASE

The statement that age is an (or the most) important risk factor for a disease is widespread with respect to several late-onset diseases of complex causation. Just as one relatively recent example of this conventional-wisdom view, Kirkwood (2008) stated, "Age is by far the biggest risk factor for a wide range of clinical conditions that are prevalent today." While the notion of "age as a risk factor" is generally accepted, Costa and McCrae (1980) noted: "on a little reflection, it becomes clear that chronological age is not in itself an explanatory variable, but rather a kind of index, backdrop, or dummy variable which is used to stand for the process or processes which causally underlie the universal, progressive and deleterious changes which we call aging." However, in an editorial titled "There is no such thing as aging," Peto and Doll (1997) questioned the usefulness for the study of causal disease mechanisms, in particular with respect to cancer, of the very notion of aging process: "Before asking whether 'aging itself' has any direct effects on the development of disease, it may be useful to consider whether there is any fundamental biological process that can usefully be labelled aging." In a letter, Powell (1998) objected to the editorial's apparently circular and merely semantic argument.[2] To which Doll and Peto (1998) replied: "Our claim is that there is no good reason to believe that...age related changes arise from a single common mechanism that could usefully be termed ageing—hence the title of our editorial." In this respect, Peto and Doll (1997) used reasoning consistent with the evolutionary theory of aging: "What the major diseases of adult life have shared for tens of millions of years is a common set of evolutionary pressures tending to relegate them to old age, but such relegation is likely to involve many different mechanisms."

The subtitle of Peto and Doll's (1997) editorial reads "Old age is associated with disease, but does not cause it"; hence, the provocative title also seems to reflect a more

---

[2] At the end of the letter, Powell (1998) disclosed, "Conflict of interest: I am aged."

general uneasiness with the notion of age as a risk factor for disease. If so, the rhetorical "There is no such thing as aging" is not in the least at odds with our work; in fact, it may be seen as a validation. In our causation model, there is no need to consider chronological age as a component cause because age's effect emerges from the time-to-event distributions of each and all component causes as combined in sufficient causes. Ultimately, then, age's effect emerges from the time-to-event distributions of the sufficient causes. Thus, from the perspective of our causation model, age is implicitly represented in all component causes rather than being a cause in itself, such that the "effect of age" on the development of disease becomes a property of the time-to-event distributions of the sufficient causes. (A similar reasoning within our causation model could be applied to the commonsense idea that age is a risk factor for death.)

The way age's effect emerges in our causation model is compatible with Korn et al.'s (1997) argument for using age instead of follow-up time (time-on-study) as the time scale in the analysis of time-to-event data. These authors refer in particular to longitudinal studies following individuals sampled in a large-scale health survey for the development of diseases or death, analyzed using Cox proportional hazards models. For other studies such as randomized clinical trials and natural history studies, time-on-study (time since randomization and time since diagnosis/symptom onset or baseline evaluation, respectively) is typically used as the time scale in time-to-event analyses. In those contexts, age is often included as an independent variable in regression models such as the Cox model; that is, age is treated as a risk factor but mostly for the purposes of adjustment or prediction. For example, one of us (G.L.) is "guilty" of extensively treating age as a risk factor in the course of conducting research on the clinical progression and development of dementia in Parkinson's disease (Levy, 2007; Levy et al., 2000, 2002, 2005).

Although our causation model rejects the widespread notion of age as a risk factor, which in the first place is only vaguely understood, the index of aging-relatedness offers a replacement that can be interpreted in more concrete terms. Counter to Korn et al.'s (1997) argument, if we consider the common use of the Cox proportional hazards model with follow-up time as the time scale in the analysis of studies following individuals for the development of disease, a significant association between age at start of follow-up and disease simply implies an increasing hazard rate of the disease with increasing age. It does not imply any particular form for the increasing hazard rate, since no parametric family of probability distributions is assumed for the survival times, and while the model is based on the assumption of proportional hazards, no particular form is assumed for the baseline hazard function. Thus, the strength and statistical significance of the Cox regression coefficient for age in relation to a specific disease do not give information about the particular form of the increasing hazard rate with age. In our mixture statistical model, the mixture parameter π is attached to a distribution characterized by an exponentially increasing hazard function (as opposed to a distribution with power hazard function), and the index of aging-relatedness thus gives quantitative information with respect to such exponential increase. In this sense, the notion of aging-relatedness as applied to complex diseases is more restrictive than the notion of age as a risk factor.

5.3   ARE AGING-RELATED DISEASES AN INTEGRAL PART OF AGING?

In the appendix of an essay on "the aging-disease dichotomy," Blumenthal (2003) listed 29 quotes of authors expressing a diversity of opinions classified according whether they were in accord with, or in opposition to (or ambiguous about), an aging-disease dichotomy. A reading of these quotes clearly shows that the question in this section's title has been addressed from multiple perspectives and using quite varied reasons. We only mean to narrowly address this question here from one specific perspective. A common meaning of "aging-related diseases being an integral part of aging" in the gerontology literature is that aging-related diseases are caused by the physiological aging process or that aging-related diseases and aging share proximate mechanisms, along the lines of Ritchie and Kildea's (1995) definition of "ageing-related disorder" and Brody and Schneider's (1986) definition of "age-dependent diseases" (reviewed in Chapter 1). In this sense, the following two authors argued, even if indirectly, that aging and aging-related diseases are separate entities. Mann (1997) described the following reasoning as fallacious: "Common disorders such as cardiovascular disease, cancer, stroke, dementia, and diabetes become increasingly prevalent in later life. It is tempting to ascribe these to the body 'wearing out'—a viewpoint supported by the frequent finding in many old, but otherwise healthy, people of low levels of the same kind of tissue changes generally associated with certain diseases when present in higher amounts. These diseases have been popularly equated with 'normal aging,' and the idea that in diseased individuals this normal process of aging may have become 'exaggerated' or have 'accelerated' out of control has often been put forward."[3] Hayflick (2000) argued that "Ageing is not a disease and the distinction is central to an understanding of why the resolution of the leading causes of death in old age—cardiovascular disease, stroke and cancer—will tell us little about the fundamental biology of age changes."

However, even those who subscribe to the view that aging and aging-related diseases are separate entities often admit to a relation between the two, in which the aging process acts as a sort of active backdrop on which aging-related diseases develop. For instance, as put by Mann (1997), "disease in old age may represent an additional burden of tissue damage superimposed on other ongoing alterations common perhaps to all cell types in the body and applicable, to a greater or lesser extent, to all individuals. These basic changes set the stage on which the disorders of old age can be played out."[4] Hayflick (2004), in a debate with Holliday (2004a) about how close the "relationship between biological aging and age-associated pathologies in humans" is, conceded: "There is no denying a close relationship between the aging process and age-associated diseases. ...I believe that the two phenomena are distinct in that an advancing aging process simply increases vulnerability to age-associated diseases or to pathology." Holliday's (2004b) response seems to suggest that the views of these

---

[3] Reproduced from *British Medical Journal*, **315**, Mann, D. M., Molecular biology's impact on our understanding of aging, pages 1078–1081, Copyright 1997, with permission from BMJ Publishing Group Ltd.
[4] Idem.

two authors are actually not far from each other: "I would argue that increased vulnerability is simply that a given amount of damage or disorder has accumulated throughout adult life, and therefore an additional increment may precipitate disease late in life." Still, Holliday's (2004a) view does differ from those of Hayflick (2004) and Mann (1997) in that he believes that "The distinction between age-related changes that are not pathological and those that are pathological is not at all fundamental."

As contrasted with the opposing views in the preceding text, which are mostly concerned with pathological tissue changes but indirectly refer to the underlying proximate mechanisms, in Masoro's (2006) review titled "Are age-associated diseases an integral part of aging?," the argument is rooted in evolutionary reasoning: "The most compelling reason to consider age-associated diseases as an integral part of aging comes from our understanding of the evolutionary basis of aging. Specifically, aging is believed to occur because of a progressive age-associated decrease in the force of natural selection; thus, deleterious traits expressed only at advanced ages do not tend to be eliminated by natural selection. Because age-associated diseases do not exhibit deleterious consequences until advanced ages, even if they begin at an early age, current views of the evolutionary basis of aging lead to the conclusion that such diseases are exactly what one would predict to be an integral part of aging." Yet Masoro (2006) is also suggesting that because the evolutionary explanations of aging and aging-related diseases are the same, the proximate mechanisms of both processes are likely to be shared. This is reinforced by his account of specific biochemical mechanisms in common between each of two "age-associated disease processes" (atherosclerosis and neoplasia) and the aging process.

Our causation model and the index of aging-relatedness are based on the notion (as discussed toward the end of Section 2.2) that aging and aging-related diseases result from the same general evolutionary process, that is, the attenuation of natural selection at later ages. However, this does not necessarily imply that they share proximate mechanisms. From this perspective, while some mechanisms may be shared between aging and aging-related diseases, as well as among different aging-related diseases, aging-related diseases are not an integral part of aging in the sense of *necessarily or completely* sharing proximate mechanisms.

5.4   BIOLOGICAL VERSUS CHRONOLOGICAL AGING

The distinction between biological and chronological age is an important theme in gerontology. Other synonymous terms for *biological age* in gerontology are *functional age* and *physiological age*. The term *functional age* was introduced in the 1950s and came to be used interchangeably with *biological age* later on (Costa and McCrae, 1980). *Chronological age* is simply "a record of time elapsed since birth" (Ries and Pöthig, 1984). While no uniform or generally accepted definition of biological age can be found in the gerontological literature, Ries and Pöthig (1984) offered the following definition: "Biological age is a term used to describe the general condition of an individual at a certain time of his chronological age, which is marked by orthological ['normal'] and pathological characteristics." According to Karasik et al. (2004), "Biological age estimates the functional status of an individual in reference to his or her chronological age." The concept of biological aging underlying these and other definitions was described by Costa and McCrae (1980) as follows: "The concept of functional age which has been developed has been alternatively phrased, but seems to rest primarily on the notion of differential rates of aging in individuals. Building on the appealing commonsense idea that some people 'burn themselves out' rapidly while others are 'well preserved,' and on the observation of individual differences in longevity, this formulation has postulated that the variation of performance around a cohort mean is due to the different rates of aging of individuals. At any given point in time, those who age rapidly will be closer to death than those who age slowly, and they will, on the average, perform less well on age-related measures of functioning. These rapidly aging individuals will be 'functionally old' in comparison with their chronological age peers."

In gerontological research, the distinction between biological and chronological age has entailed the search for "biomarkers of aging," with the purpose of measuring biological age and ultimately assessing interventions that may retard the aging process. As defined by Baker and Sprott (1988), "A biomarker of aging is a biological parameter of an organism that either alone or in some multivariate composite will, in the absence of disease, better predict functional capability at some late age than will chronological age." Most proposed measures of biological age involve batteries of tests, encompassing a large number of biochemical, physical, mental, and functional parameters; regression analysis of several such biomarkers has traditionally been used to obtain a measure of an individual's functioning relative to an individual's chronological peers (Karasik et al., 2004). Costa and McCrae (1980) listed the following variables used for functional age prediction in four different studies: grayness of hair, expected age of retirement, hearing loss, visual acuity, hemoglobin concentration, plasma urea nitrogen, plasma cholesterol, forced expiratory volume, systolic blood pressure, resting ECG, grasping power, tapping rate, hand dynamometry, reaction time, etc. Still, despite a call by the World Health Organization dating back to 1963 "to find suitable methods of determining the biological age in man" (Ries and Pöthig, 1984) and a concerted initiative by the U.S. National Institute on Aging (Baker and Sprott, 1988), the search for biomarkers of aging has not overall been successful. According to Warner (2004), "so far, a definitive panel of biomarkers to predict mortality risk has not been obtained, even though many traits that vary with age have been identified."

At the same time that efforts to identify measures of biological age have proceeded, some have questioned the methods of this research effort and the very concept of biological aging. In addition to empirical issues, Costa and McCrae (1980) questioned what they considered one of the central tenets of biological age, namely, that individuals have characteristic rates of aging that can be measured in a number of different domains or systems. The supposed effects of their critique on research prompted a defense of the concept of biological aging by Dean and Morgan (1988) (response in Costa and McCrae (1988)). Adelman (1980, 1987) also put into question the existence of a consensus regarding the meaning of biological aging in gerontology and the ultimate significance of research related to the identification of biomarkers of aging. A more recent balanced defense of the effort to identify biomarkers of aging is given in Miller (2001). He clearly identifies "the objection that biomarkers cannot measure aging because there is no such thing as aging," meaning that "there is no core process for which a biomarker can serve as a surrogate." That is, many researchers "view aging as a more-or-less parallel progression of multiple degenerative processes, some of which lead to cancer, others to alterations of connective tissue, still others to neu-rodegeneration, and yet others to muscle wasting. From this viewpoint, processes of this sort could potentially exert overlapping effects on several cell types and organ systems, but none of them serves as a 'master clock' that synchronizes these delete-rious changes." While Miller (2001) enlists himself among those who do believe that there is a core process that justifies the continued effort to find biomarkers of aging, he admits, "The discipline of gerontobiomarkerology [sic] faces a long uphill climb, with too little to show, so far, for the many miles behind us."

Our index of aging-relatedness estimated from intrinsic mortality data can be thought of as *a measure of biological aging at the population level*. In this case, pop-ulation biological aging would be formulated in terms of an exponential increase in age-specific mortality rates. Population biological aging is not only a more restrictive notion than chronological aging or the "mere passage of time" for the population, but there is an intermediate layer between population biological and chronological aging given by the reliability notion of aging (Barlow and Proschan, 1981, pp. 53–56). The reliability notion of aging is defined by increasing age-specific mortality (or failure or hazard) rates; it excludes mortality rates that are constant (i.e., the exponential survival distribution) or decreasing with increasing age. In the reliability literature, a failure rate function that is initially decreasing, then constant, and then increasing with increasing age is said to have a "bathtub shape." The increasing failure rate phase in the bathtub-shaped failure rate function is called "wearout" (Barlow and Proschan, 1981, pp. 55–56). Thus, we also refer here to the reliability notion of aging as wearout. While wearout excludes population chronological aging characterized by nonincreas-ing age-specific mortality rates, our formulation of population biological aging excludes wearout characterized by mortality rates increasing as a power function of age. This is schematically represented in Figure 5.1.

The following are remarks about our formulation of population biological aging. First, given the role played by the extreme dependence of human offspring in the evo-lutionary rationale for our causation model, our formulation of population biological aging applies to humans and other social species that show a similar dependence of their offspring. Second, although the gerontological concept of biological aging is at the level of the individual, in terms of functional or physiological status, and our for-mulation of biological aging is at the population level, the term *biological aging* is appropriate for our formulation in a way that it is not for the gerontological concept of biological aging. Given the evolutionary rationale for our causation model and the interpretation of the index of aging-relatedness in terms of genetic contribution to mortality, our formulation is fundamentally at the level of evolutionary biology and genetics. The central role of functional and physiological status in the gerontology context would make the use of the terms *functional age* or *physiological age* more

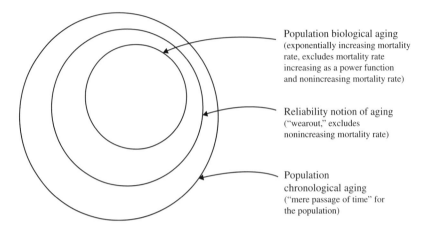

FIGURE 5.1 Population biological aging in relation to the reliability notion of aging and population chronological aging. The use of a Venn diagram to represent population biological aging as a distinct subset of the reliability notion of aging or wearout, which in turn is a subset of chronological aging in the population, serves the purpose of illustrating that each is a more restrictive notion (i.e., the "points" or elements of the sets are conceptual).

appropriate than *biological age*. Indeed, several authors have preferred to use these terms (Baker and Sprott, 1988; Costa and McCrae, 1980; Graham et al., 1999). Third, in the context of the concept of biological aging in gerontology, biological age has been used as an alternative phenotype to survival measures for estimating the heritability of aging (Karasik et al., 2005). For instance, Karasik et al. (2004), using data from the Framingham Study and a measure of biological age based only on an osseographic score applied to hand radiographs (instead of the more usual comprehensive battery of tests), obtained an estimate of heritability of 57%. If we think of the index of aging-relatedness as a measure of biological aging at the population level, the question about genetic versus environmental contributions to biological aging is moot. That is, biological aging in our formulation is by definition genetic in the sense of related to sufficient causes containing LOGE in the absence of EREF, and the index of aging-relatedness may be said to represent the contribution of biological aging to the overall (genetic and nongenetic) aging in the population.

5.5   THE PUBLIC HEALTH NOTION OF COMPRESSION OF MORBIDITY

In 1980, Fries proposed the notion of *compression of morbidity*, with public health and health policy implications. This notion involved predictions that the average period of diminished physical vigor among older persons would decrease, that chronic disease would occupy a smaller proportion of the life span, and that the need for medical care in later life would decrease. Fries (1980) considered that survival curves for the U.S. population had assumed an ever more rectangular form during the twentieth century, as a result of improvements in general living conditions, diet, sanitation, and control of infectious disease. At the same time, the average length of life increased, and chronic disease superseded acute disease as the predominant set of medical problems in the United States. A first premise of Fries' (1980) predictions was that the rectangularization of the survival curve would continue together with the continued elimination of "premature deaths," and this would result in a *compression of mortality*: "The serial data allow calculation of the position and shape of a survival curve if all premature death were eliminated: an ideally 'rectangular' survival curve." However, as pointed out by Schneider and Brody (1983), Fries (1980) took this argument to an extreme by assuming that there was a biological limit to life span ("the length of life is fixed"), based on the limited *in vitro* replicative ability of cultured human cells (the so-called Hayflick limit) and on actuarial observations.

A second premise of Fries' (1980) predictions was that there would be a postponement of the onset of chronic diseases through preventive approaches such as smoking cessation and lifestyle changes. It would follow that "The amount of disability can decrease as morbidity is compressed into the shorter span between the increasing age at onset of disability and the fixed occurrence of death. The end of the period of adult vigor will come later than it used to. Postponement of chronic illness thus results in rectangularization not only of the mortality curve but also of the morbidity curve." However, this quote does not clearly distinguish between morbidity and disability; disability resulting from morbidity depends not only on the onset of chronic diseases but also on their progression, severity, duration, and impact on functional status. As parenthetically stated by Verbrugge (1991), "It should be noted that the compression of disability is really a separate concept from compression of morbidity, although it is seldom distinguished." Two alternative views concerning trends in the relations among morbidity, disability, and mortality have been formulated (Robine and Michel, 2004; Tu and Chen, 1994). One view has been called the "expansion of morbidity hypothesis" (Olshansky et al., 1991) and originated in Gruenberg (1977) and Kramer (1980); it postulates that improvements in survival in recent years have occurred by increasing the duration of time that members of the population survive with a disease or disability, so that they are spending the additional years in poor health. The other view, called "dynamic equilibrium," proposes that an increased prevalence of chronic diseases has been counterbalanced by a decrease in the severity of the same diseases, a scenario that falls between the compression and expansion of morbidity scenarios (Manton, 1982).

The debate in the specialized literature about Fries' (1980) notion of compression of morbidity included Brody's (1985) commentary subtitled "The ageing populations of industrialized societies are more likely to be encumbered by increasing morbidity than some optimistic arguments would suggest." Some empirical evidence supports this view. For instance, McKinlay et al. (1989) found that morbidity was not declining in the United States during the twentieth century in a manner congruent with mortality and was actually increasing for some subgroups. They also found evidence that although overall life expectancy had increased over several decades, most of this increase was in years of disability. Crimmins et al. (1989) compared changes in total life expectancy to changes in disability-free life expectancy between 1970 and 1980 in the United States. They concluded that mortality had declined remarkably, but the direction of changes in disability rates and thus disability-free life expectancy was less clear. In answering their main question, "Are Americans living longer healthy lives as well as longer lives?", they reasoned: "If the definition [of health] includes an ability to participate fully in the normal activities of everyday life, the answer is that Americans are not living longer healthy lives. Additions to life expectancy between 1970 and 1980 were concentrated in the disabled years—primarily years of long-term disability. On the other hand, if we limit our definition of ill health to days spent in bed, we conclude that, below age 85, most of the increase in life expectancy has been in nondisabled years, not years spent in bed."[5]

Olshansky et al. (1991) postulated two mechanisms for explaining why declining mortality can lead to worsening health, based on a distinction between two groups of "diseases of old age": "fatal diseases," from which most people die (e.g., heart disease, stroke, and cancer), and "nonfatal diseases," which are responsible for a substantial portion of all disability (e.g., arthritis, dementia, sensory impairments, and osteoporosis). The first postulated mechanism is related to the development of new medical technologies, which have led to improvements in the medical management of the complications associated with fatal diseases and have permitted longer survival with the disability than was the case for previous cohorts. The second mechanism involves the declining mortality from fatal diseases in the population leading to a shift in the distribution of causes of disability from fatal to nonfatal diseases of aging, which would entail longer periods of disability.

Verbrugge (1991) discussed the relations among morbidity, disability, and mortality based on three scenarios defined in terms of where prevention efforts for chronic conditions are directed. In the description of these scenarios here, mortality, disability, and morbidity curves refer to the plots of the survival function for the respective outcomes of death, disability, and diseases; a curve is said to move or shift "outward" in the sense of the plot of the survival function moving higher and toward the right as a result of lower mortality or incidence rates. In the scenario of tertiary prevention —"saving people at the brink of death by costly medical measures that (a) maintain basic life processes (this is called heroic care) or (b) cure or avert fatal complications of certain diseases"— the mortality curve moves outward just a little, because relatively few people in the population are benefited, without any change in the disability and morbidity curves. Secondary prevention refers to "controlling chronic diseases so that they advance less rapidly," which comes about "(a) by more efficacious treatment procedures at any or all disease stages and (b) by earlier diagnosis of disease and thus earlier initiation of treatment." It can potentially benefit many people and thus have a large impact on shifting the mortality curve outward, but the effect on the morbidity and disability curves is uncertain due to possible opposing forces. The author contended that secondary prevention had dominated the "past several decades" of the prevention

---

[5] Reproduced from *Population and Development Review*, **15**, Crimmins, E. M., Saito, Y., and Ingegneri, D., Changes in life expectancy and disability-free life expectancy in the United States, pages 235–267, Copyright 1989, with permission from Wiley.

efforts for chronic conditions, accounting for the observed rise in morbidity and disability combined with declines in mortality rates at older ages.

Lastly, under the scenario of primary prevention —"keeping people free of a disease (a) for their entire lifetimes by disease eradication or (b) until late in life by delayed onset"— all three survival curves shift outward, resulting in more years free of morbidity, disability, and death. According to Verbrugge (1991), the notion of compression of morbidity is but one version of this scenario, premised on morbidity gains exceeding mortality gains, such that the area between the morbidity and mortality curves is "compressed" over time. He also argued that the notion of an intrinsic limit to life expectancy, resulting from Fries' (1980) assumption of a biological limit to life span, was not a necessary prerequisite for compression of morbidity, yet compression of morbidity was not "near at hand": "The ultimate scenario he [Fries (1980)] describes is possible only if we know disease risk factors thoroughly and convince people to avoid such risks throughout their lives; that is a tall order." While the three aforementioned scenarios of tertiary, secondary, and primary prevention are not mutually exclusive, in the next section we will discuss the potential population health benefits in the twenty-first century from a prevention effort directed at primary prevention, with a view to approaching such an admittedly "tall order."

Toward that end, our mixture statistical model and its interpretation on evolutionary grounds provides a new way of thinking about the notions of compression of morbidity and mortality. Even if we do not share Fries' (1980) assumption of a fixed limit to life span, we consider that the Gompertz component of the mixture model fitted to intrinsic mortality data can be seen as a benchmark of the biological aging process (from the approximate end of prepubertal development in human ancestors at age 10 years to the supposed onset of late life at about 90 years), along the lines of the meaning of the Gompertz parameter as a "biological constant" with respect to aging discussed in Section 5.1. Then, the estimated Gompertz component of the mixture distribution may be viewed as a target of rectangularization of the mortality curve (wherein all deaths are caused by sufficient causes containing LOGE in the absence of EREF), achieved through the elimination of premature deaths (i.e., deaths caused by sufficient causes containing EREF). This is illustrated in Figure 5.2, which shows plots of the survival function of the Gompertz and Weibull components of the fitted mixture distribution and the survival function of the mixture distribution, for our analysis of intrinsic mortality overall and in never and ever smokers. In these plots, the potential (theoretical) compression of mortality that could be achieved between ages 10 and 90 years in this population is represented by the area between the gray and solid black lines, corresponding, respectively, to the fitted mixture distribution and the Gompertz component. As one would expect, the potential compression of mortality that could be achieved for ever smokers (lower right panel) is quite a bit larger than that for never smokers (lower left panel). We also note that the Gompertz component appears to remain approximately fixed when we compare never to ever smokers; it is the mixture survival function and the Weibull component that appear to move the most. The same can be observed for the corresponding density functions in Figure 4.10 (lower panels).

By examining the plots of the survival function for the analysis of intrinsic mortality overall (Fig. 5.2, upper panel), we notice that a visible decline in the survival

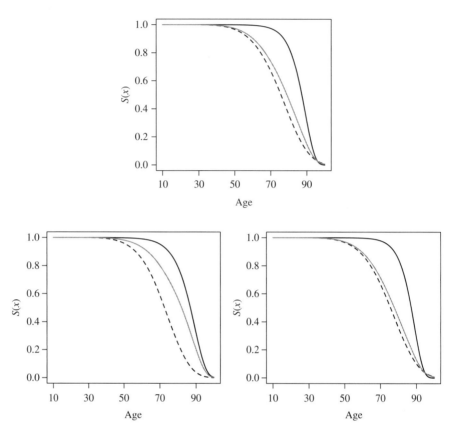

FIGURE 5.2 Plots of the survival function of the Gompertz (solid black line) and Weibull (dashed black line) components of the mixture distribution and the survival function of the mixture distribution (gray line), for the analysis of intrinsic mortality overall (upper) and in never (lower left panel) and ever (lower right panel) smokers.

function starts at about age 40 years for the fitted mixture distribution and at about age 65 years for the Gompertz component. At age 85 years, approximately 25% and 50% of the population is alive according to the mixture distribution and the Gompertz component, respectively. Overall, the survival function for the Gompertz component does not decline much up to about age 75 years and then shows a steep decline between ages 75 and 90 years, approaching a rectangular form. (Given the very wide CIs for the parameters of the mixture model in our analysis, this can only be taken as a rough numerical suggestion.) In relation to this steep decline, the corresponding plots in Figure 4.10 (upper panel) show that the density of the Gompertz component is more peaked than, and to the right of, the density of the Weibull component. This supports our reasoning earlier regarding premature deaths. More broadly, since there is no constraint to that effect in our survival mixture model, this serves as an indirect piece of evidence in favor of the evolutionary rationale for our model of causation.

For the analysis of disease incidence, rectangularization of the morbidity curve can similarly be thought of in terms of moving the survival function of the mixture model in the direction of the Gompertz component. Unlike compression of mortality, compression of morbidity can be gauged from the area between the morbidity and mortality curves based on the mixture model, and the theoretical limit of the attainable compression of morbidity on evolutionary grounds would be the area between the rectangularized (i.e., Gompertz component of the mixture model) morbidity and mortality curves. In principle, the mixture model can also be applied to a disability outcome in order to obtain disability-free survival functions, and the same reasoning can be extended to compression of disability: rectangularization of the disability curve can be thought of in terms of moving the survival function of the mixture model in the direction of the Gompertz component; compression of disability can be gauged from the area between the disability and mortality curves; and the theoretical limit of the attainable compression of disability is the area between the rectangularized disability and mortality curves.

5.6   A PICTURE OF AGING FOR THE TWENTY-FIRST CENTURY

Omran (1971) conceived a theory of the epidemiology of population change ("the epidemiologic transition") relevant to the process of modernization culminating in the twentieth century: "An epidemiologic transition has paralleled the demographic and technologic transitions in the now developed countries of the world and is still underway in less-developed societies. Ample evidence may be cited to document this transition in which degenerative and man-made diseases displace pandemics of infection as the primary causes of morbidity and mortality."[6] The theory contemplates three stages, characterized as follows: in The Age of Pestilence and Famine, which "represents for all practical purposes an extension of the pre-modern pattern of health and disease," mortality is high and fluctuating, precluding sustained population growth; leading causes of death are "the epidemic scourges, endemic, parasitic and deficiency diseases, pneumonia-diarrhea-malnutrition complex in children, and tuberculosis-puerperal-malnutrition complex in females"; and life expectancy at birth varies between 20 and 40 years. In The Age of Receding Pandemics, mortality declines progressively, mostly through improvements in sanitation and standards of living but also due to medical and public health measures (e.g., immunization and development of new therapies); population growth becomes sustained; and life expectancy increases to about 50 years. In The Age of Degenerative and Man-Made Diseases, mortality approaches stability at a relatively low level; chronic degenerative diseases such as heart disease, cancer, and stroke replace infection as the major killers; and life expectancy exceeds 50 years. Figure 5.3 shows semilog mortality plots by age at different levels of life expectancy, as presented by Omran (1971). By examining these plots, we

[6] Reproduced from *The Milbank Memorial Fund Quarterly*, **49**, Omran, A. R., The epidemiologic transition: A theory of the epidemiology of population change, pages 509–538, Copyright 1971, with permission from Wiley.

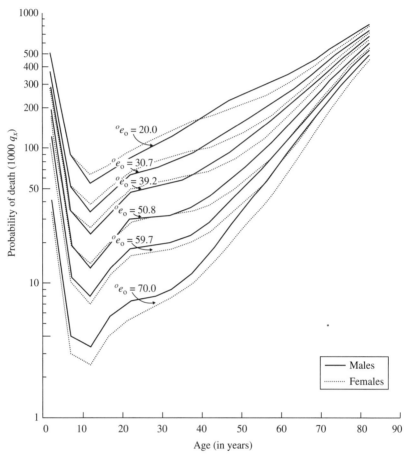

FIGURE 5.3 Semilog plots of mortality rates by age and sex and at different levels of life expectancy at birth (reproduced from *The Milbank Memorial Fund Quarterly*, **49**, Omran, A. R., The epidemiologic transition: A theory of the epidemiology of population change, pages 509–538, Copyright 1971, with permission from Wiley).

can see that the increase in life expectancy described by the epidemiologic transition, apart from relying heavily on a decrease in infantile and childhood mortality, can be pictured as a decreasing value of the Makeham parameter in the Gompertz–Makeham equation (see Fig. 2.12), pointing to the additional importance of the receding extrinsic causes of death at older ages, especially in young adults.

The increase in life expectancy during the epidemiologic transition is commensurate with degenerative diseases killing at older ages than infectious diseases do, thus causing a redistribution of deaths from the young to the old. Building on Omran's (1971) theory, Olshansky and Ault (1986) described a fourth stage of the epidemiologic transition, in which "the major degenerative causes of death that prevailed during the third stage of the transition remain with us as the major killers, but the risk of dying from these diseases is redistributed to older ages." Since this stage is characterized mostly by a substitution of the ages at which the major determinants of death tend to kill, the authors refer to it as The Age of Delayed Degenerative Diseases. (Equivalently, one might characterize this stage as a gradual replacement of heart disease, cancer, and stroke with later-onset neurodegenerative diseases such as Alzheimer's disease as causes of death.) The authors identified several factors that contributed to this "new era in our epidemiologic history," starting with the mortality transition that occurred during The Age of Receding Pandemics and the accompanying change in the age structure of the population: "This fundamental change in the age structure, with rapidly increasing proportions of successive birth cohorts surviving into advanced ages, literally created an entirely new segment of the population with unique health care needs and demands that were tied to chronic degenerative diseases and age-associated physiological impairments." Other contributing factors include advances in medical technology and reductions in some major risk factors for degenerative diseases, such as "declines in smoking, more exercise, and improved dietary habits." Based on U.S. data from the twentieth century, Olshansky and Ault (1986) projected that, while life expectancy at birth reached approximately 70 years of age in the third stage of the epidemiologic transition, The Age of Delayed Degenerative Diseases would propel life expectancy "into and perhaps beyond eight decades."

Our work provides a new prism through which one can see the mechanics and potential for better health in the current era. It starts with the proposition that the modern social and economic forces that improved population health and drove the major gains in life expectancy in the twentieth century also had negative effects, in the form of environmental factors brought about by industrialization and changes in lifestyle. Omran (1971) hinted at one aspect of this trade-off by noting that in The Age of Degenerative and Man-Made Diseases, "People become extremely conscious of nutrition, especially that of children and mothers. There is, however, a tendency to overnutrition including consumption of rich and high-fat foods which may increase the risk of heart and metabolic diseases." These unanticipated adverse effects of modernization do not nullify the prodigious health benefits that were obtained, but arguably point the way ahead. Consistent with the notion of "delaying degenerative diseases," our causation model implies that by identifying and acting on those environmental factors that we characterized as evolutionarily recent, we may delay disease onset and prevent premature deaths. On the other hand, this also implies that calling the current era The Age of Delayed Degenerative Diseases is, in a sense, misleading. Under the surface of the major gains in life expectancy due to a reduction in extrinsic causes of death, environmental factors introduced by industrialization and the modern lifestyle entailed an earlier age-of-onset distribution of the main present causes of death, compared to what it would have been in the absence of such environmental factors. This intimates a scenario—in which the age of onset of chronic diseases is solely the result of late age-specific genetic effects—that has never been evident because it has always been hidden by the predominance of extrinsic causes of death. Thus, progress in the current era can actually be seen as restoring the age-of-onset distribution of degenerative diseases to its previously undisclosed evolutionary benchmark.

While the transition described by Omran (1971) involved shifting deaths "from the young to the old" through a wide age range, thus affording a large impact on life expectancy, the transition in The Age of Delayed Degenerative Diseases involves shifting deaths within the older ages, with a much smaller impact on the number of years of life gained for each individual. Thus, the returns of improving population health in the current stage in terms of gains in life expectancy are much more limited. Such situation was described by Keyfitz (1978) as a predicament underlying "the slow health progress of recent years despite ever increasing numbers of medical personnel, better equipped hospitals, and larger expenditures on research." Using cancer deaths as an example, he noted that even if a general cure for cancer were discovered, the impact on life expectancy would be relatively small because most of the cases of cured cancer would be among older people (i.e., at the ages at which cancer predominantly occurs), who were prone to succumb to other causes of death in the short run, especially "the cardiovascular renal group." He then remarked: "Since 1900, the expectation of life at birth has risen 25 years, due mostly to the virtual elimination of acute infectious diseases. … We cannot expect the large payoff in life expectancy from advances against cancer that followed the conquest of diphtheria and tuberculosis."

Despite these low expectations, our analysis of intrinsic mortality data from Israeli males spanning the second half of the twentieth century and beginning of the twenty-first century suggests a brighter outlook in terms of potential life expectancy gains. The life expectancy at age 10 years obtained from the mixture model is 67.3 years, and the life expectancy at 10 years based on the Gompertz component of the mixture model is 76.1 years. Thus, if as discussed in the previous section the Gompertz component represents the counterfactual situation achieved through the elimination of premature deaths (i.e., deaths caused by sufficient causes containing EREF), measures to control environmental factors brought about by industrialization and relatively recent changes in lifestyle would potentially increase the life expectancy at 10 years by 8.8 years. However, note that these results can only be taken at face value as a representation of the *intrinsic mortality experience* of the population (or in the hypothetical scenario in which extrinsic causes of death have been completely eliminated). By excluding extrinsic mortality, which tends to occur predominantly in early adult life, the analysis overestimates life expectancies with respect to the total mortality experience of the population. Moreover, not only is eliminating all EREF possibly unachievable, but people who give up one unhealthy lifestyle choice may substitute another one for it, such that the life expectancy gains in the preceding text represent an upper bound. We must also keep in mind the very wide CIs for the mixture model parameters, based on whose estimates the aforementioned calculations of life expectancies were made.

However, perhaps a more appropriate gauge of the improving population health would nowadays be the absolute and relative number of prevented premature deaths. In fact, Olshansky et al. (2001) asserted that "the measure of life expectancy is no longer a reliable barometer of the health of a nation." Based on the estimated index of aging-relatedness in our analysis, the relative number of premature deaths that might be prevented is as high as 77% in the whole population, 85% in ever smokers, and 42% in never smokers (but we warn again against putting too much weight on these results due to the lack of precision of the parameter estimates). To estimate the number of preventable or premature deaths in the United States, Danaei et al. (2009) conducted a population-level comparative risk assessment for 12 risk factors including smoking, overweight–obesity, physical inactivity, and dietary factors. For each risk factor and each disease associated with it, they calculated the proportional reduction in disease-specific deaths that would occur if risk factor exposure were eliminated or reduced to an alternative level (i.e., the population attributable fraction), based on the best available evidence regarding the population distribution of risk factor exposure, the effect of risk factor exposures on disease-specific mortality, and the total number of disease-specific deaths in the population. They found that of the close to 2.5 million deaths in the United States in 2005 (four most common underlying causes: ischemic heart disease, lung cancer, stroke, and chronic obstructive pulmonary disease), smoking was responsible for nearly half a million deaths (20%), overweight–obesity and physical inactivity for approximately 200,000 (8%) each, and individual dietary factors for about 100,000 (4%) each or less. However, they cautioned that the combined attributable fraction of the examined risk factors could not be obtained by simply summing these proportions, because they may act together in causing disease-specific deaths or the effect of one risk factor may be mediated though another. Still, these findings suggest that interventions on known modifiable risk factors could avert a large number of premature deaths in the United States.

From this perspective, a positive development in population health would be characterized by an increasing index of aging-relatedness achieved through the prevention of premature deaths. At the end of Chapter 4, we considered that estimating the index of aging-relatedness across geographical areas or across time in the same area might provide useful or interesting information. With respect to the analysis across time in countries that underwent early industrialization starting in the eighteenth or nineteenth century, we can advance the following predictions. First, we would expect that the index of aging-relatedness for intrinsic mortality decreased during the nineteenth and first half of the twentieth century, due to new exposures to synthetic chemicals and industrial toxins, changes in diet, and other lifestyle factors. Second, in those countries undergoing major antitabagism campaigns during the second half of the twentieth century, we would expect a reversal of that trend, with a stable and then increasing index of aging-relatedness. This can be indirectly envisaged by the estimated index of aging-relatedness in our analysis being 0.15 for ever smokers and 0.58 for never smokers. Third, we might expect a negative reversal with a decreasing index of aging-relatedness more recently due to a stagnation of the tobacco smoking decline and an increase in overweight–obesity. Yet a positive development might ensue with renewed efforts aimed at environmental control.

The progress in preventing premature deaths would likely also improve functional performance in the aging population, by inherently delaying aging phenotypes that have an impact on quality as well as quantity of life. That is, one would "add life to the years" at the same time that one would add years to life, along the lines of the notion of "successful aging" (Havighurst, 1961). Bearing on the distinction between "usual" and successful aging among nondiseased elderly, Rowe and Kahn (1987) argued that the observed heterogeneity within normal or healthy (i.e., nondiseased) aging with respect to physiological and cognitive characteristics can be largely explained by the so-called extrinsic factors: "the modifying effects of diet, exercise, personal habits, and psychosocial factors." It follows that "To the extent that maintenance and recovery of function can be explained in terms of extrinsic factors, it becomes reasonable to think of increasing the proportion of the successful elderly." In support of this, in a cohort of adults aged 36–64 years who completed a follow-up questionnaire when they were 65 years and older (average follow-up of 26 years), a higher body mass index in middle age was associated with a poorer health-related quality of life (an individual's physical, mental, and social well-being) in older age (Daviglus et al., 2003). In a British civil service-based cohort study, participants free of major disease at baseline were followed for 17 years to assess successful aging, defined as being free of major disease and in the top tertile of physical and cognitive functioning. In addition to early life factors, socioeconomic position, and psychosocial factors, midlife health behaviors including smoking, diet, and physical activity were associated with successful aging; the overall effect of midlife health behaviors was stronger than the effects of early life and psychosocial factors (Britton et al., 2008).[7]

Such an ultimate goal—of allowing each member of the population to "live life to the fullest" (meaning for us "to the limits established by the evolutionary process") in both a quantitative and qualitative dimension—provides a reasonable and achievable directive for public health in the twenty-first century. Since the prevention of premature deaths would bring the survival experience of the population closer to the Gompertz component of our mixture model, the index of aging-relatedness applied to intrinsic mortality data is the measure par excellence of the quantitative dimension of this public health directive. Thus, just as a decreasing Makeham parameter in a Gompertz–Makeham model partly expresses the major gains in life expectancy in the twentieth century, an increasing index of aging-relatedness in our mixture model provides a hopeful picture of aging for the twenty-first century. In semilog plots of mortality rates by age, this would be visualized as curves that straighten up as they fall successively beneath each other, by virtue of decreasing mortality rates along a wide range of adult ages. This is shown in Figure 5.4 using parameter estimates from our data analysis (Section 4.5). The qualitative dimension of this public health directive, which can also be expressed as an increase in health span (as opposed to life span) or "the maintenance of full function as nearly as possible to the end of life" (Rowe and Kahn, 1987), might be assessed by the index of aging-relatedness applied to a low-threshold

---

[7] Perhaps surprisingly, the pioneer of the evolutionary theory of aging also has something relevant to say here. In an article titled "The future of life expectancy," Medawar (1985) stated: "no one entertains the ambition to populate the world with decrepit old dotards: what is hoped for is a readjustment to the tempo of aging such that a person of 90…has the same vigor and address to life as present-day 70-year-olds, and so proportionately at other ages." Medawar's (1985) article, published in *Clinical Orthopaedics and Related Research*, was introduced by a biographical note written by his former student Eugene M. Lance, M.D., Ph.D., who had asked him to write "an essay of a philosophical cast." In this biographical note, it was communicated that one week after submitting the article, Sir Peter Medawar suffered a severe cerebral hemorrhage, from which he was recovering. He died in 1987, at age 72 years (*Encyclopaedia Britannica*, 1990, 15th ed., vol. 7, pages 997–998).

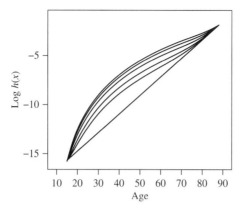

FIGURE 5.4 Semilog plots of mortality rates by age. Uppermost curve shows mixture model fitted to overall intrinsic mortality data, using $\hat{\pi} = 0.23$ and other parameter estimates given in Table 4.5 (first column). Other curves use successively, from top to bottom, $\hat{\pi} = 0.40, 0.60, 0.80$, 0.90, and 1.0 and the same values of the other four parameter estimates.

disability outcome that captured functional impairment even in the absence of morbidity. Based on the definition of a "frailty" phenotype (Fried et al., 2001; Rockwood et al., 2007), a dichotomous frailty outcome might alternatively be appropriate for that purpose.

However, the hope of maximizing the period of full function late in life presupposes the more basic scenario of compression of morbidity (or disability). Although this was characterized in Section 5.5 as a tall order, there is evidence that it is potentially attainable through primary prevention. For instance, in a longitudinal study of white adults under the age of 70 years with 9-year follow-up, lifestyle factors (cigarette smoking, alcohol consumption, physical exercise, hours of sleep per night, and weight in relation to height) were significantly associated with a health status measure taking into account disability, chronic conditions or impairments, and symptoms (Wiley and Camacho, 1980). Vita et al. (1998) conducted a longitudinal study of cumulative disability in relation to three levels of "health risk" defined on the basis of smoking, body mass index, and exercise. Subjects with high health risks had twice the cumulative disability of those with low health risks, and the age of onset of "minimal disability" was postponed by approximately 7 years in the low-risk group compared to the high-risk group. In a cohort of healthy middle-aged adults followed for 26 years, Willis et al. (2012) found that cardiorespiratory fitness was significantly associated with a lower risk of developing chronic disease outcomes (a summary measure of eight chronic conditions, including congestive heart failure, ischemic heart disease, stroke, diabetes mellitus, chronic obstructive pulmonary disease, chronic kidney disease, Alzheimer disease, and colon or lung cancer). Compared to subjects with lower midlife fitness, those with higher midlife fitness spent a greater proportion of their final 5 years of life with a low burden of chronic conditions. Moreover, among deceased subjects, higher midlife fitness was associated with a delay in the development of chronic conditions to a greater extent than the extension of the life span.

In what follows, we briefly consider an approach that may help further identify modifiable risk factors and thus enhance the potential of compression of morbidity through primary prevention.

Coming full circle with the evolutionary basis of this work, our causation model is consistent with the framework of "evolutionary health promotion," through the shared notion that there is a mismatch between the human genetic makeup, which was selected in past environments, and modern life, in which exposure to noxious substances and lifestyle factors (e.g., nutrition, sedentarism) represent a dramatic departure from those past environments (Boyd Eaton and Konner, 1985; Boyd Eaton et al., 1988, 2002b; Cordain et al., 2005). This mismatch fosters the "diseases of civilization," for which the long-term (backward-looking) evolutionary perspective offers the following prescription: "In order to regain relative freedom from these illnesses, we need to take a step backward in time. For each disorder, we may anticipate increasingly sophisticated and effective treatments, but the crucial corrective measure will almost certainly be prevention. This will entail reintroduction of essential elements from the lifestyle of our Paleolithic ancestors" (Boyd Eaton et al., 1988).[8] Under evolutionary health promotion, Boyd Eaton et al. (2002b) proposed guidelines for informing a research agenda and, ultimately, public policy: "(1) Better characterize differences between ancient and modern life patterns. (2) Identify which of these affect the development of disease. (3) Integrate epidemiological, mechanistic, and genetic data with evolutionary principles to create an overarching formulation upon which to base persuasive, consistent, and effective recommendations." That is to say, even as it is neither possible nor desirable to revert back to the time of our ancestors, we can benefit from characterizing differences in lifestyle and environmental exposures between past and modern times, identifying those factors that are associated with disease, and meticulously acting on them.

While emphasizing that preventive recommendations must ultimately rest on conventional epidemiological and experimental studies, Konner and Boyd Eaton (2010) restated the "discordance hypothesis" in general lines that seem unassailable: our genome evolved to adapt to conditions that no longer exist; the change has occurred too rapidly for adequate genetic adaptation (i.e., cultural evolution has outpaced genetic evolution); and the resulting mismatch contributes to the causation of common chronic diseases. Still, strong criticism has been leveled against evolutionary health promotion, in particular against some forms of "Paleolithic diets" (Zuk, 2013). This criticism involves the following main points: (i) species are never perfectly adapted to their concurrent environments, and given the continuity of evolution, there is no reason for a particular human ancestor to have especially good adaptation; (ii) Paleolithic environments are heterogeneous and our knowledge about them is incomplete; and (iii) species can and do evolve quite rapidly, such that adaptations in the last 10,000 years since the end of the Paleolithic period are possible. To the extent that this criticism can also be used to more broadly undermine the notion of mismatch,

---

[8] Reproduced from *The American Journal of Medicine*, **84**, Boyd Eaton, S., Konner, M., and Shostak, M., Stone agers in the fast lane: Chronic degenerative diseases in evolutionary perspective, pages 739–749, Copyright 1988, with permission from Elsevier.

it can be offset by the following counterarguments: (i) just because all species are somewhat mismatched to their environments, it does not follow that they are all equally mismatched; (ii) our incomplete knowledge about the Paleolithic (or more recent) environments still allows us to recognize some marked differences with the modern environment; and (iii) examples of rapid evolution for some traits do not preclude the existence of persistent mismatch for others (Boyd Eaton et al., 2002a; Deaner and Winegard, 2013). In our causation model, we are primarily concerned with the mismatch that has occurred over the last 200–300 years since the industrial revolution, rather than the about 10,000 years since the introduction of agriculture, and "No one proposes that genetic adaptations could have caught up with dietary and lifestyle changes over the past 2 centuries" (Konner and Boyd Eaton, 2010).

The approach advocated here in light of our causation model is in keeping with Geoffrey Rose's "population strategy" of disease prevention, which "seeks to control the determinants of incidence in the population as a whole," as contrasted with the "'high-risk' strategy," which "seeks to identify high-risk susceptible individuals and to offer them some individual protection" (Rose, 1985). The population strategy is regarded by Rose (1985) as radical in that it attempts to remove the underlying causes that make the disease common; it has a large potential to benefit the population as a whole even as it offers a relatively small benefit to each individual. Within the population strategy, Rose (1985) described a particular approach that resonates with ours : "the restoration of biological normality by the removal of an abnormal exposure (e.g., stopping smoking, controlling air pollution, moderating some of our recently-acquired dietary deviations)." What is not explicitly recognized by Rose (1985), and modern epidemiology in general, is that exposures are not abnormal in and of themselves. On the evolutionary view, what makes modern life exposures "abnormal" is the lack of human adaptation to their effects or the mismatch between the human genetic makeup and modern life. In our times, the promise of this approach can also be fulfilled with the help of epigenetics. This could come about from advances in understanding epigenetic mechanisms, as suggested by Lamb (1994) ("Studies of EISs [epigenetic inheritance systems] should help us to understand how environmental variables influence longevity and aging"), or along the lines suggested by Cooney (2007) ("The current challenge is to identify environmental factors that influence or direct epigenetics to the benefit and maintenance of health as well as those that damage or misdirect epigenetics to cause disease and dysfunction").

Returning to Figure 5.2 (upper panel), by viewing the Gompertz component of our mixture model as a benchmark of biological aging, as described in the previous section, and considering that a steep decline of the Gompertz component's survival function only starts after about age 75 years, this would suggest that natural selection has been more effective in weeding out late-onset deleterious mutations in human populations over evolutionary history than one would imagine on the basis of—in the words of Perks (1932) as quoted at the end of Section 3.1—"all the roughnesses in our data referable to errors of observation and an ever-changing environment." Yet this can also be seen to imply that improvements in the health of the aging population beyond a certain point are only achievable through altering the fundamental genetic mechanisms of aging. Indeed, referring to a supposed "intrinsic ceiling" in life expectancy, Keyfitz (1978) asked what would be needed "to break through the barrier that now seems to be set at about 80 years..." He then suggested that beyond attacking individual diseases as causes of death, "future research should focus on what underlies them all—the deterioration and senescence of the cells of the human body." Along the same lines, Olshansky et al. (1991) considered that "To extend life expectancy beyond 85 years, it will be necessary for medical science to alter the fundamental rate of aging by manipulating 'aging' genes through techniques developed in molecular biology."

Although Olshansky et al.'s (1990, 2001) broad life expectancy projections one decade apart did not show any substantial changes, Olshansky et al. (2002a) basically reiterated the same argument as in the preceding text but pushed the supposed biological limit of life expectancy a little further: "Even with precipitous declines in mortality at middle and older ages from those present today, life expectancy at birth is unlikely to exceed 90 years (males and females combined) in the twenty-first century without scientific advances that permit the modification of the fundamental processes of aging." Irrespective of what the value of such biological limit of life expectancy may be, our analysis suggests that there is still nonnegligible room to improve life expectancy through the elimination of environmentally induced premature deaths in human populations—and even if the effect on life expectancy may be relatively small, the effect on the proportion of premature deaths that are prevented, all the while enhancing quality of life, is potentially very large. As such, despite the calls to rather invest in the understanding and modification of the fundamental processes of aging, it seems to us that the continuation and intensification of the efforts directed at primary prevention are presently justified. Consistent with that, while recognizing that gains in life expectancy in the twenty-first century will be limited, Bonneux et al. (1998) considered that "Opportunities for slowing the rate of senescence are to be sought in decreasing the rate of accumulation of damage, which is identical to a familiar concept to public health practitioners and epidemiologists: diminishing exposure to risk factors."

In fact, by considering across-the-board effects of risk factor modification on several diseases representing the present major causes of death, not only are the potential returns in preventing premature deaths substantial (Danaei et al., 2009), but even the prospect for life expectancy gains looks more promising. Schatzkin (1980) characterized Keyfitz's (1978) argument earlier about the life expectancy gains from a hypothetical cure for cancer as a "competing causes" argument, based on the scenario that one cause of death is eliminated at a time. He opposed to that the more realistic "common risk factors" scenario, in which case simultaneous/multiple-cause elimination is possible through public health interventions on risk factors associated with several diseases (e.g., smoking and animal fat consumption). As life expectancy gains in this scenario are considerably greater, Schatzkin (1980) argued: "To increase life expectancy in this period, we should marshal our resources not toward aging per se, our protoplasmic limitations, but *primarily* toward the *reversible* social determinants of the leading causes of death that keep us from reaching nine and perhaps ten decades of vigorous, healthy life." Motivated by Keyfitz's (1978, 1980) and Schatzkin's (1980) commentaries, Olshansky (1985) compared longevity gains under a single-cause elimination model to those resulting from preventive measures leading to 5-year delay in major cardiovascular diseases, diabetes mellitus, and some cancers; these simultaneous delays produced projected gains in life expectancy equal to or greater than those obtained through the hypothetical elimination of some single major causes of death. Thus, Olshansky (1985) concluded: "the extension of years-to-life *and* life-to-years is an appropriate goal for the allocation of research and service funds. These data indicate that preventive health care measures should be a prime target."

As stated by Brody (1985) not so long ago, we are "far short of reaching the potential of better health and quality of life in later years. Two vehicles offer promise: health promotion through the improvement of personal health practices throughout life, and major research efforts to understand and postpone the ageing processes…" Although the health-promotion and postponed-aging strategies are not mutually exclusive and may well run in parallel, evolutionary theory, by implying that hundreds of biochemical pathways and hundreds or thousands of genes play a role in aging (Rose, 2004; Rose et al., 2012), suggests that the postponed-aging strategy will remain a challenging and unfruitful endeavor for many years to come. This is supported by experimental studies in *Drosophila melanogaster* indicating that the number of genetic loci that underlie aging is at least in the hundreds (Rose and Long, 2002; Rose and Burke, 2011). Moreover, in a "Genome-wide analysis of a long-term evolution experiment with *Drosophila*," Burke et al. (2010) showed that for a life history character (development time), adaptation was not associated with "hard sweeps," in which newly arising, highly advantageous mutations become fixed; instead, the findings supported the "soft sweep model," in which preexisting intermediate-frequency genetic variants become more common. In a review, Pritchard et al. (2010) noted that studies using large genome-wide datasets have generally evidenced few examples of hard sweeps in recent human evolution. Based on the view that the evolution of aging results from a failure of adaptation involving a large number of genetic variants and biochemical pathways, one may even be led to "regard the slowing of human aging as an essentially intractable problem" (Rose, 2009).

Indeed, early in the development of the evolutionary theory of aging, Williams (1957) stated that its implication of a large number of physiological processes involved in aging "banishes the 'fountain of youth' to the limbo of scientific impossibilities where other human aspirations, like the perpetual motion machine and Laplace's 'superman' have already been placed by other theoretical considerations." Wallace (1967) similarly noted that it is "futile to waste time searching for a single root cause of ageing and its cure, an elixir vitae." Notwithstanding, the search for the fountain of youth has long existed, and its appeal in our times has not subsided (Kirkwood, 1999, chapter 15; Olshansky et al., 2002b). Whether or not the skeptics will eventually be proven wrong, the broad public health implication of our work is even more relevant given the enduring difficulties faced by the postponed-aging strategy. What emerges from this work is that aging (in the sense of population biological aging) should be seen as a target to be achieved rather than to be defeated. The control of environmental factors brought about by industrialization and relatively recent changes in lifestyle may currently be a practical and productive strategy for improving the health of our aging population.

APPENDIX A

PROOFS OF RESULTS IN SECTION 2.1.2 WITH SOME EXTENSIONS

Proof of Corollary to Theorem 2. If the survival function $S(x)$ is infinitely differentiable or C^∞ at x_0 but is not analytic, the Taylor expansion of $S(x)$ about x_0 converges to $S(x)$ only at x_0. We assume to the contrary that there exists a Taylor expansion of $S(x)$ about x_0 with a positive radius of convergence. To study the limiting behavior of the expression in the left-hand side of Equation 2.32, we express $S(x)$ as the Taylor series about x_0:

$$S(x) = \sum_{i=0}^{\infty} \frac{S^{(i)}(x_0)}{i!}(x-x_0)^i = 1 + \sum_{i=1}^{\infty} \frac{S^{(i)}(x_0)}{i!}(x-x_0)^i. \tag{A.1}$$

Letting $C_p = -S^{(p)}(x_0)$ and assuming there exists a smallest finite $p \geq 1$ with $C_p \neq 0$, then from Equation A.1,

$$1 - S(x) = \frac{C_p}{p!}(x-x_0)^p + \frac{C_{p+1}}{(p+1)!}(x-x_0)^{p+1} + \frac{C_{p+2}}{(p+2)!}(x-x_0)^{p+2} + \cdots \tag{A.2}$$

Using the power series representation $-\log(1-x) = x + x^2/2 + x^3/3 + \cdots$ for $|x| < 1$, we obtain the following three expressions. If p>1,

---

The Biostatistics of Aging: From Gompertzian Mortality to an Index of Aging-Relatedness,
First Edition. Gilberto Levy and Bruce Levin.
© 2014 John Wiley & Sons, Inc. Published 2014 by John Wiley & Sons, Inc.

$$-\log S(x) = 1 - S(x) + \frac{[1-S(x)]^2}{2} + \frac{[1-S(x)]^3}{3} + \cdots = \left[\frac{C_p}{p!}(x-x_0)^p + \frac{C_{p+1}}{(p+1)!}(x-x_0)^{p+1} + \cdots\right]$$

$$+ \frac{\left[\frac{C_p}{p!}(x-x_0)^p + \frac{C_{p+1}}{(p+1)!}(x-x_0)^{p+1} + \cdots\right]^2}{2} + \cdots \qquad (A.3)$$

$$\frac{d}{dx}[-\log S(x)] = \frac{C_p}{(p-1)!}(x-x_0)^{p-1} + \frac{C_{p+1}}{p!}(x-x_0)^p + \cdots + \frac{C_p^2}{(p-1)!p!}(x-x_0)^{2p-1}$$

$$+ C_p C_{p+1}\left[\frac{1}{p!^2} + \frac{1}{(p-1)!(p+1)!}\right](x-x_0)^{2p} + \cdots \qquad (A.4)$$

$$\frac{d^2}{dx^2}[-\log S(x)] = \frac{C_p}{(p-2)!}(x-x_0)^{p-2} + \frac{C_{p+1}}{(p-1)!}(x-x_0)^{p-1} + \cdots + \frac{(2p-1)C_p^2}{(p-1)!\,p!}(x-x_0)^{2p-2}$$

$$+ 2pC_p C_{p+1}\left[\frac{1}{p!^2} + \frac{1}{(p-1)!(p+1)!}\right](x-x_0)^{2p-1} + \cdots \qquad (A.5)$$

The expressions in Equations A.2, A.4, and A.5 allow us to re-express the limit in the left-hand side of Equation 2.32 as follows:

$$\lim_{x \downarrow x_0} \frac{\left[\frac{C_p}{p!}(x-x_0)^p + \frac{C_{p+1}}{(p+1)!}(x-x_0)^{p+1} + \cdots\right]\left[\frac{C_p}{(p-2)!}(x-x_0)^{p-2} + \frac{C_{p+1}}{(p-1)!}(x-x_0)^{p-1} + \cdots\right]}{\left[\frac{C_p}{(p-1)!}(x-x_0)^{p-1} + \frac{C_{p+1}}{p!}(x-x_0)^p + \cdots\right]^2}$$

$$= \lim_{x \downarrow x_0} \frac{\frac{C_p^2}{(p-2)!p!}(x-x_0)^{2p-2} + C_p C_{p+1}\left[\frac{1}{(p-1)!p!} + \frac{1}{(p-2)!(p+1)!}\right](x-x_0)^{2p-1} + \cdots}{\frac{C_p^2}{(p-1)!^2}(x-x_0)^{2p-2} + \frac{2C_p C_{p+1}}{(p-1)!\,p!}(x-x_0)^{2p-1} + \cdots}$$

$$= \lim_{x \downarrow x_0} \frac{(x-x_0)^{2p-2}\left\{\frac{C_p^2}{(p-2)!\,p!} + C_p C_{p+1}\left[\frac{1}{(p-1)!\,p!} + \frac{1}{(p-2)!(p+1)!}\right](x-x_0) + \cdots\right\}}{(x-x_0)^{2p-2}\left[\frac{C_p^2}{(p-1)!^2} + \frac{2C_p C_{p+1}}{(p-1)!\,p!}(x-x_0) + \cdots\right]}$$

$$= \frac{C_p^2/(p-2)!\,p!}{C_p^2/(p-1)!^2} = \frac{(p-1)!^2}{(p-2)!\,p!} = \frac{p-1}{p} = 1 - \frac{1}{p} \neq 1. \qquad (A.6)$$

If p=1, Equation A.6 is easily seen to equal 0 directly. This shows that the limit in Equation 2.32 is not equal to 1, and thus Equation 2.32 cannot hold for any finite p. Thus, if $S(x)$ satisfies the von Mises condition, all its derivatives at x_0 must equal 0. If the Taylor series about x_0 in Equation A.1 had a nonzero radius of convergence, then $S(x)$ would equal 1 for some $x > x_0$, contradicting the assumption that $S(x) < 1$ for all $x > x_0$. Hence, $S(x)$ is not analytic at x_0. This concludes the proof of the corollary.

Proof of Theorem 6. Since $F(x_0) = 0$ and $F(x) > 0$ for $x > x_0$, we have that $\phi(x) = -\log F(x) \to \infty$ as $x \to x_0$, $\phi'(x) = -f(x)/F(x) \le 0$, and $\psi(x) = -1/\phi'(x) = F(x)/f(x) \ge 0$ for $x > x_0$. By assumption, $\phi'(x) \to -\infty$ as $x \to x_0$, that is, $\psi(x) \to 0$ as $x \to x_0$, so define $\psi(x_0) = 0$. From Equation 2.22, if the von Mises sufficient condition for the minimum is met, $\lim_{x \downarrow x_0} \psi'(x) = 0$. Suppose to the contrary that $\lim_{x \downarrow x_0} \psi'(x) = \psi'(x_0) = \lim_{x \downarrow x_0} \frac{\psi(x) - \psi(x_0)}{x - x_0} = c$ with $0 < c < \infty$. Then, there exists an $x^* > x_0$ such that for $x_0 < x < x^*$,

$$\frac{\psi(x) - \psi(x_0)}{x - x_0} = \frac{\psi(x)}{x - x_0} > \frac{c}{2} > 0, \tag{A.7}$$

but then for $x < x^*$, using $\psi(x) = -1/\phi'(x) \Rightarrow \phi'(x) = -1/\psi(x)$,

$$\phi(x) = \int_x^{x^*} \frac{1}{\psi(u)} du + \text{const} = \int_x^{x^*} \frac{du}{(u - x_0)[\psi(u)/(u - x_0)]} + \text{const} < \frac{2}{c} \int_x^{x^*} \frac{du}{(u - x_0)} + \text{const}$$

$$= \frac{2}{c} \log (u - x_0)\Big|_x^{x^*} + \text{const} = -\frac{2}{c} \log (x - x_0) + \text{const}, \tag{A.8}$$

so that

$$F(x) = \exp[-\phi(x)] > k \exp\left[\frac{2}{c} \log (x - x_0)\right] = k(x - x_0)^{2/c}, \tag{A.9}$$

where k is a positive constant. We show that this implies that $F(x)$ does not have all derivatives at $x = x_0$ equal to 0. Let $r = \lceil 2/c \rceil$ be the smallest integer greater than or equal to $2/c$, so that $r = 2/c + \varepsilon$ with $0 \le \varepsilon < 1$. If $F^{(j)}(x_0) \ne 0$ for some $j = 0, ..., r - 1$, we are done, so assume $F^{(j)}(x_0) = 0$ for $j = 0, ..., r - 1$ and consider $F^{(r)}(x_0)$. Then, by L'Hospital's rule,

$$\frac{F^{(r)}(x_0)}{r!} = \lim_{x \downarrow x_0} \frac{F(x)}{(x - x_0)^r} \ge k \lim_{x \downarrow x_0} (x - x_0)^{2/c - r} = k \lim_{x \downarrow x_0} (x - x_0)^{-\varepsilon}$$

$$\Rightarrow F^{(r)}(x_0) \ge r! k \lim_{x \downarrow x_0} (x - x_0)^{-\varepsilon} > 0, \tag{A.10}$$

since $\lim_{x \downarrow x_0} (x - x_0)^{-\varepsilon} = 1$ for $\varepsilon = 0$ and $\lim_{x \downarrow x_0} (x - x_0)^{-\varepsilon} = \infty$ for $\varepsilon > 0$.

Suppose now that $\lim_{x \downarrow x_0} \psi'(x)$ exists but is infinite. Then, there exists an $x^{**} > x_0$ such that for $x_0 < x < x^{**}$,

$$\frac{\psi(x) - \psi(x_0)}{x - x_0} = \frac{\psi(x)}{x - x_0} > 1, \tag{A.11}$$

but then for $x < x^{**}$,

$$\phi(x) = \int_x^{x^{**}} \frac{1}{\psi(u)} du + \mathrm{const} = \int_x^{x^{**}} \frac{du}{(u - x_0)[\psi(u)/(u - x_0)]} + \mathrm{const} < \int_x^{x^{**}} \frac{du}{(u - x_0)} + \mathrm{const}$$

$$= \log (u - x_0)\big|_x^{x^{**}} + \mathrm{const} = - \log (x - x_0) + \mathrm{const}, \tag{A.12}$$

so that

$$F(x) = \exp[-\phi(x)] > k \exp[\log (x - x_0)] = k(x - x_0), \tag{A.13}$$

in which case $F(x)$ does not have the first derivative at $x = x_0$ equal to 0, since $F'(x_0) = \lim_{x \downarrow x_0} F(x)/(x - x_0) \geq k > 0$. In all cases, then, under the assumption that $\psi'(x)$ is continuous at x_0, if the von Mises sufficient condition for the minimum is not met, $F(x)$ is not flat at the lower endpoint of the distribution. It follows that under the assumption that $\psi'(x)$ is continuous at x_0, if $F(x)$ is flat at the lower endpoint of the distribution, the von Mises sufficient condition for the minimum is met. This concludes the proof of Theorem 6.

Proof of Proposition. First consider the case of integer ρ, say, $\rho = p \geq 1$. Then, by L'Hospital's rule used repeatedly,

$$L(0) = \lim_{x \downarrow 0} \frac{F(x)}{x^p} = \lim_{x \downarrow 0} \frac{F^{(p)}(x)}{p!} = 0. \tag{A.14}$$

Now for $x > 0$, $L'(x) = x^{-p} F'(x) - p x^{-(p+1)} F(x)$, and using L'Hospital's rule on each term, we have

$$\lim_{x \downarrow 0} \frac{F'(x)}{x^p} = \lim_{x \downarrow 0} \frac{F^{(p+1)}(x)}{p!} = 0, \tag{A.15}$$

$$\lim_{x \downarrow 0} \frac{-p F(x)}{x^{p+1}} = -p \lim_{x \downarrow 0} \frac{F^{(p+1)}(x)}{(p+1)!} = 0, \tag{A.16}$$

whence $L'(0) = \lim_{x \downarrow 0} L'(x) = 0$. In general, the rth derivative of $L(x)$ is, writing $p^{[0]} = 1$ and $p^{[i]} = p(p + 1) \cdots (p + i - 1)$ for $i \geq 1$,

$$L^{(r)}(x) = \sum_{i=0}^{r} (-1)^i \binom{r}{i} p^{[i]} x^{-(p+i)} F^{(r-i)}(x). \tag{A.17}$$

Applying L'Hospital's rule to each term,

$$\lim_{x\downarrow 0}(-1)^i \binom{r}{i} p^{[i]} x^{-(p+i)} F^{(r-i)}(x) = (-1)^i \binom{r}{i} p^{[i]} \lim_{x\downarrow 0} \frac{F^{(r-i)}(x)}{x^{p+i}}$$

$$= (-1)^i \binom{r}{i} p^{[i]} \lim_{x\downarrow 0} \frac{F^{(r+p)}(x)}{(p+i)!} = 0, \qquad (A.18)$$

whence $L^{(r)}(0) = \lim_{x\downarrow 0} L^{(r)}(x) = 0$. For noninteger ρ, write $\rho = p - \varepsilon$ where $p = \lceil \rho \rceil$, $0 < \varepsilon < 1$. Then, for any term of the form $(-1)^i \binom{r}{i} \rho^{[i]} x^{-(\rho+i)} F^{(r-i)}(x)$, $(-1)^i \binom{r}{i} \rho^{[i]}$ is just a constant and

$$\lim_{x\downarrow 0} \frac{F^{(r-i)}(x)}{x^{\rho+i}} = \lim_{x\downarrow 0} \frac{F^{(r-i)}(x)}{x^{p-\varepsilon+i}} = \lim_{x\downarrow 0} \frac{x^\varepsilon F^{(r-i)}(x)}{x^{p+i}} = \lim_{x\downarrow 0} x^\varepsilon \lim_{x\downarrow 0} \frac{F^{(r-i)}(x)}{x^{p+i}}$$

$$= \lim_{x\downarrow 0} x^\varepsilon \lim_{x\downarrow 0} \frac{F^{(r+p)}(x)}{(p+i)!} = 0, \qquad (A.19)$$

so in all cases,

$$L^{(r)}(0) = \lim_{x\downarrow 0} L^{(r)}(x) = 0. \qquad (A.20)$$

This concludes the proof of the proposition.

Proof of Theorem 7. Karamata (1930) deduced from the representation in Equation 2.63 the following property of slowly varying functions at infinity:

$$\lim_{x\to\infty} x^p Z(x) = \infty \quad \text{and} \quad \lim_{x\to\infty} x^{-p} Z(x) = 0 \quad \text{for any } p > 0. \qquad (A.21)$$

This property is given as a fundamental result concerning slowly varying functions by Adamovic (1966), and a simpler proof of Equation 2.63 and the property in Equation A.21 is given by Korevaar et al. (1949). Using the reciprocal transformation, we obtain the analogous property of slowly varying functions at 0, which is Equation 1.4 in Qualls and Watanabe (1972):

$$\lim_{x\downarrow 0} x^{-p} L(x) = \infty \quad \text{and} \quad \lim_{x\downarrow 0} x^p L(x) = 0 \quad \text{for any } p > 0. \qquad (A.22)$$

By taking $p = 1$, it immediately follows from Equation A.22 that if $L(x)$ is slowly varying at 0 with $L(0) = 0$ and $L(x) > 0$ for $x > 0$, then $\lim_{x\downarrow 0} L(x)/x = L'(0) = \infty$; hence, $L(x)$ is not flat at 0. This concludes the proof of Theorem 7.

Some Particular Results in the i.i.d. Case Concerning the Prototypical Flat Functions. We state a lemma concerning flat functions with $\psi(x)$ decreasing as x^p as x decreases to 0.

Lemma. Let $F(x)$ be a c.d.f. with $F(0) = 0$ and $F(x) > 0$ for $x > 0$, which is differentiable in a right-neighborhood of 0. Let $\phi(x) = -\log F(x)$ and $\psi(x) = -1/\phi'(x)$ for $\phi'(x) \neq 0$. Assume $F(x)$ is such that for some real number $p > 1$,

$$\psi(x) = cx^p + o(x^p) \text{ as } x \to 0 \text{ with } c > 0. \tag{A.23}$$

Then, there are constants $a_n > 0$ and $b_n > 0$ such that, with $W_n = \min\{X_1, X_2, ..., X_n\}$ and $X_i \sim$ iid F, we have $P[W_n > a_n x + b_n] \to \exp(-e^x)$ as $n \to \infty$, for any fixed $-\infty < x < \infty$. In fact, we may take $b_n = F^{-1}(1/n)$ and $a_n = cb_n^p$.

Proof of Lemma. We use x here instead of w^* as in the main text for typographical convenience. $P[W_n > a_n x + b_n] = [1 - nF(a_n x + b_n)/n]^n \to \exp(-e^x)$ as $n \to \infty$ iff $nF(a_n x + b_n) = e^x + o(1)$ as $n \to \infty$ or, equivalently,

$$\log n - \phi(a_n x + b_n) = x + o(1) \text{ as } n \to \infty. \tag{A.24}$$

Take $b_n = F^{-1}(1/n)$ so that $\log n - \phi(a_n x + b_n) = x$ exactly at $x = 0$; that is, $\phi(b_n) = \log n$. Now write $\phi(a_n x + b_n) = \phi(b_n) + \phi'(b_n + a_n x t_n)a_n x$ for some $0 < t_n < 1$ using the mean value theorem (MVT) or, equivalently,

$$\log n - \phi(a_n x + b_n) = \frac{x a_n}{\psi(b_n + a_n x t_n)}. \tag{A.25}$$

Thus, to show Equation A.24, it suffices to show that $a_n/\psi(b_n + a_n x t_n) = 1 + o(1)$ as $n \to \infty$. Taking $a_n = cb_n^p$ and using assumption (Eq. A.23), we have

$$\frac{a_n}{\psi(b_n + a_n x t_n)} = \frac{a_n}{c(b_n + a_n x t_n)^p + o[(b_n + a_n x t_n)^p]} = \frac{cb_n^p}{c(b_n + cb_n^p x t_n)^p + o[(b_n + cb_n^p x t_n)^p]}$$

$$= \frac{cb_n^p}{cb_n^p\left(1 + cb_n^{p-1}x t_n\right)^p + o\left[b_n^p\left(1 + cb_n^{p-1}x t_n\right)^p\right]}$$

$$= \frac{1}{\left(1 + cb_n^{p-1}x t_n\right)^p + o(1)} = 1 + o(1) \text{ as } n \to \infty, \tag{A.26}$$

since $p > 1$ and $b_n \to 0$ as $n \to \infty$. This concludes the proof of the Lemma.

Remark A.1. For $\psi(x) = cx^p$ with $c > 0$ and $p > 1$, $\phi'(x) = -1/\psi(x) = -x^{-p}/c$, and

$$\phi(x) = \int_x^\omega \frac{du}{\psi(u)} + \text{const} = \int_x^\omega \frac{du}{cu^p} + \text{const} = \frac{u^{1-p}}{c(1-p)}\Big|_x^\omega + \text{const} = \frac{x^{1-p}}{c(p-1)} + \frac{\omega^{1-p}}{c(1-p)} + \text{const}.$$

Then,

$$F(x) = \exp[-\phi(x)] = K \exp\left[\frac{-x^{1-p}}{c(p-1)}\right], \tag{A.27}$$

where K is such that $F(\omega) = 1 \Rightarrow K = \exp\{\omega^{1-p}/[c(p-1)]\}$ and $F(x)$ is flat at 0 for $p > 1$. Our prototype example (Eq. 2.59) of a flat function at 0 is the case $c = 1$ and $p = 2$, so that $\psi(x) = x^2$, $\phi(x) = 1/x$, and $F(x) = e^{-1/x}$. In this case, we can choose $b_n = F^{-1}(1/n) = 1/\log n$ and $a_n = cb_n^p = b_n^2 = 1/(\log n)^2$. More generally, for the family of flat functions $F(x) = e^{-(\sigma/x)^\rho}$, where $\sigma > 0$ and $\rho > 0$ are scale and shape parameters, respectively, we have $p = \rho + 1$ and $c = 1/(\rho\sigma^\rho)$, so we can choose $b_n = \sigma/(\log n)^{1/\rho}$ and $a_n = \sigma/[\rho(\log n)^{(\rho+1)/\rho}]$.

Remark A.2. The functional form of $\psi(x)$ is not important so long as $\psi(0) = 0$ and $\psi'(x) \to 0$ as $x \to 0$. Note that in the proof of the Lemma, all we needed to show was that $a_n/\psi(b_n + a_n x t_n) \to 1$ as $n \to \infty$. Using the MVT again, this time on $\psi(x)$ instead of $\phi(x)$ (so here we need to assume that $F(x)$ is twice differentiable in a right-neighborhood of 0), we write

$$\psi(b_n + a_n x t_n) = \psi(b_n) + \psi'\left(b_n + a_n x t_n t_n^*\right) a_n x t_n \quad \text{for some } 0 < t_n^* < 1, \tag{A.28}$$

and dividing both sides by a_n, we obtain an expression for $[a_n/\psi(b_n + a_n x t_n)]^{-1}$,

$$\frac{\psi(b_n + a_n x t_n)}{a_n} = \frac{\psi(b_n)}{a_n} + \psi'\left(b_n + a_n x t_n t_n^*\right) x t_n. \tag{A.29}$$

If we define $a_n = \psi(b_n)$ and use the von Mises condition (Eq. 2.22), this expression approaches 1 in the limit as n approaches infinity, because $\left(b_n + a_n x t_n t_n^*\right) \to 0$ (since $b_n \to 0$, $a_n = \psi(b_n) \to \psi(0) = 0$, x is a constant, and t_n and t_n^* are bounded), and it follows that $\psi'\left(b_n + a_n x t_n t_n^*\right) x t_n \to 0$. In fact, with $b_n = F^{-1}(1/n)$, we can choose a_n more generally as $a_n = \psi(b_n) + o[\psi(b_n)]$ since then $\psi(b_n)/a_n$ and $\psi(b_n + a_n x t_n)/a_n$ approach 1 as well.

We now turn to some non-i.i.d. versions of the Lemma.

Proof of Theorem 8. We consider the case of continuous σ; the proof of the discrete case is similar. Taking negative logs on both sides of $P[W_n > a_n x + b_n] = \prod_{i=1}^n [1 - F_i(a_n x + b_n)]$ and using the power series representation $-\log(1-x) = x + x^2/2 + x^3/3 + \cdots$, we obtain

$$-\log P[W_n > a_n x + b_n] = -\sum_{i=1}^n \log[1 - F_i(a_n x + b_n)]$$

$$= \sum_{i=1}^n F_i(a_n x + b_n) + O\left[\sum_{i=1}^n F_i^2(a_n x + b_n)\right] \quad \text{as } n \to \infty. \tag{A.30}$$

Thus, we wish to show that, for suitable a_n and b_n, $\sum_{i=1}^{n} F_i(a_n x + b_n) \to e^x$ for any x, while $\sum_{i=1}^{n} F_i^2(a_n x + b_n) = o(1)$ as $n \to \infty$:

$$\sum_{i=1}^{n} F_i(a_n x + b_n) = \sum_{i=1}^{n} \exp[-\phi_i(a_n x + b_n)]$$

$$= \sum_{i=1}^{n} \exp\left[-\phi_i(b_n) + \frac{a_n x}{\psi_i(b_n + a_n x t_{n,i})}\right] \quad \text{for some } 0 < t_{n,i} < 1, \text{ by the MVT}$$

$$= \sum_{i=1}^{n} \exp\left[-\phi_i(b_n) + \frac{a_n x}{\psi_i(b_n) + \psi'_i\left(b_n + a_n x t_{n,i} t_{n,i}^*\right) a_n x t_{n,i}}\right]$$

for some $0 < t_{n,i}^* < 1$, again by the MVT

$$= \sum_{i=1}^{n} \exp\left[-\phi_i(b_n) + \frac{x}{\psi_i(b_n)/a_n + \psi'_i\left(b_n + a_n x t_{n,i} t_{n,i}^*\right) x t_{n,i}}\right]. \tag{A.31}$$

By the von Mises condition, $\psi'_i(b_n + a_n x t_{n,i} t_{n,i}^*) x t_{n,i} = o(1)$ as $n \to \infty$, so we want

$$\sum_{i=1}^{n} \exp\left[-\phi_i(b_n) + \frac{x}{\psi_i(b_n)/a_n}\right] \to e^x \quad \text{as } n \to \infty. \tag{A.32}$$

Now specializing to $F_i(x) = \exp[-(\sigma_i/x^\rho)] = \exp(-\tau_i/x^\rho)$, with $\tau_i = \sigma_i^\rho$, we have $\phi_i(x) = \tau_i x^{-\rho}$, $\phi'_i(x) = -\rho\tau_i x^{-(\rho+1)}$, and $\psi_i(x) = x^{\rho+1}/\rho\tau_i$, so that

$$\sum_{i=1}^{n} \exp\left[-\phi_i(b_n) + \frac{a_n x}{\psi_i(b_n)}\right] = \sum_{i=1}^{n} \exp\left[\frac{-\tau_i}{b_n^\rho} + \frac{a_n x \rho \tau_i}{b_n^{\rho+1}}\right]. \tag{A.33}$$

Letting $u = i/n$ $(i = 1, \ldots, n)$ and assuming there exists a continuous function $\tau : [0,1] \to \mathfrak{R}^+$ such that $\tau_i = \tau(i/n) = \tau(u)$,

$$\sum_{i=1}^{n} \exp\left[\frac{-\tau_i}{b_n^\rho} + \frac{a_n x \rho \tau_i}{b_n^{\rho+1}}\right] = n \sum_{u=1/n}^{n/n} \exp\left[\frac{-\tau(u)}{b_n^\rho} + \frac{a_n x \rho \tau(u)}{b_n^{\rho+1}}\right] \frac{1}{n}$$

$$\approx n \int_0^1 \exp\left[\frac{-\tau(u)}{b_n^\rho} + \frac{a_n x \rho \tau(u)}{b_n^{\rho+1}}\right] du = n \int_0^1 \exp\left[\left(\frac{-1}{b_n^\rho} + \frac{a_n x \rho}{b_n^{\rho+1}}\right) \tau(u)\right] du$$

$$= n \int_{\tau_0}^{\infty} \exp\left[\left(\frac{-1}{b_n^\rho} + \frac{x \rho a_n}{b_n^{\rho+1}}\right) \tau\right] dG(\tau), \tag{A.34}$$

where we changed variables from u to τ. Then, by taking $a_n = b_n^{\rho+1}/(\rho\tau_0)$,

$$n\int_{\tau_0}^{\infty} \exp\left[\left(\frac{-1}{b_n^\rho} + \frac{x\rho a_n}{b_n^{\rho+1}}\right)\tau\right]dG(\tau) = n\int_{\tau_0}^{\infty} \exp\left[\left(\frac{-1}{b_n^\rho} + \frac{x}{\tau_0}\right)(\tau-\tau_0+\tau_0)\right]dG(\tau)$$

$$= \frac{nb_n^\rho \exp\left((-\tau_0/b_n^\rho)+x\right)\int_{\tau_0}^{\infty} \exp\left[\left((-1/b_n^\rho)+(x/\tau_0)\right)(\tau-\tau_0)\right]dG(\tau)}{b_n^\rho}. \quad (A.35)$$

Letting $h_n(\tau) = \exp\left[\left((-1/b_n^\rho)+(x/\tau_0)\right)(\tau-\tau_0)\right]/b_n^\rho$ and breaking the integral into two pieces,

$$nb_n^\rho e^{(-\tau_0/b_n^\rho)+x}\int_{\tau_0}^{\infty} h_n(\tau)dG(\tau) = nb_n^\rho e^{(-\tau_0/b_n^\rho)+x}\left[\int_{\tau_0}^{\tau_0+\varepsilon} h_n(\tau)dG(\tau) + \int_{\tau_0+\varepsilon}^{\infty} h_n(\tau)dG(\tau)\right]$$

$$= nb_n^\rho e^{(-\tau_0/b_n^\rho)+x}\left[\int_{\tau_0}^{\tau_0+\varepsilon} h_n(\tau)g(\tau)d\tau + \int_{\tau_0+\varepsilon}^{\infty} h_n(\tau)dG(\tau)\right]$$

$$\leq nb_n^\rho e^{(-\tau_0/b_n^\rho)+x}\left[\sup_{\tau_0\leq\tau\leq\tau_0+\varepsilon} g(\tau)\int_{\tau_0}^{\tau_0+\varepsilon} h_n(\tau)d\tau + \sup_{\tau>\tau_0+\varepsilon} h_n(\tau)\right]$$

$$= nb_n^\rho e^{(-\tau_0/b_n^\rho)+x}\sup_{\tau_0\leq\tau\leq\tau_0+\varepsilon} g(\tau)[1+o(1)]$$

$$= nb_n^\rho e^{(-\tau_0/b_n^\rho)}\sup_{\tau_0\leq\tau\leq\tau_0+\varepsilon} g(\tau)e^x + o(1) \quad as\ n\to\infty, \quad (A.36)$$

because $\displaystyle\int_{\tau_0}^{\tau_0+\varepsilon} h_n(\tau)d\tau = \int_{\tau_0}^{\tau_0+\varepsilon}\frac{e^{[(-1/b_n^\rho)+(x/\tau_0)](\tau-\tau_0)}}{b_n^\rho}d\tau = \int_0^{\varepsilon}\frac{e^{[(-1/b_n^\rho)+(x/\tau_0)]\tau'}}{b_n^\rho}d\tau' =$

$\displaystyle\frac{e^{[(-1/b_n^\rho)+(x/\tau_0)]\tau'}}{[-1+(xb_n^\rho/\tau_0)]}\bigg|_0^{\varepsilon} = \frac{1-e^{[(-1/b_n^\rho)+(x/\tau_0)]\varepsilon}}{[1-(xb_n^\rho/\tau_0)]} = 1+o(1)$ as $n\to\infty$ and $\sup_{\tau>\tau_0+\varepsilon} h_n(\tau) =$

$e^{[(-1/b_n^\rho)+(x/\tau_0)]\varepsilon}/b_n^\rho = o(1)$ as $n\to\infty$, since $e^{-1/x}/x\to 0$ as $x\to 0$. Similarly, Equation A.35 is $\geq nb_n^\rho e^{(-\tau_0/b_n^\rho)}\inf_{\tau_0\leq\tau\leq\tau_0+\varepsilon} g(\tau)e^x + o(1)$, and since ε was arbitrary, Equation A.35 is equal to $nb_n^\rho e^{(-\tau_0/b_n^\rho)}g(\tau_0)e^x + o(1)$ as $n\to\infty$. Then, by taking b_n such that $nb_n^\rho e^{(-\tau_0/b_n^\rho)}g(\tau_0) = 1$ or, equivalently,

$$\log n + \log b_n^\rho - \frac{\tau_0}{b_n^\rho} + \log g(\tau_0) = 0, \quad (A.37)$$

Equation A.32 is satisfied. Finally, to show that $\sum_{i=1}^{n} F_i^2(a_n x + b_n) = o(1)$ as $n\to\infty$, we write

$$\sum_{i=1}^{n} F_i^2(a_n x + b_n) \le \left[\sum_{i=1}^{n} F_i(a_n x + b_n)\right] \sup_i F_i(a_n x + b_n) \to 0 \quad \text{as } n \to \infty, \quad \text{(A.38)}$$

because $\sum_{i=1}^{n} F_i(a_n x + b_n) \to e^x$ and

$$\sup_i F_i(a_n x + b_n) = \exp\left[-\inf_i \frac{\tau_i}{(a_n x + b_n)^\rho}\right] \le \exp\left[\frac{-\tau_0}{(a_n x + b_n)^\rho}\right] \to 0 \quad \text{as } n \to \infty.$$

$$\text{(A.39)}$$

This concludes the proof of Theorem 8.

Remark A.3. As examples, if $G(\tau)$ is the uniform distribution over the interval $[\tau_0, \ \tau_1]$, such that $g(\tau) = 1/(\tau_1 - \tau_0)$, we take from Equation A.30 b_n to satisfy $\log[n/(\tau_1 - \tau_0)] + \log b_n^\rho - (\tau_0/b_n^\rho) = 0$, and if $G(\tau)$ is the exponential distribution for $\tau > \tau_0$, such that $g(\tau) = \lambda e^{-\lambda(\tau - \tau_0)}$ and $g(\tau_0) = \lambda$, we take b_n to satisfy $\log(\lambda n) + \log b_n^\rho - (\tau_0/b_n^\rho) = 0$.

Remark A.4. The same result as in Theorem 8 would follow if we started with the assumption that $\{\tau_i\}$ is a realization of an i.i.d. sequence from the distribution function $G(\tau)$ with the same properties as in the theorem (proof omitted). Instead of specifying $G(\tau)$, we may equivalently specify a distribution for σ and let $G(\tau)$ be the distribution induced via the transformation $\tau = \sigma^\rho$.

Remark A.5. The exact c.d.f. of W_n displayed in Figure 2.9 in the case of varying τ_i arrayed in a uniform grid centered on τ_m is remarkably close to the exact c.d.f. of W_n in the i.i.d. case with constant $\tau_i = \tau_m$ (Fig. 2.7). See Figure A.1, which shows the two exact distributions for $n = 100, \ 500,$ and 1000. We explain why this should be so here, but note in passing that this already shows that under certain conditions, the limiting Gompertz distribution of W_n in the non-i.i.d. case can clearly be very close to that in the i.i.d. case.

For fixed n, τ_0, τ_1, and ρ, let $\tau_m = (\tau_0 + \tau_1)/2$ be the midpoint of the interval of support $[\tau_0, \tau_1]$ for G, and let w_{med} denote the median age at death in the i.i.d. case with $\tau = \tau_m$. From $P[W_n > w_{\text{med}}|\tau_m] = [1 - \exp(-\tau_m/w_{\text{med}}^\rho)]^n = 1/2$, we have $\exp(-\tau_m/w_{\text{med}}^\rho) = 1 - (1/2)^{1/n}$ and, explicitly, $w_{\text{med}} = \{\tau_m/-\log[1 - (1/2)^{1/n}]\}^{1/\rho}$. Also, let $\delta = \tau_1 - \tau_0$, so that $\tau_0 = \tau_m - \delta/2$, $\tau_1 = \tau_m + \delta/2$, and $\tau_i = \tau_0 + i(\delta/n)$ for $i = 1, \ldots, n$.

Now consider the ratio of survival probabilities in the uniform grid case to those in the i.i.d. case:

$$R_n(w) = \frac{P[W_n > w|\tau_i = \tau_0 + i\delta/n]}{P[W_n > w|\tau_i = \tau_m]} = \frac{\prod_{i=1}^{n}\left(1 - e^{-\tau_i/w^\rho}\right)}{(1 - e^{-\tau_m/w^\rho})^n}$$

$$= \prod_{i=1}^{n}\left(\frac{1 - e^{-\tau_i/w^\rho}}{1 - e^{-\tau_m/w^\rho}}\right) = \prod_{i=1}^{n}\left(1 - \frac{e^{-\tau_i/w^\rho} - e^{-\tau_m/w^\rho}}{1 - e^{-\tau_m/w^\rho}}\right). \quad \text{(A.40)}$$

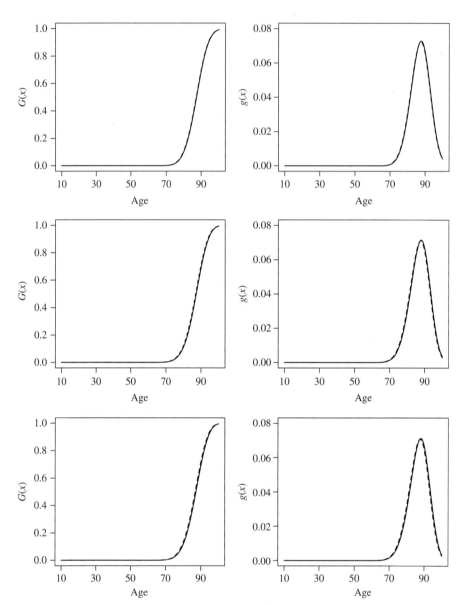

FIGURE A.1 Exact distributions of the minimum of i.i.d. (solid line) and nonidentically distributed (dashed line) random variables, whose parent distributions belong to a family of flat functions, for $n = 100$, 500, and 1000 (first, second, and third rows of graphs, respectively). Column of graphs at the left gives the c.d.f. and at the right gives the p.d.f.

Taking logs and assuming that $\exp(-\tau_0/w^\rho)$ is small, we have

$$-\log R_n(w) = \sum_{i=1}^{n} -\log\left(1 - \frac{e^{-\tau_i/w^\rho} - e^{-\tau_m/w^\rho}}{1 - e^{-\tau_m/w^\rho}}\right) \approx \sum_{i=1}^{n} \frac{e^{-\tau_i/w^\rho} - e^{-\tau_m/w^\rho}}{1 - e^{-\tau_m/w^\rho}},$$

ignoring higher-order terms, or

$$-\log R_n(w) \approx \left\{\frac{ne^{-\tau_m/w^\rho}}{1 - e^{-\tau_m/w^\rho}}\right\}\left\{\frac{1}{n}\sum_{i=1}^{n}\left[e^{-(\tau_i - \tau_m)/w^\rho} - 1\right]\right\}. \qquad (A.41)$$

Consider the first factor in braces at the median, $w = w_{\mathrm{med}}$. By definition of w_{med}, this factor equals $n(1 - (\tfrac{1}{2})^{1/n})/(\tfrac{1}{2})^{1/n} = n\,(2^{1/n} - 1) = n\{\exp[(\log 2)/n] - 1\} \approx \log 2$ for large n. The second factor in braces can be approximated by the integral $\int_{\tau_0}^{\tau_1}\left[e^{-(\tau - \tau_m)/w^\rho_{\mathrm{med}}} - 1\right]d\tau/\delta$. Changing variables to $u = (\tau - \tau_m)/\delta$ and letting $C = \delta/w^\rho_{\mathrm{med}}$, the integral equals

$$\int_{-1/2}^{1/2}\left[e^{-uC} - 1\right]du = \frac{e^{C/2} - e^{-C/2}}{C} - 1 = \frac{C^2}{24} + \frac{C^4}{1920} + \cdots + \frac{C^{2j}}{2^{2j}(2j+1)!} + \cdots \qquad (A.42)$$

This is a rapidly convergent series that is small if C^2 is not too large, say, less than 1.

In Figure A.1, the median residual age at death after 10 years is approximately $w_{\mathrm{med}} = 77.3$ years in each panel, and the values of C are 0.995, 1.316, and 1.455 for $n = 100$, 500, and 1000, respectively. So even though C^2 is not small, the integral is approximately $C^2/24 = 0.0413$, 0.0722, and 0.0882, respectively; $-\log R_n(w_{\mathrm{med}}) \approx \log 2 \cdot C^2/24$ is approximately 0.0286, 0.0500, and 0.0611, respectively; and $R_n(w_{\mathrm{med}}) = \exp[-\log R_n(w_{\mathrm{med}})]$ is approximately 0.972, 0.951, and 0.941, respectively. The exact values of $R_n(w_{\mathrm{med}})$ are 0.975, 0.951, and 0.940, respectively, suggesting that the i.i.d. a_n and b_n provide a reasonable approximation. The ratio $R_n(w_{\mathrm{med}})$ moves away from 1 as n increases in this illustration because selecting τ_m and ρ so as to keep the approximating Gompertz distribution fixed with a support width of $\delta = 0.2\tau_m$ causes C to increase.

In general, as w increases above w_{med}, the first term in braces increases, and for large w approximately linearly so, since the first factor is approximately $n(1 - \tau_m/w^\rho)/(\tau_m/w^\rho) = n[(w^\rho/\tau_m) - 1]$, while the second term decreases as $w^{-2\rho}$, whence $-\log R_n(m) \to 0$ for large w. As w decreases below w_{med}, the first term in braces decreases exponentially as $ne^{-\tau_m/w^\rho}$, while the second term grows as $w^\rho e^{\delta/w^\rho}/\delta$. So if $\tau_m \geq \delta$, the product decreases as $w^\rho e^{-(\tau_m - \delta)/w^\rho}$ as $w \to 0$, hence $-\log R_n(w) \to 0$ as $w \to 0$.

The preceding calculation implies that the absolute difference between the two c.d.f.'s at the median is not more than about 0.03, hardly noticeable in the graph, with smaller differences elsewhere.

Remark A.6. Although Theorem 8 demonstrates convergence of $(W_n - b_n)/a_n$ to a Gumbel distribution, there is no reason to believe that the particular choice of a_n and b_n given in the theorem is the best choice to approximate the exact c.d.f. $P[W_n \le w]$. In fact, Remark A.5 showed that the exact c.d.f. of W_n in the case of a uniform grid of τ, namely, $\tau_i = \tau_0 + i(\tau_1 - \tau_0)/n$, is remarkably well approximated by the exact c.d.f. of W_n in the i.i.d. case with $\tau = \tau_m = (\tau_1 + \tau_0)/2$ so long as $(\tau_1 - \tau_0)/w_{med}^\rho$ is small. This suggests that the choice of a_n and b_n for the i.i.d. case may, under certain circumstances, provide a better approximation of the exact c.d.f. in the uniform grid case, and Figure 2.8 and Figure 2.9 show this to be the case.

To see this in somewhat greater generality, consider any family of flat distributions parameterized by τ such that $\phi_\tau(x) = -\log F_\tau(x) = \tau\phi(x)$ for some fixed function $\phi(x)$ with $\phi'(x) \to -\infty$ and with $\psi(x) = -1/\phi'(x)$, $\psi'(x) \to 0$ as $x \to 0$. Suppose that the distribution G of τ is supported on a bounded interval $[\tau_0, \tau_1]$ with $\tau_0 > 0$ and width $\delta = \tau_1 - \tau_0$. Let $E\tau = \int_{\tau_0}^{\tau_0 + \delta} \tau dG(\tau)$ denote the mean value of τ under G, and analogous to the previous definition, let w_{med} denote the median age at death in the i.i.d. case with τ fixed at value $E\tau$. (In the development given previously, $\phi(x) = 1/x^\rho$, G was uniform on $[\tau_0, \tau_1]$, and we used the midpoint $E\tau = \tau_m$; the exact median age at death w_{med} in the i.i.d. case with τ fixed at value $E\tau$ was approximately equal to that of the approximating Gompertz distribution.)

Then, in place of Equation A.34, we have the approximation

$$-\log P[W_n > w] \approx n \int_{\tau_0}^{\tau_1} \exp\left\{ \left[-\phi(b_n) + \frac{xa_n}{\psi(a_n)} \right] \tau \right\} dG(\tau). \qquad (A.43)$$

Now take $a_n = \psi(b_n)/E\tau$, in which case the approximation becomes

$$-\log P[W_n > w] \approx n \int_{\tau_0}^{\tau_1} \exp\left\{ [-E\tau \cdot \phi(b_n) + x] \frac{\tau}{E\tau} \right\} dG(\tau). \qquad (A.44)$$

Change variables to $u = (\tau - E\tau)/\delta$ to re-express the approximation as

$$-\log P[W_n > w] \approx n \int_{u_0}^{u_1} \exp\left\{ [-E\tau \cdot \phi(b_n) + x] \left(1 + \frac{\delta}{E\tau} u \right) \right\} dG(E\tau + \delta u)$$

$$= \{ n \exp[-E\tau \cdot \phi(b_n)] \} e^x \int_{u_0}^{u_1} \exp(-Cu) dG(E\tau + \delta u), \qquad (A.45)$$

where $C = [E\tau \cdot \phi(b_n) - x](\delta/E\tau)$, $u_0 = (\tau_0 - E\tau)/\delta < 0$, and $u_1 = (\tau_1 - E\tau)/\delta > 0$. Note that $u_1 - u_0 = 1$. Now choose b_n such that the leading term in braces equals 1, that is, such that $E\tau \cdot \phi(b_n) = \log n$, in which case

$$C = [(\log n) - x]\frac{\delta}{E\tau}. \qquad (A.46)$$

Finally, expanding $\exp(-Cu)$ and integrating term by term, we have

$$\int_{u_0}^{u_1} \exp(-Cu)dG(E\tau + \delta u) = \int_{u_0}^{u_1}\left(1 - Cu + \frac{C^2u^2}{2} + \cdots\right)dG(E\tau + \delta u)$$

$$= 1 + \frac{(C^2/2)(\mathrm{Var}\tau)}{\delta^2} + \cdots \qquad (A.47)$$

since $u_1 - u_0 = 1$, $\displaystyle\int_{u_0}^{u_1} udG(E\tau + \delta u) = \int_{\tau_0}^{\tau_1}(\tau - E\tau)/\delta dG(\tau) = 0$, and $\displaystyle\int_{u_0}^{u_1} u^2 dG(E\tau + \delta u) =$

$\displaystyle\int_{\tau_0}^{\tau_1}[(\tau - E\tau)/\delta]^2 dG(\tau) = (\mathrm{Var}\tau)/\delta^2$. Thus, if C is small, say, $C < 1$, the integral will

be approximately equal to 1, and so we conclude that $-\log P[W_n > w] \approx e^x$ as desired. Note that in all cases, $(\mathrm{Var}\,\tau)/\delta^2 \le 1/4$ by Popoviciu's inequality (Popoviciu, 1935); $(\mathrm{Var}\,\tau)/\delta^2 = 1/12$ for uniformly distributed τ.

When is C small enough for a reasonable approximation in the scenario portrayed in Figure 2.9? In these graphs, $b_n = 79.193$ and $a_n = 5.294$. Thus, for values of $w > 79.2$, we have $x > 0$, and since we chose $\delta/E\tau = 0.2$, from Equation A.46, we see that C is no greater than about 1.4. Because $(C^2/2)(\mathrm{Var}\,\tau)/\delta^2 = C^2/24$, the relative error is no greater than about 8%. At the median age $w_{\mathrm{med}} = 77.3$, C is no greater than about 1.45, and the relative error is no greater than about 9%. For values of w below w_{med}, the relative error grows, but the absolute error is maximized at about 0.04 around age 75. Note that by definition of w_{med}, $\left(1 - e^{-E\tau \cdot \phi(w_{\mathrm{med}})}\right)^n = 1/2$, so that

$$E\tau = \frac{-\log\left[1 - (1/2)^{1/n}\right]}{\phi(w_{\mathrm{med}})} = \frac{-\log\{1 - \exp[-(\log 2)/n]\}}{\phi(w_{\mathrm{med}})} \approx \frac{\log(n/\log 2)}{\phi(w_{\mathrm{med}})}, \qquad (A.48)$$

in which case $C = \delta\dfrac{(\log n) - x}{E\tau} \approx \delta\phi(w_{\mathrm{med}})\dfrac{(\log n) - x}{(\log n) - \log\log 2} \approx \delta\phi(w_{\mathrm{med}})$ for w

around w_{med} (because x is approximately log log 2 there) or for n large enough for x and log log 2 to be negligible compared to log n. Thus, $C < 1$ roughly when the width of the support interval satisfies $\delta < 1/\phi(w_{\mathrm{med}})$. Finally, we observe that if C is not small, then the scaling and centering constants a_n and b_n given by Theorem 8 may provide the better approximation.

Proof of Theorem 9. $P[W_n > a_n x + b_n] = \left[1 - \dfrac{nF_1(a_n x + b_n)}{n}\right]^{np_1 + o(n)} \times$

$\left[1 - \dfrac{nF_2(a_n x + b_n)}{n}\right]^{n(1-p_1)+o(n)}$. We take $b_n = F_1^{-1}(1/n)$ and $a_n = \psi_1(b_n)$, so that, from the Lemma, the first term approaches a Gumbel-type limiting distribution of the form $\exp(-p_1 e^x)$ as $n \to \infty$. Here, we have used the fact that $[1-(e^x+o(1))/n]^{o(n)} \to 1$ as $n \to \infty$, which can easily be seen by taking logarithms and noting that $\lim_{n\to\infty} (o(n)/n)n\log [1-(e^x+o(1))/n]$. is the product of two limits, one zero and the other finite. So we have to show that $nF_2(a_n x + b_n)$ is $o(1)$ as $n \to \infty$ or, equivalently,

$$\log n - \phi_2(a_n x + b_n) \to -\infty \text{ as } n \to \infty. \tag{A.49}$$

Using the MVT,

$$\log n - \phi_2(a_n x + b_n) = \log n - \phi_2(b_n) + \frac{a_n x}{\psi_2(b_n + a_n x t_n)} \quad \text{for some } 0 < t_n < 1. \tag{A.50}$$

Using the MVT again, we write

$$\psi_2(b_n + a_n x t_n) = \psi_2(b_n) + \psi_2'\left(b_n + a_n x t_n t_n^*\right) a_n x t_n \quad \text{for some } 0 < t_n^* < 1, \tag{A.51}$$

where the second term goes to 0 as $n \to \infty$ by the von Mises condition. Thus, as $n \to \infty$,

$$\log n - \phi_2(a_n x + b_n) \approx \log n - \phi_2(b_n) + \frac{a_n x}{\psi_2(b_n)} = \phi_1(b_n) - \phi_2(b_n) + x\frac{\psi_1(b_n)}{\psi_2(b_n)}. \tag{A.52}$$

If $\rho_2 > \rho_1$, $F_i(x) = \exp(-\tau_i/x^{\rho_i})$, $\phi_i(x) = \tau_i x^{-\rho_i}$, $\phi_i'(x) = -\rho_i \tau_i x^{-(\rho_i+1)}$, and $\psi_i(x) = x^{\rho_i+1}/\rho_i \tau_i$. Since $b_n = F_1^{-1}(1/n) = (\tau_1/\log n)^{1/\rho_1}$ and $\tau_1 b_n^{-\rho_1} = \log n$, the first two terms on the right-hand side of Equation A.52 become

$$\phi_1(b_n) - \phi_2(b_n) = \tau_1 b_n^{-\rho_1} - \tau_2 b_n^{-\rho_2} = \log n - \tau_2 \tau_1^{\rho_1/\rho_2}\left(\tau_1 b_n^{-\rho_1}\right)^{\rho_2/\rho_1}$$

$$= \log n - \tau_2 \tau_1^{\rho_1/\rho_2}(\log n)^{\rho_2/\rho_1}, \tag{A.53}$$

and the third term becomes

$$x\frac{\psi_1(b_n)}{\psi_2(b_n)} = x\frac{b_n^{\rho_1+1}}{\rho_1\tau_1}\frac{\rho_2\tau_2}{b_n^{\rho_2+1}} = x\frac{\rho_2\tau_2}{\rho_1\tau_1}b_n^{\rho_1-\rho_2} = x\frac{\rho_2\tau_2}{\rho_1\tau_1}\left(b_n^{-\rho_1}\right)^{(\rho_2/\rho_1)-1}$$

$$= x\frac{\rho_2\tau_2}{\rho_1\tau_1}\left(\frac{\log n}{\tau_1}\right)^{(\rho_2/\rho_1)-1}. \tag{A.54}$$

Putting Equations A.53 and A.54 together, Equation A.52 becomes

$$\phi_1(b_n) - \phi_2(b_n) + x\frac{\psi_1(b_n)}{\psi_2(b_n)} = \log n - \tau_2\tau_1^{\rho_1/\rho_2}(\log n)^{(\rho_2/\rho_1)} + x\frac{\rho_2\tau_2}{\rho_1\tau_1}\left(\frac{\log n}{\tau_1}\right)^{(\rho_2/\rho_1)-1}.$$

$$(A.55)$$

Since $\rho_2 > \rho_1$, Equation A.55 goes to $-\infty$ as $n \to \infty$, because $\rho_2/\rho_1 > \rho_2/\rho_1 - 1$ and $\rho_2/\rho_1 > 1$. This concludes the proof of Theorem 9.

Proof of Theorem 10. $P[W_n > a_n x] = [1 - F_1(a_n x)]^{np_1 + o(n)}[1 - F_2(a_n x)]^{n(1-p_1) + o(n)}$. If we take $a_n = F_1^{-1}(1/n)$ and use the fact that the regularly varying function $F_i(x)$ meets the necessary and sufficient condition for an initial distribution to be in minimum domain of attraction of the Weibull-type limiting distribution (Eq. 2.21), we can write

$$[1 - F_1(a_n x)]^{np_1 + o(n)}[1 - F_2(a_n x)]^{n(1-p_1) + o(n)} = \left[1 - \frac{F_1(a_n x)}{F_1(a_n)}F_1(a_n)\right]^{np_1 + o(n)}$$

$$\times \left[1 - \frac{F_2(a_n x)}{F_2(a_n)}F_2(a_n)\right]^{n(1-p_1) + o(n)}$$

$$= \left[1 - \frac{x^{\rho_1} + o(1)}{n}\right]^{np_1 + o(n)}\left[1 - \frac{x^{\rho_2} + o(1)}{n}nF_2(a_n)\right]^{n(1-p_1) + o(n)}. \qquad (A.56)$$

The first term $[1 - (x^{\rho_1} + o(1))/n]^{np_1 + o(n)} = \{[1 - (x^{\rho_1} + o(1))/n]^n\}^{p_1 + o(1)} \to \exp(-p_1 x^{\rho_1})$ as $n \to \infty$. So we want the second term $[1 - ((x^{\rho_2} + o(1))/n) \, nF_2(a_n)]^{n(1-p_1) + o(n)} \to \exp(0) = 1$, for which it suffices to show that $F_2(a_n) = o(1/n)$ as $n \to \infty$. Now we write

$$F_2(x) = x^{\rho_2}L(x) = x^{\rho_2 - \rho_1}x^{\rho_1}L(x) = x^{\rho_2 - \rho_1}F_1(x). \qquad (A.57)$$

From taking $a_n = F_1^{-1}(1/n)$,

$$F_2(a_n) = a_n^{\rho_2 - \rho_1}F_1(a_n) = \frac{a_n^{\rho_2 - \rho_1}}{n}, \qquad (A.58)$$

which is $o(1/n)$ as $n \to \infty$ because $a_n \to 0$ for n sufficiently large and $\rho_2 > \rho_1$. This concludes the proof of Theorem 10.

APPENDIX B

DERIVATION OF HAMILTON'S EQUATION FOR THE FORCE OF NATURAL SELECTION ON MORTALITY

We start with a derivation of the Euler–Lotka equation, which was developed for describing population growth (Lotka, 1907, 1913). Crow and Kimura (1970, pp. 3–20) defined four deterministic models of population growth: discrete nonoverlapping generations (model 1); continuous random births and deaths (model 2); overlapping generations, discrete time intervals (model 3); and overlapping generations, continuous change (model 4). The Euler–Lotka equation pertains to model 4, in which, unlike in model 3, the process of population change occurs in a continuum of time and, unlike in model 2, individuals are not regarded as equally likely to die or reproduce at all times. We consider how the Malthusian parameter m relates to a measure of fitness applicable to the simple model of population growth for discrete nonoverlapping generations or model 1 (Crow and Kimura, 1970, pp. 5–6). Let N_t be the number of individuals in the population at time t, measured in generations, and w or the Darwinian fitness be the average number of progeny per individual. The population number in generation t can be expressed in terms of the number in the previous generation, $t - 1$, by $N_t = wN_{t-1}$. The relation between N_{t-1} and N_{t-2} is the same as that between N_t and N_{t-1}. If w remains constant, we can write $N_t = w(wN_{t-2}) = w^2 N_{t-2}$. Continuing this process, we obtain

$$N_t = N_0 w^t, \tag{B.1}$$

The Biostatistics of Aging: From Gompertzian Mortality to an Index of Aging-Relatedness,
First Edition. Gilberto Levy and Bruce Levin.
© 2014 John Wiley & Sons, Inc. Published 2014 by John Wiley & Sons, Inc.

where N_0 is the population size in generation 0. In a model of population growth occurring in a continuum of time (e.g., model 2), N_t is the number of individuals in the population at continuous time t, and m represents the instantaneous rate of increase in population size; that is, $dN_t/dt = mN_t$. This implies that the rate of growth of the population is proportional to the population size at any given moment and gives

$$N_t = N_0 e^{mt}, \tag{B.2}$$

where N_0 is the population size at time 0. From Equations B.1 and B.2, the relation between w and m is $w = e^m \Rightarrow m = \log w$ (Crow and Kimura, 1970, pp. 7–11).

We now consider model 4. Equation B.2 is applicable to model 4 when the population has achieved age distribution stability, and N_0 is the population size after enough time has elapsed to achieve a stable age distribution. Following Crow and Kimura (1970, pp. 17–20), if $l(x)$ is the probability of survival from birth to age x (i.e., the survival function) and $b(x)$ is the instantaneous birth rate (or rate of reproduction) at age x, the probability of reproducing during the infinitesimal age interval from x to $x + dx$ is $b(x)dx$, and the probability of living to age x and reproducing during the next time interval dx is $l(x)b(x)dx$. The expected number of offspring per individual for the whole lifetime is this quantity summed over all ages, which is called the net reproduction rate and denoted R_0 (Charlesworth, 1994, p. 29; Roff, 2008):

$$R_0 = \int_0^\infty l(x)b(x)dx. \tag{B.3}$$

Now, let the number of births occurring in the infinitesimal interval dt be $B(t)dt$; that is, $B(t)$ is the instantaneous birth rate at time t. Of the population alive at time t, those of age x were born at time $t - x$, when the birth rate was $B(t - x)$. Of those born at that time, a fraction $l(x)$ will still be alive, and of these, a fraction $b(x)dx$ will give birth during the interval dx. Thus, the current birth rate of persons of age x at time t will be $B(t - x)l(x)b(x)$, and this summed over all ages is the total birth rate at time t:

$$B(t) = \int_0^\infty B(t-x)l(x)b(x)dx. \tag{B.4}$$

A population with a constant set of age-specific birth and death rates eventually achieves a stable age distribution, and in this state, the population size will increase or decrease at a constant rate (Lotka, 1922). If the population has achieved a stable age distribution, its size (and therefore its birth rate) is increasing at the instantaneous rate m. In x years, the birth rate will have increased by a factor e^{mx} (see Eq. B.2). Thus, the rate x years ago was a fraction e^{-mx} of the current rate:

$$B(t-x) = B(t)e^{-mx}. \tag{B.5}$$

Substituting this in Equation B.4 and canceling $B(t)$ on both sides of the equation, we obtain the Euler–Lotka equation,

$$\int_0^\infty e^{-mx} l(x) b(x) dx = 1, \tag{B.6}$$

whose analogue for discrete age classes is

$$\sum_{x=1}^\infty e^{-mx} l(x) b(x) = 1. \tag{B.7}$$

A similar derivation, following Stearns (1992, p. 24) and Roff (2002, p. 68), can be given in terms of the total number of newborns at time t to females in a population, denoted $N(t)$. The number of newborns contributed by females of age x can be obtained by the product of the number of newborn females at time $t - x$, their probability of survival to age x, and the probability of reproducing during an infinitesimal interval dx, which gives $N(t-x) l(x) b(x) dx$. We can then obtain the total number of newborns at time t by summing over all ages:

$$N(t) = \int_0^\infty N(t-x) l(x) b(x) dx. \tag{B.8}$$

If the population is growing exponentially at a constant rate m,

$$N(t) = N(t-x) e^{mx} \Rightarrow N(t-x) = N(t) e^{-mx}. \tag{B.9}$$

Substituting this in Equation B.8, and canceling $N(t)$ on both sides, gives again Equation B.6.

We now derive Hamilton's equation for the force of natural selection on mortality. Defining the survival function $l(x)$ as $l(x) = p(0)p(1)p(2) \cdots p(x-1)$, where $p(x)$ gives the proportion of population members who have already reached age x who then reach age $x + 1$, we see that the age-specific $p(x)$ values act multiplicatively to determine $l(x)$; hence, they act additively on $\log l(x)$:

$$\log l(x) = \sum_{j=0}^{x-1} \log p(j) \Rightarrow l(x) = e^{\sum_{j=0}^{x-1} \log p(j)}. \tag{B.10}$$

Substituting this in the Euler–Lotka equation for discrete age classes (Eq. B.7), we obtain

$$\sum_{x=1}^\infty e^{-mx + \sum_{j=0}^{x-1} \log p(j)} b(x) = 1, \tag{B.11}$$

which defines m as an implicit function of $\log p(j)$. Then, the partial derivative of m with respect to the logarithm of $p(x)$ at a given age a can be obtained as follows:

$$\frac{\partial}{\partial \log p(a)} \left[\sum_{x=1}^{\infty} e^{-mx + \sum_{j=0}^{x-1} \log p(j)} b(x) \right] = 0$$

$$\Rightarrow \sum_{x=1}^{\infty} \left[e^{-mx} \frac{\partial}{\partial \log p(a)} e^{\sum_{j=0}^{x-1} \log p(j)} b(x) + e^{\sum_{j=0}^{x-1} \log p(j)} \frac{\partial}{\partial \log p(a)} e^{-mx} b(x) \right] = 0$$

$$\Rightarrow \sum_{x=a+1}^{\infty} e^{-mx} l(x) b(x) + \sum_{x=1}^{\infty} e^{\sum_{j=0}^{x-1} \log p(j)} \frac{\partial}{\partial m} e^{-mx} \frac{\partial m}{\partial \log p(a)} b(x) = 0$$

$$\Rightarrow \sum_{x=a+1}^{\infty} e^{-mx} l(x) b(x) - \sum_{x=1}^{\infty} x e^{-mx} l(x) b(x) \frac{\partial m}{\partial \log p(a)} = 0$$

$$\Rightarrow \frac{\partial m}{\partial \log p(a)} = \frac{\sum_{x=a+1}^{\infty} e^{-mx} l(x) b(x)}{\sum_{x=1}^{\infty} x e^{-mx} l(x) b(x)}. \tag{B.12}$$

The age-specific survival probabilities $p(x)$ at age a depend on the instantaneous death rates (or the force of mortality), denoted $\mu(x)$ in the notation of life tables, between ages a and $a + 1$, through the equation

$$p(a) = \exp\left[-\int_a^{a+1} \mu(x) dx \right] = \exp[-\bar{\mu}(a)], \tag{B.13}$$

where $\bar{\mu}(a)$ is the average mortality in the interval between ages a and $a + 1$ (Baudisch, 2005). This gives $\log p(a) = -\bar{\mu}(a)$ and implies that Equation B.12 can also be expressed as

$$-\frac{\partial m}{\partial \bar{\mu}(a)} = \frac{\sum_{x=a+1}^{\infty} e^{-mx} l(x) b(x)}{\sum_{x=1}^{\infty} x e^{-mx} l(x) b(x)}. \tag{B.14}$$

The corresponding formula for the continuous case, given in Charlesworth (2000), is

$$-\frac{\partial m}{\partial \mu(a)} = \frac{\int_a^{\infty} e^{-mx} l(x) b(x) dx}{\int_0^{\infty} x e^{-mx} l(x) b(x) dx}. \tag{B.15}$$

APPENDIX C

SOME PROPERTIES OF THE GOMPERTZ AND WEIBULL DISTRIBUTIONS

Here, $\lambda > 0$ and θ are parameters of the Gompertz distribution, and $\alpha > 0$ and $\gamma > 0$ are parameters of the Weibull distribution. The hazard and cumulative hazard functions of the Gompertz distribution are given by, respectively,

$$h_G(x) = \lambda e^{\theta x}, \tag{C.1}$$

$$H_G(x) = \int_0^x h_G(y)dy = \int_0^x \lambda e^{\theta y} dy = \frac{\lambda}{\theta}\left(e^{\theta x} - 1\right). \tag{C.2}$$

Then, the Gompertz survival function, c.d.f., and p.d.f. are, respectively,

$$S_G(x) = \exp[-H_G(x)] = \exp\left[-\frac{\lambda}{\theta}\left(e^{\theta x} - 1\right)\right], \tag{C.3}$$

$$F_G(x) = 1 - S_G(x) = 1 - \exp\left[-\frac{\lambda}{\theta}\left(e^{\theta x} - 1\right)\right], \tag{C.4}$$

$$f_G(x) = h_G(x)S_G(x) = \lambda e^{\theta x}\exp\left[-\frac{\lambda}{\theta}\left(e^{\theta x} - 1\right)\right]. \tag{C.5}$$

The hazard and cumulative hazard functions of the Weibull distribution are, respectively,

The Biostatistics of Aging: From Gompertzian Mortality to an Index of Aging-Relatedness,
First Edition. Gilberto Levy and Bruce Levin.
© 2014 John Wiley & Sons, Inc. Published 2014 by John Wiley & Sons, Inc.

$$h_W(x) = \alpha \gamma x^{\gamma - 1},$$
(C.6)

$$H_W(x) = \alpha x^\gamma.$$
(C.7)

The Weibull survival function, c.d.f., and p.d.f. are, respectively,

$$S_W(x) = \exp(-\alpha x^\gamma),$$
(C.8)

$$F_W(x) = 1 - \exp(-\alpha x^\gamma),$$
(C.9)

$$f_W(x) = \alpha \gamma x^{\gamma - 1} \exp(-\alpha x^\gamma).$$
(C.10)

The life expectancy or mean survival time of the Gompertz distribution can be obtained using the following steps:

$$E_G[X] = \int_0^\infty x f_G(x) dx = \int_0^\infty x \lambda e^{\theta x} \exp\left[-\frac{\lambda}{\theta}\left(e^{\theta x} - 1\right)\right] dx = \lambda e^{\lambda/\theta} \int_0^\infty x e^{\theta x} e^{-(\lambda/\theta)e^{\theta x}} dx$$

(by substituting $y = (\lambda/\theta)e^{\theta x} \Rightarrow dy/dx = \lambda e^{\theta x} \Rightarrow dy/\lambda = e^{\theta x} dx$ and $y = (\lambda/\theta)e^{\theta x} \Rightarrow x = (1/\theta)\log[(\theta/\lambda)y]$, which also changes the lower limit of integration)

$$= \lambda e^{\lambda/\theta} \int_{\lambda/\theta}^\infty \frac{1}{\theta} \log\left(\frac{\theta}{\lambda} y\right) e^{-y} \frac{dy}{\lambda} = \frac{e^{\lambda/\theta}}{\theta} \int_{\lambda/\theta}^\infty \log\left(\frac{\theta}{\lambda} y\right) e^{-y} dy$$

(by integration by parts with $u = \log[(\theta/\lambda)y] \Rightarrow du = (1/y)dy$ and $dv = e^{-y} dy \Rightarrow v = -e^{-y}$)

$$= \frac{e^{\lambda/\theta}}{\theta} \left\{ \left[\log\left(\frac{\theta}{\lambda} y\right)(-e^{-y})\right]_{y=\lambda/\theta}^{y=\infty} + \int_{\lambda/\theta}^\infty e^{-y} \frac{1}{y} dy \right\} = \frac{e^{\lambda/\theta}}{\theta} \int_{\lambda/\theta}^\infty y^{-1} e^{-y} dy.$$
(C.11)

The integral in the formula is the exponential integral, which is tabulated for different values of the lower limit of integration (represented by λ/θ in Eq. C.11) by Abramowitz and Stegun (1972, chapter 5). The median survival time of the Gompertz distribution is obtained by setting $S_G(x_{50})$ equal to 1/2, which gives

$$x_{50} = \frac{1}{\theta} \log\left(1 + \frac{\theta}{\lambda} \log 2\right).$$
(C.12)

We can similarly obtain the mean and median of the Weibull distribution as, respectively,

$$E_W[X] = \alpha^{-1/\gamma} \Gamma\left(\gamma^{-1} + 1\right),$$
(C.13)

$$x_{50} = \left(\frac{1}{\alpha} \log 2\right)^{1/\gamma},$$
(C.14)

where $\Gamma(x) = \int_0^\infty y^{x-1} e^{-y} dy$ is the gamma function.

A commonly used quantity of interest for the Gompertz distribution with $\theta > 0$ is the MRDT, which is measured in the same unit as x. By setting

$$\frac{h_G(x + \text{MRDT})}{h_G(x)} = \frac{\lambda e^{\theta(x + \text{MRDT})}}{\lambda e^{\theta x}} = 2 \Rightarrow \exp[\theta(x + \text{MRDT} - x)] = 2$$

$$\Rightarrow \text{MRDT} = \frac{\log 2}{\theta}.$$

(C.15)

Hence, the mortality rate doubles after $(\log 2)/\theta$ units of time. Note that the MRDT depends on θ but not on λ or x. An analogous quantity for the Weibull distribution with $\gamma > 1$ would be given by the solution to

$$\frac{h_W(x + \text{MRDT})}{h_W(x)} = \frac{\alpha\gamma(x + \text{MRDT})^{\gamma-1}}{\alpha\gamma x^{\gamma-1}} = 2 \Rightarrow \frac{(x + \text{MRDT})^{\gamma-1}}{x^{\gamma-1}} = 2$$

$$\Rightarrow \text{MRDT} = x\left(2^{1/(\gamma-1)} - 1\right),$$

(C.16)

which depends on γ and x.

An important property of the Gompertz distribution is that truncating a Gompertz distribution at x_0 and setting the origin at x_0 leaves the form of the distribution unchanged, except for λ, which changes to $\lambda' = \lambda e^{\theta x_0}$ (Garg et al., 1970). That is, if X is distributed as Gompertz (λ, θ), $X' = X - x_0$ is distributed as Gompertz $\left(\lambda' = \lambda e^{\theta x_0}, \theta\right)$, because

$$\frac{S_G(x)}{S_G(x_0)} = \frac{\exp\left[-(\lambda/\theta)\left(e^{\theta x} - 1\right)\right]}{\exp\left[-(\lambda/\theta)\left(e^{\theta x_0} - 1\right)\right]} = \exp\left[-\frac{\lambda}{\theta}\left(e^{\theta x} - e^{\theta x_0}\right)\right]$$

$$= \exp\left[-\frac{\lambda e^{\theta x_0}}{\theta}\left(e^{\theta(x - x_0)} - 1\right)\right] = \exp\left[-\frac{\lambda'}{\theta}\left(e^{\theta x'} - 1\right)\right] = S_G(x'),$$

(C.17)

where $x' = x - x_0$ and $\lambda' = \lambda e^{\theta x_0}$. On the other hand, unlike for the Gompertz distribution, if X is distributed as Weibull (α, γ), $X' = X - x_0$ does not have a Weibull distribution, because

$$\frac{S_W(x)}{S_W(x_0)} = \frac{\exp(-\alpha x^\gamma)}{\exp(-\alpha x_0^\gamma)} = \exp\left[-\alpha(x^\gamma - x_0^\gamma)\right],$$

(C.18)

which cannot be put in the form of the Weibull survival function.

The point of inflection of the Gompertz survival function is obtained by taking the second derivative of Equation C.3 and setting it equal to 0:

$$\frac{d^2 S_G(x)}{dx^2} = -\lambda \exp\left[\theta x - \frac{\lambda}{\theta}\left(e^{\theta x} - 1\right)\right]\left(\theta - \lambda e^{\theta x}\right),$$

(C.19)

which is equal to 0 if and only if the third multiplicative term is equal to 0 or

$$\theta = \lambda e^{\theta \tilde{x}}, \tag{C.20}$$

where $\tilde{x}$ is the point of inflection. There is no solution for Equation C.20 in terms of $\tilde{x}$ if $\theta \le 0$, so there is no point of inflection if $\theta \le 0$. If $\theta > 0$, the point of inflection occurs at

$$\tilde{x} = \frac{1}{\theta} \log\left(\frac{\theta}{\lambda}\right). \tag{C.21}$$

From Equation C.21, since x cannot be negative, there is no point of inflection if $\theta < \lambda$. Thus, there only exists a point of inflection if $\theta > \lambda$ and, from Equation C.20, the hazard rate at the point of inflection is θ (Garg et al., 1970). Moreover, from $S'(x) = -f(x)$ and $S''(x) = -f'(x)$,

$$S''(\tilde{x}) = 0 \Rightarrow f'(\tilde{x}) = 0; \tag{C.22}$$

that is, the point of inflection of the survival function corresponds to the mode of the distribution. This shows that θ is the hazard rate at the point of inflection of the Gompertz survival function as well as at the modal age of the distribution, as we also demonstrate in Section 5.1.

To obtain the point of inflection of the Weibull survival function, we take the second derivative of Equation C.8:

$$\frac{d^2 S_W(x)}{dx^2} = -\alpha \gamma \exp(-\alpha x^\gamma) \left[x^{2\gamma - 2}(-\alpha \gamma) + x^{\gamma - 2}(\gamma - 1) \right], \tag{C.23}$$

which is equal to 0 if and only if the term in square brackets is equal to 0 or

$$\tilde{x}^{2\gamma - 2}(-\alpha \gamma) + \tilde{x}^{\gamma - 2}(\gamma - 1) = 0, \tag{C.24}$$

where $\tilde{x}$ is the point of inflection. There is no solution for Equation C.24 in terms of $\tilde{x}$ if $0 < \gamma \le 1$, so there is no point of inflection if $0 < \gamma \le 1$. If $\gamma > 1$, the point of inflection occurs at

$$\tilde{x} = \left(\frac{\gamma - 1}{\alpha \gamma}\right)^{1/\gamma}. \tag{C.25}$$

Note also that, from Equation C.25,

$$\alpha \gamma \tilde{x}^{\gamma - 1} = \frac{\gamma - 1}{\tilde{x}}; \tag{C.26}$$

that is, the hazard rate at the point of inflection for the Weibull distribution depends on γ and on the value of the point of inflection itself (which in turn depends on α and γ).

Point estimation procedures for the parameters of the Gompertz and Weibull distributions are given in Appendix E.

APPENDIX D

FIRST AND SECOND PARTIAL DERIVATIVES OF THE MIXTURE LOG-LIKELIHOOD FUNCTION

To present the formulas for the first and second partial derivatives of the mixture log-likelihood function (Eq. 4.24) with respect to the five parameters μ, θ, β, γ, and Λ, we initially obtain, from the general form of the likelihood function

$$L(\mu,\theta,\beta,\gamma,\Lambda) = \prod_{i=1}^{n} \left\{ f(x_i)^{\delta_i} S(x_i)^{1-\delta_i} / S(a_i) \right\},$$

$$\log L(\mu,\theta,\beta,\gamma,\Lambda) = \sum_{i=1}^{n} \left\{ \delta_i \log f(x_i) + (1-\delta_i) \log S(x_i) - \log S(a_i) \right\}. \qquad \text{(D.1)}$$

Then, using the notation $f_\mu(x) = \partial f(x)/\partial\mu$, $f_\theta(x) = \partial f(x)/\partial\theta$, ...,

$$\frac{\partial \log L(\mu,\theta,\beta,\gamma,\Lambda)}{\partial \mu} = \sum_{i=1}^{n} \left\{ \delta_i \frac{f_\mu(x_i)}{f(x_i)} + (1-\delta_i) \frac{S_\mu(x_i)}{S(x_i)} - \frac{S_\mu(a_i)}{S(a_i)} \right\}, \qquad \text{(D.2)}$$

$$\frac{\partial \log L(\mu,\theta,\beta,\gamma,\Lambda)}{\partial \theta} = \sum_{i=1}^{n} \left\{ \delta_i \frac{f_\theta(x_i)}{f(x_i)} + (1-\delta_i) \frac{S_\theta(x_i)}{S(x_i)} - \frac{S_\theta(a_i)}{S(a_i)} \right\}, \qquad \text{(D.3)}$$

and similarly for the partial derivatives of the log-likelihood function with respect to β, γ, and Λ. For the second partial derivatives, using the notation $f_{\mu\mu}(x) = \partial^2 f(x)/\partial\mu\partial\mu$, $f_{\mu\theta}(x) = \partial^2 f(x)/\partial\mu\partial\theta$, ...,

The Biostatistics of Aging: From Gompertzian Mortality to an Index of Aging-Relatedness,
First Edition. Gilberto Levy and Bruce Levin.
© 2014 John Wiley & Sons, Inc. Published 2014 by John Wiley & Sons, Inc.

$$\frac{\partial^2 \log L(\mu,\theta,\beta,\gamma,\Lambda)}{\partial \mu^2} = \sum_{i=1}^{n}\left\{\delta_i\left[\frac{f_{\mu\mu}(x_i)}{f(x_i)} - \left(\frac{f_\mu(x_i)}{f(x_i)}\right)^2\right] + (1-\delta_i)\left[\frac{S_{\mu\mu}(x_i)}{S(x_i)} - \left(\frac{S_\mu(x_i)}{S(x_i)}\right)^2\right]\right.$$

$$\left. - \left[\frac{S_{\mu\mu}(a_i)}{S(a_i)} - \left(\frac{S_\mu(a_i)}{S(a_i)}\right)^2\right]\right\}, \tag{D.4}$$

$$\frac{\partial^2 \log L(\mu,\theta,\beta,\gamma,\Lambda)}{\partial \mu \partial \theta} = \sum_{i=1}^{n}\left\{\delta_i\left[\frac{f_{\mu\theta}(x_i)}{f(x_i)} - \frac{f_\mu(x_i)f_\theta(x_i)}{f(x_i)^2}\right] + (1-\delta_i)\left[\frac{S_{\mu\theta}(x_i)}{S(x_i)} - \frac{S_\mu(x_i)S_\theta(x_i)}{S(x_i)^2}\right]\right.$$

$$\left. - \left[\frac{S_{\mu\theta}(a_i)}{S(a_i)} - \frac{S_\mu(a_i)S_\theta(a_i)}{S(a_i)^2}\right]\right\}, \tag{D.5}$$

and similarly for the other 13 second partial derivatives.

Thus, for ease of presentation and implementation, $f(x)$, $S(x)$, and their first and second partial derivatives with respect to the five parameters can be seen as the building blocks of the first and second partial derivatives of the log-likelihood function. We present the formulas for the first and second partial derivatives of $f(x)$ and $S(x)$ here, but we first note that $f_{\mu\beta}(x) = S_{\mu\beta}(x) = 0$, $f_{\mu\gamma}(x) = S_{\mu\gamma}(x) = 0$, $f_{\theta\beta}(x) = S_{\theta\beta}(x) = 0$, and $f_{\theta\gamma}(x) = S_{\theta\gamma}(x) = 0$. Hence, for the four corresponding second partial derivatives of the log-likelihood function, the first terms in the square brackets in Equation D.5 are equal to 0, and the analogous formula reduces to

$$\frac{\partial^2 \log L(\mu,\theta,\beta,\gamma,\Lambda)}{\partial \mu \partial \beta} = \sum_{i=1}^{n}\left\{-\delta_i\frac{f_\mu(x_i)f_\beta(x_i)}{f(x_i)^2} - (1-\delta_i)\frac{S_\mu(x_i)S_\beta(x_i)}{S(x_i)^2} + \frac{S_\mu(a_i)S_\beta(a_i)}{S(a_i)^2}\right\}$$

$$\tag{D.6}$$

and similarly for the other three second partial derivatives.

Using parameters μ, θ, β, γ, and Λ, $f(x)$ and $S(x)$ in our mixture model are given by

$$f(x) = \frac{e^\Lambda}{1+e^\Lambda}e^{\theta x}\exp\left[\mu - \frac{e^\mu}{\theta}\left(e^{\theta x}-1\right)\right] + \frac{1}{1+e^\Lambda}\gamma x^{\gamma-1}\exp\left(\beta - e^\beta x^\gamma\right), \tag{D.7}$$

$$S(x) = \frac{e^\Lambda}{1+e^\Lambda}\exp\left[-\frac{e^\mu}{\theta}\left(e^{\theta x}-1\right)\right] + \frac{1}{1+e^\Lambda}\exp\left(-e^\beta x^\gamma\right). \tag{D.8}$$

The first partial derivatives of $f(x)$ and $S(x)$ are

$$f_\mu(x) = \frac{e^\Lambda}{1+e^\Lambda}e^{\theta x}\exp\left[\mu - \frac{e^\mu}{\theta}\left(e^{\theta x}-1\right)\right]\left[1 - \frac{e^\mu}{\theta}\left(e^{\theta x}-1\right)\right], \tag{D.9}$$

$$f_\theta(x) = \frac{e^\Lambda}{1+e^\Lambda} e^{\theta x} \exp\left[\mu - \frac{e^\mu}{\theta}(e^{\theta x}-1)\right]\left\{x - \frac{e^\mu}{\theta}\left[xe^{\theta x} - \frac{(e^{\theta x}-1)}{\theta}\right]\right\},$$ (D.10)

$$f_\beta(x) = \frac{1}{1+e^\Lambda}\gamma x^{\gamma-1}\exp(\beta - e^\beta x^\gamma)(1 - e^\beta x^\gamma),$$ (D.11)

$$f_\gamma(x) = \frac{1}{1+e^\Lambda}x^{\gamma-1}\exp(\beta - e^\beta x^\gamma)\left[1 + \gamma\log x(1 - e^\beta x^\gamma)\right],$$ (D.12)

$$f_\Lambda(x) = \frac{e^\Lambda}{(1+e^\Lambda)^2}\left\{e^{\theta x}\exp\left[\mu - \frac{e^\mu}{\theta}(e^{\theta x}-1)\right] - \gamma x^{\gamma-1}\exp(\beta - e^\beta x^\gamma)\right\},$$ (D.13)

$$S_\mu(x) = \frac{e^\Lambda}{1+e^\Lambda}\exp\left[\mu - \frac{e^\mu}{\theta}(e^{\theta x}-1)\right]\left[-\frac{(e^{\theta x}-1)}{\theta}\right],$$ (D.14)

$$S_\theta(x) = \frac{e^\Lambda}{1+e^\Lambda}\exp\left[-\frac{e^\mu}{\theta}(e^{\theta x}-1)\right]\left\{-\frac{e^\mu}{\theta}\left[xe^{\theta x} - \frac{(e^{\theta x}-1)}{\theta}\right]\right\},$$ (D.15)

$$S_\beta(x) = \frac{1}{1+e^\Lambda}\exp(\beta - e^\beta x^\gamma)(-x^\gamma),$$ (D.16)

$$S_\gamma(x) = \frac{1}{1+e^\Lambda}\exp(-e^\beta x^\gamma)(-e^\beta x^\gamma\log x),$$ (D.17)

$$S_\Lambda(x) = \frac{e^\Lambda}{(1+e^\Lambda)^2}\left\{\exp\left[-\frac{e^\mu}{\theta}(e^{\theta x}-1)\right] - \exp(-e^\beta x^\gamma)\right\}.$$ (D.18)

The second partial derivatives of $f(x)$, excluding those that are equal to 0, are

$$f_{\mu\mu}(x) = \frac{e^\Lambda}{1+e^\Lambda}e^{\theta x}\exp\left[\mu - \frac{e^\mu}{\theta}(e^{\theta x}-1)\right]\left\{\left[1 - \frac{e^\mu}{\theta}(e^{\theta x}-1)\right]^2 - \frac{e^\mu}{\theta}(e^{\theta x}-1)\right\},$$ (D.19)

$$f_{\theta\theta}(x) = \frac{e^\Lambda}{1+e^\Lambda}e^{\theta x}\exp\left[\mu - \frac{e^\mu}{\theta}(e^{\theta x}-1)\right]\left\{-\frac{e^\mu}{\theta}\left\{\left[xe^{\theta x} - \frac{(e^{\theta x}-1)}{\theta}\right]\right.\right.$$

$$\left.\left.\left\{-\frac{e^\mu}{\theta}\left[xe^{\theta x} - \frac{(e^{\theta x}-1)}{\theta}\right] + 2x - \frac{2}{\theta}\right\}x^2 e^{\theta x}\right\} + x^2\right\},$$ (D.20)

$$f_{\beta\beta}(x) = \frac{1}{1+e^\Lambda}\gamma x^{\gamma-1}\exp(\beta - e^\beta x^\gamma)\left[(1 - e^\beta x^\gamma)^2 - e^\beta x^\gamma\right],$$ (D.21)

$$f_{\gamma\gamma}(x) = \frac{1}{1+e^\Lambda}x^{\gamma-1}\exp(\beta - e^\beta x^\gamma)\left\{-e^\beta x^\gamma\log x\left[\gamma\log x(3 - e^\beta x^\gamma) + 2\right]\right.$$

$$\left. + \log x(\gamma\log x + 2)\right\},$$ (D.22)

$$f_{\Lambda\Lambda}(x) = \frac{e^\Lambda(1-e^\Lambda)}{(1+e^\Lambda)^3}\left\{e^{\theta x}\exp\left[\mu-\frac{e^\mu}{\theta}(e^{\theta x}-1)\right]-\gamma x^{\gamma-1}\exp(\beta-e^\beta x^\gamma)\right\},\tag{D.23}$$

$$f_{\mu\theta}(x) = \frac{e^\Lambda}{1+e^\Lambda}e^{\theta x}\exp\left[\mu-\frac{e^\mu}{\theta}(e^{\theta x}-1)\right]\left\{-\frac{e^\mu}{\theta}\left[xe^{\theta x}-\frac{(e^{\theta x}-1)}{\theta}\right]\left[2-\frac{e^\mu}{\theta}(e^{\theta x}-1)\right]\right.$$
$$\left.+x\left[1-\frac{e^\mu}{\theta}(e^{\theta x}-1)\right]\right\},\tag{D.24}$$

$$f_{\beta\gamma}(x) = \frac{1}{1+e^\Lambda}x^{\gamma-1}\exp(\beta-e^\beta x^\gamma)\left\{-e^\beta x^\gamma\left[\gamma\log x(3-e^\beta x^\gamma)+1\right]+\gamma\log x+1\right\},\tag{D.25}$$

$$f_{\mu\Lambda}(x) = \frac{e^\Lambda}{(1+e^\Lambda)^2}e^{\theta x}\exp\left[\mu-\frac{e^\mu}{\theta}(e^{\theta x}-1)\right]\left[1-\frac{e^\mu}{\theta}(e^{\theta x}-1)\right],\tag{D.26}$$

$$f_{\theta\Lambda}(x) = \frac{e^\Lambda}{(1+e^\Lambda)^2}e^{\theta x}\exp\left[\mu-\frac{e^\mu}{\theta}(e^{\theta x}-1)\right]\left\{x-\frac{e^\mu}{\theta}\left[xe^{\theta x}-\frac{(e^{\theta x}-1)}{\theta}\right]\right\},\tag{D.27}$$

$$f_{\beta\Lambda}(x) = \frac{e^\Lambda}{(1+e^\Lambda)^2}(-\gamma x^{\gamma-1})\exp(\beta-e^\beta x^\gamma)(1-e^\beta x^\gamma),\tag{D.28}$$

$$f_{\gamma\Lambda}(x) = \frac{e^\Lambda}{(1+e^\Lambda)^2}(-x^{\gamma-1})\exp(\beta-e^\beta x^\gamma)\left[1+\gamma\log x(1-e^\beta x^\gamma)\right].\tag{D.29}$$

Finally, the second partial derivatives of $S(x)$, excluding those that are equal to 0, are

$$S_{\mu\mu}(x) = \frac{e^\Lambda}{1+e^\Lambda}\exp\left[-\frac{e^\mu}{\theta}(e^{\theta x}-1)\right]\left\{\left[-\frac{e^\mu}{\theta}(e^{\theta x}-1)\right]^2-\frac{e^\mu}{\theta}(e^{\theta x}-1)\right\},\tag{D.30}$$

$$S_{\theta\theta}(x) = \frac{e^\Lambda}{1+e^\Lambda}\exp\left[-\frac{e^\mu}{\theta}(e^{\theta x}-1)\right]\left\{-\frac{e^\mu}{\theta}\left\{\left[xe^{\theta x}-\frac{(e^{\theta x}-1)}{\theta}\right]\right.\right.$$
$$\left.\left.\left\{-\frac{e^\mu}{\theta}\left[xe^{\theta x}-\frac{(e^{\theta x}-1)}{\theta}\right]-\frac{2}{\theta}\right\}+x^2 e^{\theta x}\right\}\right\},\tag{D.31}$$

$$S_{\beta\beta}(x) = \frac{1}{1+e^\Lambda}\exp(-e^\beta x^\gamma)\left[(-e^\beta x^\gamma)^2-e^\beta x^\gamma\right],\tag{D.32}$$

$$S_{\gamma\gamma}(x) = \frac{1}{1+e^\Lambda}\exp(-e^\beta x^\gamma)\left[-e^\beta x^\gamma(\log x)^2\right](1-e^\beta x^\gamma),\tag{D.33}$$

$$S_{\Lambda\Lambda}(x) = \frac{e^\Lambda(1-e^\Lambda)}{(1+e^\Lambda)^3}\left\{\exp\left[-\frac{e^\mu}{\theta}(e^{\theta x}-1)\right]-\exp(-e^\beta x^\gamma)\right\},\tag{D.34}$$

$$S_{\mu\theta}(x) = \frac{e^\Lambda}{1+e^\Lambda} \exp\left[\mu - \frac{e^\mu}{\theta}\left(e^{\theta x}-1\right)\right]\left(-\frac{1}{\theta}\right)\left[xe^{\theta x} - \frac{\left(e^{\theta x}-1\right)}{\theta}\right]\left[1 - \frac{e^\mu}{\theta}\left(e^{\theta x}-1\right)\right],$$

$$\tag{D.35}$$

$$S_{\beta\gamma}(x) = \frac{1}{1+e^\Lambda} \exp\left(\beta - e^\beta x^\gamma\right)\left(-x^\gamma \log x\right)\left(1 - e^\beta x^\gamma\right), \tag{D.36}$$

$$S_{\mu\Lambda}(x) = \frac{e^\Lambda}{(1+e^\Lambda)^2} \exp\left[\mu - \frac{e^\mu}{\theta}\left(e^{\theta x}-1\right)\right]\left[-\frac{\left(e^{\theta x}-1\right)}{\theta}\right], \tag{D.37}$$

$$S_{\theta\Lambda}(x) = \frac{e^\Lambda}{(1+e^\Lambda)^2} \exp\left[-\frac{e^\mu}{\theta}\left(e^{\theta x}-1\right)\right]\left\{-\frac{e^\mu}{\theta}\left[xe^{\theta x} - \frac{\left(e^{\theta x}-1\right)}{\theta}\right]\right\}, \tag{D.38}$$

$$S_{\beta\Lambda}(x) = \frac{e^\Lambda}{(1+e^\Lambda)^2} \exp\left(\beta - e^\beta x^\gamma\right)x^\gamma, \tag{D.39}$$

$$S_{\gamma\Lambda}(x) = \frac{e^\Lambda}{(1+e^\Lambda)^2} \exp\left(-e^\beta x^\gamma\right)e^\beta x^\gamma \log x. \tag{D.40}$$

APPENDIX E

EXPECTATION–CONDITIONAL MAXIMIZATION (ECM) ALGORITHM

The expectation-maximization (EM) algorithm is a widely applied iterative method in modern statistics for finding maximum likelihood estimates (MLEs) (Dempster et al., 1977; McLachlan and Krishnan, 2008). The EM algorithm is numerically stable (i.e., it monotonically increases the likelihood function), but it can be extremely slow to converge in certain situations. Even before the article by Dempster et al. (1977), estimation for mixture models had been recognized as a natural application of the EM algorithm (McLachlan and Peel, 2000, pp. 47–48; Redner and Walker, 1984). If we interpret our mixture model as an incomplete-data problem and let y_i denote the "missing" group indicator ($y_i = 1$ for an observation arising from the Gompertz distribution and $y_i = 0$ for an observation arising from the Weibull distribution), such that the hypothetical complete data for subject i is given by the vector $(a_i, \delta_i, x_i, y_i)$, the complete-data likelihood function taking right-censoring into account and conditioning on age at entry into the study is, from $P[(\delta_i, x_i, y_i)|a_i] = P[y_i|a_i] \times$ likelihood for δ_i, x_i given y_i and a_i,

$$L_c(\lambda, \theta, \alpha, \gamma, \pi) = \prod_{i=1}^{n} P[Y_i = y_i|a_i] \left[\frac{f_G(x_i)^{\delta_i} S_G(x_i)^{1-\delta_i}}{S_G(a_i)} \right]^{y_i} \left[\frac{f_W(x_i)^{\delta_i} S_W(x_i)^{1-\delta_i}}{S_W(a_i)} \right]^{1-y_i},$$

(E.1)

The Biostatistics of Aging: From Gompertzian Mortality to an Index of Aging-Relatedness,
First Edition. Gilberto Levy and Bruce Levin.
© 2014 John Wiley & Sons, Inc. Published 2014 by John Wiley & Sons, Inc.

where

$$P[Y_i = y_i | a_i] = \frac{P[X_i > a_i | Y_i = y_i] P[Y_i = y_i]}{P[X_i > a_i | Y_i = 1] P[Y_i = 1] + P[X_i > a_i | Y_i = 0] P[Y_i = 0]}$$

$$= \frac{\pi^{y_i}(1-\pi)^{1-y_i} S_G(a_i)^{y_i} S_W(a_i)^{1-y_i}}{\pi S_G(a_i) + (1-\pi) S_W(a_i)}. \tag{E.2}$$

By introducing a function denoted $\pi(a_i)$, involving the five parameters and age at entry into the study for each subject,

$$\pi(a_i) = \frac{\pi S_G(a_i)}{\pi S_G(a_i) + (1-\pi) S_W(a_i)}, \tag{E.3}$$

we can express the complete-data likelihood and log-likelihood functions as follows:

$$L_c(\lambda,\theta,\alpha,\gamma,\pi) = \prod_{i=1}^{n} \pi(a_i)^{y_i} [1-\pi(a_i)]^{1-y_i} \left[\frac{f_G(x_i)^{\delta_i} S_G(x_i)^{1-\delta_i}}{S_G(a_i)} \right]^{y_i} \left[\frac{f_W(x_i)^{\delta_i} S_W(x_i)^{1-\delta_i}}{S_W(a_i)} \right]^{1-y_i}, \tag{E.4}$$

$$\log L_c(\lambda,\theta,\alpha,\gamma,\pi) = \sum_{i=1}^{n} \{ y_i \log \pi(a_i) + (1-y_i) \log [1-\pi(a_i)]$$

$$+ y_i [\delta_i \log f_G(x_i) + (1-\delta_i) \log S_G(x_i) - \log S_G(a_i)]$$

$$+ (1-y_i)[\delta_i \log f_W(x_i) + (1-\delta_i) \log S_W(x_i) - \log S_W(a_i)] \}. \tag{E.5}$$

One of the main reasons the EM algorithm is attractive is that its maximization step using the complete-data likelihood function is often computationally simple. While this is not the case for the complete-data likelihood function given in Equation E.1, the complete-data maximum likelihood estimation becomes relatively simple when conditional on (i.e., for a given value of) the function of the parameters $\pi(a_i)$, based on the log-likelihood function as expressed in Equation E.5. In this situation, an extension of the EM algorithm that retains its favorable properties called the ECM algorithm can be employed (McLachlan and Krishnan, 2008, pp. 60–75; Meng and Rubin, 1993). Like the EM algorithm, the ECM algorithm monotonically increases the likelihood function and converges to a stationary point under essentially the same conditions that guarantee the convergence of the EM algorithm (Meng and Rubin, 1993). The ECM algorithm replaces a complicated maximization step of the EM algorithm with two or more computationally simpler conditional maximization substeps, each of which maximizes the likelihood function over the parameter vector but with a function of the parameters held fixed at its current value. In many applications of the ECM algorithm, the conditional maximization substeps correspond to a partitioning of the parameter vector into subvectors (i.e., at each conditional maximization substep, the likelihood function is maximized with respect to a subvector of the parameter vector with the other parameters held fixed).

Our application of the ECM algorithm involves two conditional maximization substeps. In the first substep, we maximize the likelihood function over λ, θ, α, and γ with $\pi(a_i)$ held fixed, and in the second substep, we maximize the likelihood function over π with λ, θ, α, and γ held fixed (this second conditional maximization substep involves a simple partitioning of the parameter vector). We give the general outline of our ECM algorithm here, and we will detail and provide mathematical formulas for each step and substep in what follows. In the expectation step, Y_i is the random variable corresponding to y_i.

(i) Start with initial values for λ, θ, α, and γ obtained from fitting separate Gompertz and Weibull models to the data (i.e., assuming that the data originate from a Gompertz distribution, obtain MLEs for λ and θ, and assuming that the data originate from a Weibull distribution, obtain MLEs for α and γ); use 0.5 as the initial value for π.

(ii) Expectation step: calculate the expected value of "random variable" Y_i, using current values of λ, θ, α, γ, and π.

(iii) Maximization step: first calculate $\pi(a_i)$, using current values of λ, θ, α, γ, and π.

(iv) Conditional maximization substep: update the estimates of λ, θ, α, and γ, given current value of $\pi(a_i)$ and using current expected value of Y_i.

(v) Conditional maximization substep: update the estimate of π, given current values of λ, θ, α, and γ and using current expected value of Y_i.

(vi) If convergence criterion is satisfied, stop; otherwise, return to (ii) and iterate.

For the initial step (i), we detail the procedures for obtaining the MLEs of the parameters of the Gompertz and Weibull distributions fitted separately to the data. In order to differentiate the parameters of these separate Gompertz and Weibull models from the analogous parameters of the mixture distribution, we will denote them λ^*, θ^*, α^*, and γ^*. Note the important point corresponding to this notation distinction that while λ, θ, α, and γ are estimated based on our actual assumption that the true underlying distribution of the data is the mixture distribution, λ^* and θ^* are estimated on the working assumption that the true underlying distribution of the data is the Gompertz distribution, and α^* and γ^* are estimated on the working assumption that the true underlying distribution of the data is the Weibull distribution. Only when $\pi = 1$, $\lambda^* = \lambda$ and $\theta^* = \theta$, and only when $\pi = 0$, $\alpha^* = \alpha$ and $\gamma^* = \gamma$, because the mixture model reduces to the Gompertz model for $\pi = 1$ and to the Weibull model for $\pi = 0$. Because of the different roles played by λ^* and λ, one does not expect $\hat{\lambda}^*$ to estimate or even approximate $\hat{\lambda}$ (and similarly for the other pairs corresponding to θ, α, and γ).

The likelihood and log-likelihood functions of the Gompertz distribution taking into account right-censoring and age at entry into the study are

$$L_G(\lambda^*,\theta^*)=\prod_{i=1}^{n}\frac{f_G(x_i)^{\delta_i}S_G(x_i)^{1-\delta_i}}{S_G(a_i)}=\prod_{i=1}^{n}\frac{[h_G(x_i)S_G(x_i)]^{\delta_i}S_G(x_i)^{1-\delta_i}}{S_G(a_i)}=\prod_{i=1}^{n}\frac{h_G(x_i)^{\delta_i}S_G(x_i)}{S_G(a_i)}$$

$$=\prod_{i=1}^{n}\frac{\left(\lambda^*e^{\theta^*x_i}\right)^{\delta_i}\exp\left[-(\lambda^*/\theta^*)\left(e^{\theta^*x_i}-1\right)\right]}{\exp\left[-(\lambda^*/\theta^*)(e^{\theta^*a_i}-1)\right]}=\prod_{i=1}^{n}\left(\lambda^*e^{\theta^*x_i}\right)^{\delta_i}\exp\left[-\frac{\lambda^*}{\theta^*}\left(e^{\theta^*x_i}-e^{\theta^*a_i}\right)\right],$$

$$(E.6)$$

$$\log L_G(\lambda^*,\theta^*)=\sum_{i=1}^{n}\left[\delta_i(\log\lambda^*+\theta^*x_i)-\frac{\lambda^*}{\theta^*}\left(e^{\theta^*x_i}-e^{\theta^*a_i}\right)\right]$$

$$=D\log\lambda^*+\theta^*T_G-\frac{\lambda^*}{\theta^*}Q_G(\theta^*),\qquad(E.7)$$

where $D=\sum_{i=1}^{n}\delta_i$, $T_G=\sum_{i=1}^{n}\delta_i x_i$, and $Q_G(\theta^*)=\sum_{i=1}^{n}\left(e^{\theta^*x_i}-e^{\theta^*a_i}\right)$. By taking the first partial derivatives of Equation E.7 with respect to λ^* and θ^* and equating them to 0, we obtain

$$\hat{\lambda}^*=\frac{D\hat{\theta}^*}{Q_G(\hat{\theta}^*)},\qquad(E.8)$$

$$T_G+\frac{D}{\hat{\theta}^*}-\frac{DQ'_G(\hat{\theta}^*)}{Q_G(\hat{\theta}^*)}=0,\qquad(E.9)$$

where $Q'_G(\theta^*)=\sum_{i=1}^{n}\left(x_ie^{\theta^*x_i}-a_ie^{\theta^*a_i}\right)$. Thus, to obtain the MLEs of the parameters of the Gompertz distribution, we first solve numerically for $\hat{\theta}^*$ in Equation E.9 using Newton's method and then obtain $\hat{\lambda}^*$ from Equation E.8. We obtain an initial estimate of θ^* for an iterative solution by weighted linear regression based on the linearized form of the Gompertz hazard function, $\log h_G(x)=\log\lambda+\theta x$, in which the outcome is the log of age-specific mortality rates calculated from grouped data using 5-year age intervals, the independent variable is the midpoint of the age intervals, and the weights are the number of events in each age interval.

The likelihood and log-likelihood functions of the Weibull distribution taking into account right-censoring and age at entry into the study are

$$L_W(\alpha^*,\gamma^*)=\prod_{i=1}^{n}\frac{f_W(x_i)^{\delta_i}S_W(x_i)^{1-\delta_i}}{S_W(a_i)}=\prod_{i=1}^{n}\frac{h_W(x_i)^{\delta_i}S_W(x_i)}{S_W(a_i)}$$

$$=\prod_{i=1}^{n}\frac{\left(\alpha^*\gamma^*x_i^{\gamma^*-1}\right)^{\delta_i}\exp\left(-\alpha^*x_i^{\gamma^*}\right)}{\exp\left(-\alpha^*a_i^{\gamma^*}\right)}=\prod_{i=1}^{n}\left(\alpha^*\gamma^*x_i^{\gamma^*-1}\right)^{\delta_i}\exp\left[-\alpha^*\left(x_i^{\gamma^*}-a_i^{\gamma^*}\right)\right],$$

$$(E.10)$$

$$\log L_{\mathrm{W}}(\alpha^*, \gamma^*) = \sum_{i=1}^{n} \left\{ \delta_i \left[\log (\alpha^* \gamma^*) + (\gamma^* - 1) \log x_i \right] - \alpha^* \left(x_i^{\gamma^*} - a_i^{\gamma^*} \right) \right\}$$

$$= D \log (\alpha^* \gamma^*) + (\gamma^* - 1) T_{\mathrm{W}} - \alpha^* Q_{\mathrm{W}}(\gamma^*), \tag{E.11}$$

where $T_{\mathrm{W}} = \sum_{i=1}^{n} \delta_i \log x_i$ and $Q_{\mathrm{W}}(\gamma^*) = \sum_{i=1}^{n} \left(x_i^{\gamma^*} - a_i^{\gamma^*} \right)$. By taking the first partial derivatives of Equation E.11 with respect to α^* and γ^* and equating them to 0, we obtain

$$\hat{\alpha}^* = \frac{D}{Q_{\mathrm{W}}(\hat{\gamma}^*)}, \tag{E.12}$$

$$T_{\mathrm{W}} + \frac{D}{\hat{\gamma}^*} - \frac{D Q'_{\mathrm{W}}(\hat{\gamma}^*)}{Q_{\mathrm{W}}(\hat{\gamma}^*)} = 0, \tag{E.13}$$

where $Q'_{\mathrm{W}}(\gamma^*) = \sum_{i=1}^{n} \left(x_i^{\gamma^*} \log x_i - a_i^{\gamma^*} \log a_i \right)$. Thus, to obtain the MLEs of the parameters of the Weibull distribution, we first solve numerically for $\hat{\gamma}^*$ in Equation E.13 using Newton's method and then obtain $\hat{\alpha}^*$ from Equation E.12. We obtain an initial estimate of γ^* for an iterative solution by weighted linear regression based on the linearized form of the Weibull hazard function, $\log h_{\mathrm{W}}(x) = \log (\alpha \gamma) + (\gamma - 1)\log x$, in which the outcome is the log of age-specific mortality rates calculated from grouped data using 5-year age intervals, the independent variable is the log of the midpoint of the age intervals, and the weights are the number of events in each age interval.

In the expectation step (ii), we use the following. For those cases corresponding to events ($\delta_i = 1$), we obtain from Bayes' theorem

$$E[Y_i | X_i = x_i] = P[Y_i = 1 | X_i = x_i] = \frac{P[X_i = x_i | Y_i = 1] P[Y_i = 1]}{P[X_i = x_i | Y_i = 1] P[Y_i = 1] + P[X_i = x_i | Y_i = 0] P[Y_i = 0]}$$

$$= \frac{\pi f_{\mathrm{G}}(x_i)}{\pi f_{\mathrm{G}}(x_i) + (1 - \pi) f_{\mathrm{W}}(x_i)}, \tag{E.14}$$

and for censored cases ($\delta_i = 0$),

$$E[Y_i | X_i > x_i] = P[Y_i = 1 | X_i > x_i] = \frac{\pi S_{\mathrm{G}}(x_i)}{\pi S_{\mathrm{G}}(x_i) + (1 - \pi) S_{\mathrm{W}}(x_i)}. \tag{E.15}$$

Thus, given current values of λ, θ, α, γ, and π, this expectation is the posterior probability that subject i, with age at event or censoring x_i and event/censoring indicator δ_i, belongs to the Gompertz component of the mixture distribution. In general, the expectation step is given by

$$E[Y_i|x_i, \delta_i] = \delta_i \left[\frac{\pi f_G(x_i)}{\pi f_G(x_i) + (1-\pi)f_W(x_i)} \right] + (1-\delta_i)\left[\frac{\pi S_G(x_i)}{\pi S_G(x_i) + (1-\pi)S_W(x_i)} \right]. \quad \text{(E.16)}$$

Similarly, in the maximization step (iii) (to calculate the value of the function $\pi(a_i)$ given current values of λ, θ, α, γ, and π), we note from Equation E.3 that

$$\pi(a_i) = P[Y_i = 1|X_i > a_i] = \frac{\pi S_G(a_i)}{\pi S_G(a_i) + (1-\pi)S_W(a_i)}. \quad \text{(E.17)}$$

Thus, $\pi(a_i)$ represents the posterior probability, for given λ, θ, α, γ, and π, that subject i with age at entry into the study a_i belongs to the Gompertz component of the mixture distribution.

In the conditional maximization substep (iv), we update the estimates of λ, θ, α, and γ, given the current value of $\pi(a_i)$ and using the current expected value of Y_i in place of y_i. By taking the first partial derivatives of the complete-data log-likelihood function in Equation E.5 with respect to λ, θ, α, and γ, which also involves the partial derivatives of $\pi(a_i)$ with respect to λ, θ, α, and γ, and equating them to 0, we obtain estimating equations that are analogous to those for the separate Gompertz and Weibull models. For λ and θ,

$$\hat{\lambda} = \frac{D_{CG}\hat{\theta}}{Q_{CG}(\hat{\theta})}, \quad \text{(E.18)}$$

$$T_{CG} + \frac{D_{CG}}{\hat{\theta}} - \frac{D_{CG}Q'_{CG}(\hat{\theta})}{Q_{CG}(\hat{\theta})} = 0, \quad \text{(E.19)}$$

where $D_{CG} = \sum_{i=1}^{n} y_i\delta_i$, $T_{CG} = \sum_{i=1}^{n} y_i\delta_i x_i$, $Q_{CG}(\theta) = \sum_{i=1}^{n} \left[y_i\left(e^{\theta x_i} - 1\right) - \pi(a_i) \right.$ $\left. \left(e^{\theta a_i} - 1\right) \right]$, and $Q'_{CG}(\theta) = \sum_{i=1}^{n} \left[y_i x_i e^{\theta x_i} - \pi(a_i)a_i e^{\theta a_i} \right]$. For α and γ,

$$\hat{\alpha} = \frac{D_{CW}}{Q_{CW}(\hat{\gamma})}, \quad \text{(E.20)}$$

$$T_{CW} + \frac{D_{CW}}{\hat{\gamma}} - \frac{D_{CW}Q'_{CW}(\hat{\gamma})}{Q_{CW}(\hat{\gamma})} = 0, \quad \text{(E.21)}$$

where $D_{CW} = \sum_{i=1}^{n}(1-y_i)\delta_i$, $T_{CW} = \sum_{i=1}^{n}(1-y_i)\delta_i \log x_i$, $Q_{CW}(\gamma) = \sum_{i=1}^{n}\{(1-y_i)$ $x_i^{\gamma} - [1-\pi(a_i)]a_i^{\gamma}\}$, and $Q'_{CW}(\gamma) = \sum_{i=1}^{n}\{(1-y_i)x_i^{\gamma} \log x_i - [1-\pi(a_i)]a_i^{\gamma} \log a_i\}$. Thus, at each maximization step, λ and θ are estimated separately from α and γ. For λ and θ, we solve numerically for $\hat{\theta}$ in Equation E.19 using Newton's method and then obtain $\hat{\lambda}$ from Equation E.18, and for α and γ, we solve numerically for $\hat{\gamma}$ in Equation E.21 using Newton's method and then obtain $\hat{\alpha}$ from Equation E.20.

Lastly, in the conditional maximization substep (v), we update the estimate of π, given the current values of λ, θ, α, and γ and using the current expected value of Y_i in place of y_i. By taking the partial derivative of the complete-data log-likelihood function in Equation E.5 with respect to π and equating it to 0, we obtain

$$\sum_{i=1}^{n} [y_i - \pi(a_i)] = \sum_{i=1}^{n} \left[y_i - \frac{\hat{\pi} S_G(a_i)}{\hat{\pi} S_G(a_i) + (1-\hat{\pi}) S_W(a_i)} \right] = 0. \tag{E.22}$$

Equation E.22 can be solved for $\hat{\pi}$ using a numerical procedure. To that end, we note that Equation E.22 corresponds to the estimating equation of the following logistic regression model involving only an intercept in terms of π and an offset:

$$\log \frac{P[Y_i = 1]}{P[Y_i = 0]} = \log \frac{\pi(a_i)}{1-\pi(a_i)} = \log \frac{\pi S_G(a_i)}{(1-\pi) S_W(a_i)} = \log \frac{\pi}{1-\pi} + \log \frac{S_G(a_i)}{S_W(a_i)}$$

$$\Rightarrow \log \frac{P[Y_i = 1]}{P[Y_i = 0]} - \log \frac{S_G(a_i)}{S_W(a_i)} = \log \frac{\pi}{1-\pi}. \tag{E.23}$$

Thus, in order to obtain the estimate of π, we run a logistic regression model with outcome y_i and offset $\log[S_G(a_i)/S_W(a_i)]$. If we denote the intercept of this logistic regression model β_0, the estimate of π at each maximization step is given by

$$\hat{\pi} = \frac{\exp(\hat{\beta}_0)}{1 + \exp(\hat{\beta}_0)}. \tag{E.24}$$

APPENDIX F

R PROGRAM*

```
# Program to fit Gompertz, Weibull and mixture distributions
to data
#    using maximum likelihood estimation, in order to
calculate
#    index of aging-relatedness
#
# Input (dataset containing):
#    Event status
#    Age at event/censoring (in years)
#    Age at baseline (in years)
#
# Output:
#    Event rates by 5-year intervals
#    Iterative procedures (Newton method, expectation-
maximization algorithm, and Newton–Raphson method)
#    Log LR and LR for Weibull versus Gompertz model
#    Parameter estimates, standard errors and 95% CIs for
Gompertz, Weibull, and mixture models
#    Fitted event rates
#    Plots
```

*Available upon request from the authors. Please email GL227@caa.columbia.edu.

The Biostatistics of Aging: From Gompertzian Mortality to an Index of Aging-Relatedness,
First Edition. Gilberto Levy and Bruce Levin.
© 2014 John Wiley & Sons, Inc. Published 2014 by John Wiley & Sons, Inc.

```
# Input mortality intrinsic data
Data <- read.table("MortalityIntrinsic.dat", header = FALSE)
Event <- Data[,1]
AgeEventCensoring <- Data[,2]
AgeBaseline <- Data[,3]
n <- length(AgeEventCensoring)

# Input mortality intrinsic by smoking data
# 1 - Never, 2 - Past, 3 - Current
Data <- read.table("MortalitySmoking3.dat", header = FALSE)
Data <- subset(Data, Data[,1] == 1)
# Data <- subset(Data, Data[,1] == 2 | Data[,1] == 3)
Event <- Data[,2]
AgeEventCensoring <- Data[,3]
AgeBaseline <- Data[,4]
n <- length(AgeEventCensoring)


#### Calculation of age-specific event rates for 5-year age
intervals ####

PersonYears40to45 <- PersonYears45to50 <- PersonYears50to55 <-
PersonYears55to60 <- PersonYears60to65 <- PersonYears65to70 <-
PersonYears70to75 <- PersonYears75to80 <- PersonYears80to85 <-
PersonYears85to90 <- PersonYears90to95 <- PersonYearsOver95 <- 0
Events40to45 <- Events45to50 <- Events50to55 <- Events55to60
<- Events60to65 <- Events65to70 <- Events70to75 <-
Events75to80 <- Events80to85 <- Events85to90 <- Events90to95
<- EventsOver95 <- 0
AtRisk40to45 <- AtRisk45to50 <- AtRisk50to55 <- AtRisk55to60
<- AtRisk60to65 <- AtRisk65to70 <- AtRisk70to75 <-
AtRisk75to80 <- AtRisk80to85 <- AtRisk85to90 <- AtRisk90to95
<- AtRiskOver95 <- 0
for (i in 1:n) {
  if (AgeEventCensoring[i] > 40 && AgeEventCensoring[i] <= 45) {
    PersonYears40to45 <- PersonYears40to45 +
(AgeEventCensoring[i] - max(40, AgeBaseline[i]))
    Events40to45 <- Events40to45 + Event[i]
    AtRisk40to45 <- AtRisk40to45 + 1
  }
  if (AgeEventCensoring[i] > 45 && AgeBaseline[i] < 45) {
    PersonYears40to45 <- PersonYears40to45 + min(5, (45 -
AgeBaseline[i]))
    AtRisk40to45 <- AtRisk40to45 + 1
  }
```

```
  if (AgeEventCensoring[i] > 45 && AgeEventCensoring[i] <=
50) {
    PersonYears45to50 <- PersonYears45to50 +
(AgeEventCensoring[i] - max(45, AgeBaseline[i]))
    Events45to50 <- Events45to50 + Event[i]
    AtRisk45to50 <- AtRisk45to50 + 1
  }
  if (AgeEventCensoring[i] > 50 && AgeBaseline[i] < 50) {
    PersonYears45to50 <- PersonYears45to50 + min(5, (50 -
AgeBaseline[i]))
    AtRisk45to50 <- AtRisk45to50 + 1
  }
  if (AgeEventCensoring[i] > 50 && AgeEventCensoring[i] <= 55) {
    PersonYears50to55 <- PersonYears50to55 +
(AgeEventCensoring[i] - max(50, AgeBaseline[i]))
    Events50to55 <- Events50to55 + Event[i]
    AtRisk50to55 <- AtRisk50to55 + 1
  }
  if (AgeEventCensoring[i] > 55 && AgeBaseline[i] < 55) {
    PersonYears50to55 <- PersonYears50to55 + min(5, (55 -
AgeBaseline[i]))
    AtRisk50to55 <- AtRisk50to55 + 1
  }
  if (AgeEventCensoring[i] > 55 && AgeEventCensoring[i] <= 60) {
    PersonYears55to60 <- PersonYears55to60 +
(AgeEventCensoring[i] - max(55, AgeBaseline[i]))
    Events55to60 <- Events55to60 + Event[i]
    AtRisk55to60 <- AtRisk55to60 + 1
  }
  if (AgeEventCensoring[i] > 60 && AgeBaseline[i] < 60) {
    PersonYears55to60 <- PersonYears55to60 + min(5, (60 -
AgeBaseline[i]))
    AtRisk55to60 <- AtRisk55to60 + 1
  }
  if (AgeEventCensoring[i] > 60 && AgeEventCensoring[i] <= 65) {
    PersonYears60to65 <- PersonYears60to65 +
(AgeEventCensoring[i] - max(60, AgeBaseline[i]))
    Events60to65 <- Events60to65 + Event[i]
    AtRisk60to65 <- AtRisk60to65 + 1
  }
  if (AgeEventCensoring[i] > 65 && AgeBaseline[i] < 65) {
    PersonYears60to65 <- PersonYears60to65 + min(5, (65 -
AgeBaseline[i]))
    AtRisk60to65 <- AtRisk60to65 + 1
  }
```

```
  if (AgeEventCensoring[i] > 65 && AgeEventCensoring[i] <= 70) {
    PersonYears65to70 <- PersonYears65to70 +
(AgeEventCensoring[i] - max(65, AgeBaseline[i]))
  Events65to70 <- Events65to70 + Event[i]
  AtRisk65to70 <- AtRisk65to70 + 1
  }
  if (AgeEventCensoring[i] > 70 && AgeBaseline[i] < 70) {
    PersonYears65to70 <- PersonYears65to70 + min(5, (70 -
AgeBaseline[i]))
    AtRisk65to70 <- AtRisk65to70 + 1
  }
  if (AgeEventCensoring[i] > 70 && AgeEventCensoring[i] <= 75) {
    PersonYears70to75 <- PersonYears70to75 +
(AgeEventCensoring[i] - max(70, AgeBaseline[i]))
    Events70to75 <- Events70to75 + Event[i]
    AtRisk70to75 <- AtRisk70to75 + 1
  }
  if (AgeEventCensoring[i] > 75 && AgeBaseline[i] < 75) {
    PersonYears70to75 <- PersonYears70to75 + min(5, (75 -
AgeBaseline[i]))
    AtRisk70to75 <- AtRisk70to75 + 1
  }
  if (AgeEventCensoring[i] > 75 && AgeEventCensoring[i] <= 80) {
    PersonYears75to80 <- PersonYears75to80 +
(AgeEventCensoring[i] - max(75, AgeBaseline[i]))
    Events75to80 <- Events75to80 + Event[i]
    AtRisk75to80 <- AtRisk75to80 + 1
  }
  if (AgeEventCensoring[i] > 80 && AgeBaseline[i] < 80) {
    PersonYears75to80 <- PersonYears75to80 + min(5, (80 -
AgeBaseline[i]))
    AtRisk75to80 <- AtRisk75to80 + 1
  }
  if (AgeEventCensoring[i] > 80 && AgeEventCensoring[i] <= 85) {
    PersonYears80to85 <- PersonYears80to85 +
(AgeEventCensoring[i] - max(80, AgeBaseline[i]))
    Events80to85 <- Events80to85 + Event[i]
    AtRisk80to85 <- AtRisk80to85 + 1
  }
  if (AgeEventCensoring[i] > 85 && AgeBaseline[i] < 85) {
    PersonYears80to85 <- PersonYears80to85 + min(5, (85 -
AgeBaseline[i]))
    AtRisk80to85 <- AtRisk80to85 + 1
  }
  if (AgeEventCensoring[i] > 85 && AgeEventCensoring[i] <= 90) {
```

```
    PersonYears85to90 <- PersonYears85to90 +
(AgeEventCensoring[i] - max(85, AgeBaseline[i]))
    Events85to90 <- Events85to90 + Event[i]
    AtRisk85to90 <- AtRisk85to90 + 1
  }
  if (AgeEventCensoring[i] > 90 && AgeBaseline[i] < 90) {
    PersonYears85to90 <- PersonYears85to90 + min(5, (90 -
AgeBaseline[i]))
    AtRisk85to90 <- AtRisk85to90 + 1
  }
  if (AgeEventCensoring[i] > 90 && AgeEventCensoring[i] <= 95) {
    PersonYears90to95 <- PersonYears90to95 +
(AgeEventCensoring[i] - max(90, AgeBaseline[i]))
    Events90to95 <- Events90to95 + Event[i]
    AtRisk90to95 <- AtRisk90to95 + 1
  }
  if (AgeEventCensoring[i] > 95 && AgeBaseline[i] < 95) {
    PersonYears90to95 <- PersonYears90to95 + min(5, (95 -
AgeBaseline[i]))
    AtRisk90to95 <- AtRisk90to95 + 1
  }
  if (AgeEventCensoring[i] > 95) {
    PersonYearsOver95 <- PersonYearsOver95 +
(AgeEventCensoring[i] - max(95, AgeBaseline[i]))
    EventsOver95 <- EventsOver95 + Event[i]
    AtRiskOver95 <- AtRiskOver95 + 1
  }
}
PersonYears <- c(PersonYears40to45, PersonYears45to50,
PersonYears50to55, PersonYears55to60, PersonYears60to65,
PersonYears65to70, PersonYears70to75, PersonYears75to80,
PersonYears80to85, PersonYears85to90, PersonYears90to95,
PersonYearsOver95)
Events <- c(Events40to45, Events45to50, Events50to55,
Events55to60, Events60to65, Events65to70, Events70to75,
Events75to80, Events80to85, Events85to90, Events90to95,
EventsOver95)
AtRisk <- c(AtRisk40to45, AtRisk45to50, AtRisk50to55,
AtRisk55to60, AtRisk60to65, AtRisk65to70, AtRisk70to75,
AtRisk75to80, AtRisk80to85, AtRisk85to90, AtRisk90to95,
AtRiskOver95)
EventRate <- (Events / PersonYears)
LogEventRate <- log(EventRate)
Age<-c(42.5,47.5,52.5,57.5,62.5,67.5,72.5,77.5,82.5,87.5,
92.5,97.5)
```

```
# Right-censor data and calculate number of events
AgeRightCensoring <- 90
AtRiskRightCensoring <- EventsRightCensoring <- 0
for (i in 1:n) {
  if (AgeEventCensoring[i] > AgeRightCensoring) {
    AtRiskRightCensoring <- AtRiskRightCensoring + 1
    EventsRightCensoring <- EventsRightCensoring + Event[i]
    AgeEventCensoring[i] <- AgeRightCensoring
    Event[i] <- 0
  }
}
D <- sum(Event)

# Subtract earliest age at reproduction in the population from
age at event/censoring and age at baseline
AgeEventCensoring <- AgeEventCensoring - 10
AgeBaseline <- AgeBaseline - 10

# Output
list (n = n, Events = D, AgeRightCensoring =
AgeRightCensoring, AtRiskRightCensoring =
AtRiskRightCensoring, EventsRightCensoring =
EventsRightCensoring)
descriptive1 <- cbind(Age, AtRisk, Events, PersonYears,
EventRate, LogEventRate)
colnames(descriptive1) <- c("Age", "At risk", "Events",
"Person-years", "Event rate", "Log event rate")
descriptive1



#################### Gompertz model ####################

# Function to compute log-likelihood function
GompertzLogLik <- function(LambdaStar, ThetaStar) {
  Q_G <- sum(exp(ThetaStar * AgeEventCensoring) - exp
(ThetaStar * AgeBaseline))
  GompertzLogLikValue <- D * log(LambdaStar) + ThetaStar *
T_G - (LambdaStar / ThetaStar) * Q_G
  return(GompertzLogLikValue)
}

# Function to compute estimating equation
GompertzEquation <- function(ThetaStar) {
```

```
  Q_G <- sum(exp(ThetaStar * AgeEventCensoring) - exp
(ThetaStar * AgeBaseline))
  DerQ_G <- sum(AgeEventCensoring * exp(ThetaStar *
AgeEventCensoring) - AgeBaseline * exp(ThetaStar *
AgeBaseline))
  GompertzEquationValue <- T_G + D / ThetaStar - D * DerQ_G / Q_G
  return(GompertzEquationValue)
}

# Function to compute derivative of estimating equation
GompertzDerEquation <- function(ThetaStar) {
  Q_G <- sum(exp(ThetaStar * AgeEventCensoring) - exp
(ThetaStar * AgeBaseline))
  DerQ_G <- sum(AgeEventCensoring * exp(ThetaStar *
AgeEventCensoring) - AgeBaseline * exp(ThetaStar *
AgeBaseline))
  DerDerQ_G <- sum(AgeEventCensoring ^ 2 * exp(ThetaStar *
AgeEventCensoring) - AgeBaseline ^ 2 * exp(ThetaStar *
AgeBaseline))
  GompertzDerEquationValue <- D * ((DerQ_G / Q_G) ^ 2 -
DerDerQ_G / Q_G - ThetaStar ^ -2)
  return(GompertzDerEquationValue)
}

# Initial parameter estimates (weighted least-squares method)
for (i in 1:10)
  if (is.na(LogEventRate[i]) == FALSE && LogEventRate[i] ==
-Inf) LogEventRate[i] = NA
GompertzLeastSquaresPredictor <- Age[1:10] - 10
GompertzLeastSquares <- lm(LogEventRate[1:10] ~
GompertzLeastSquaresPredictor, weights = Events[1:10])
GompertzInterceptLeastSquares <- as.numeric(coefficients
(GompertzLeastSquares)[1])
ThetaStarLeastSquares <- as.numeric(coefficients
(GompertzLeastSquares)[2])
LambdaStarLeastSquares <- exp(GompertzInterceptLeastSquares)

# Iterative procedure (Newton method) to estimate ThetaStar
i <- 0
T_G <- sum(Event * AgeEventCensoring)
GompertzNewtonMethod <- c(i, ThetaStarLeastSquares, NA,
GompertzEquation(ThetaStarLeastSquares), GompertzLogLik
(LambdaStarLeastSquares, ThetaStarLeastSquares))
ThetaStarCurrent <- ThetaStarLeastSquares
```

```
ThetaStarPrevious <- -Inf              # To make sure it
iterates
while (i < 20 && abs(ThetaStarCurrent - ThetaStarPrevious) >
1e-10) {
  ThetaStarPrevious <- ThetaStarCurrent
  ThetaStarCurrent <- ThetaStarPrevious - GompertzEquation
(ThetaStarPrevious) / GompertzDerEquation
(ThetaStarPrevious)
  Q_G <- sum(exp(ThetaStarCurrent * AgeEventCensoring) - exp
(ThetaStarCurrent * AgeBaseline))
  LambdaStarCurrent <- D * ThetaStarCurrent / Q_G
  i <- i + 1
  GompertzNewtonMethod <- rbind(GompertzNewtonMethod,
c(i, ThetaStarCurrent, (ThetaStarCurrent -
ThetaStarPrevious), GompertzEquation(ThetaStarCurrent),
GompertzLogLik(LambdaStarCurrent, ThetaStarCurrent)))
}
ThetaStar <- ThetaStarCurrent
LambdaStar <- LambdaStarCurrent
GompertzLogLikelihood <- GompertzNewtonMethod[i+1,5]

# Standard errors and 95% CIs
DerQ_G <- sum(AgeEventCensoring * exp(ThetaStar *
AgeEventCensoring) - AgeBaseline * exp(ThetaStar *
AgeBaseline))
DerDerQ_G <- sum(AgeEventCensoring ^ 2 * exp(ThetaStar *
AgeEventCensoring) - AgeBaseline ^ 2 * exp(ThetaStar *
AgeBaseline))
SecondDerLambdaStar <- -D / LambdaStar ^ 2
# Second partial derivative of the log-likelihood function
wrt LambdaStar/LambdaStar
SecondDerLambdaStarThetaStar <- Q_G / ThetaStar ^ 2 - DerQ_G /
ThetaStar
# Second partial derivative of the log-likelihood function
wrt LambdaStar/ThetaStar
SecondDerThetaStar <- -2 * (LambdaStar / ThetaStar) * (Q_G /
ThetaStar ^ 2 - DerQ_G / ThetaStar + DerDerQ_G / 2)    # Second
partial derivative of the log-likelihood function wrt
ThetaStar/ThetaStar
FisherInformation <- -1 * matrix(c(SecondDerLambdaStar,
SecondDerLambdaStarThetaStar, SecondDerLambdaStarThetaStar,
SecondDerThetaStar), nrow = 2, ncol = 2)
GompertzVarianceMatrix <- solve(FisherInformation)
LambdaStarSE <- sqrt(GompertzVarianceMatrix[1,1])
```

```
ThetaStarSE <- sqrt(GompertzVarianceMatrix[2,2])
LambdaStarCI <- c(LambdaStar - 1.96 * LambdaStarSE,
LambdaStar + 1.96 * LambdaStarSE)
ThetaStarCI <- c(ThetaStar - 1.96 * ThetaStarSE, ThetaStar +
1.96 * ThetaStarSE)

# Fitted event rates
GompertzFittedEventRate <- LambdaStar * exp(ThetaStar * (Age
[1:10] - 10))
GompertzFittedLogEventRate <- log(GompertzFittedEventRate)

# Output for Gompertz model
summary(GompertzLeastSquares)
list(LambdaStarLeastSquares = LambdaStarLeastSquares,
ThetaStarLeastSquares = ThetaStarLeastSquares)
colnames(GompertzNewtonMethod) <- c("i", "ThetaStar",
"ThetaStar change", "Estimating equation", "Log likelihood")
print(GompertzNewtonMethod, digits = 10)
print(GompertzLogLikelihood, digits = 15)
GompertzVarianceMatrix
descriptive2 <- matrix(c(LambdaStar, LambdaStarSE,
LambdaStarCI, ThetaStar, ThetaStarSE, ThetaStarCI), nrow =
2, byrow = TRUE)
colnames(descriptive2) <- c("Parameter estimate", "Standard
error", "95% Confidence interval", " ")
rownames(descriptive2) <- c("LambdaStar", "ThetaStar")
descriptive2
descriptive3 <- cbind(Age[1:10], EventRate[1:10],
GompertzFittedEventRate, LogEventRate[1:10],
GompertzFittedLogEventRate)
colnames(descriptive3) <- c("Age", "Event rate", "Gompertz
fitted", "Log event rate", "Gompertz fitted")
descriptive3


#################### Weibull model ####################

# Function to compute log-likelihood function
WeibullLogLik <- function(AlphaStar, GammaStar) {
  Q_W <- sum(AgeEventCensoring ^ GammaStar - AgeBaseline ^
GammaStar)
  WeibullLogLikValue <- D * log(AlphaStar * GammaStar) +
(GammaStar - 1) * T_W - AlphaStar * Q_W
  return(WeibullLogLikValue)
}
```

```r
# Function to compute estimating equation
WeibullEquation <- function(GammaStar) {
  Q_W <- sum(AgeEventCensoring ^ GammaStar - AgeBaseline ^
GammaStar)
  DerQ_W <- sum(AgeEventCensoring ^ GammaStar * log
(AgeEventCensoring) - AgeBaseline ^ GammaStar * log
(AgeBaseline))
  WeibullEquationValue <- T_W + D / GammaStar - D * DerQ_W
/ Q_W
  return(WeibullEquationValue)
}

# Function to compute derivative of estimating equation
WeibullDerEquation <- function(GammaStar) {
  Q_W <- sum(AgeEventCensoring ^ GammaStar - AgeBaseline ^
GammaStar)
  DerQ_W <- sum(AgeEventCensoring ^ GammaStar * log
(AgeEventCensoring) - AgeBaseline ^ GammaStar * log
(AgeBaseline))
  DerDerQ_W <- sum(AgeEventCensoring ^ GammaStar * log
(AgeEventCensoring) ^ 2 - AgeBaseline ^ GammaStar * log
(AgeBaseline) ^ 2)
  WeibullDerEquationValue <- D * ((DerQ_W / Q_W) ^ 2 -
DerDerQ_W / Q_W - GammaStar ^ -2)
  return(WeibullDerEquationValue)
}

# Initial parameter estimates (weighted least-squares
method)
WeibullLeastSquares <- lm(LogEventRate[1:10] ~ log(Age
[1:10] - 10), weights = Events[1:10])
WeibullInterceptLeastSquares <- as.numeric(coefficients
(WeibullLeastSquares)[1])
GammaStarLeastSquares <- as.numeric(coefficients
(WeibullLeastSquares)[2] + 1)
AlphaStarLeastSquares <- exp
(WeibullInterceptLeastSquares) / GammaStarLeastSquares

# Iterative procedure (Newton method) to estimate GammaStar
i <- 0
T_W <- sum(Event * log(AgeEventCensoring))
WeibullNewtonMethod <- c(i, GammaStarLeastSquares, NA,
WeibullEquation(GammaStarLeastSquares), WeibullLogLik
(AlphaStarLeastSquares, GammaStarLeastSquares))
GammaStarCurrent <- GammaStarLeastSquares
```

```
GammaStarPrevious <- -Inf          # To make sure it iterates
while (i < 20 && abs(GammaStarCurrent - GammaStarPrevious) >
1e-10) {
  GammaStarPrevious <- GammaStarCurrent
  GammaStarCurrent <- GammaStarPrevious - WeibullEquation
(GammaStarPrevious) / WeibullDerEquation
(GammaStarPrevious)
  Q_W <- sum(AgeEventCensoring ^ GammaStarCurrent -
AgeBaseline ^ GammaStarCurrent)
  AlphaStarCurrent <- D / Q_W
  i <- i + 1
  WeibullNewtonMethod <- rbind(WeibullNewtonMethod, c(i,
GammaStarCurrent, (GammaStarCurrent - GammaStarPrevious),
WeibullEquation(GammaStarCurrent), WeibullLogLik
(AlphaStarCurrent, GammaStarCurrent)))
}
GammaStar <- GammaStarCurrent
AlphaStar <- AlphaStarCurrent
WeibullLogLikelihood <- WeibullNewtonMethod[i+1,5]

# Standard errors and 95% CIs
DerQ_W <- sum((AgeEventCensoring ^ GammaStar) * log
(AgeEventCensoring) - (AgeBaseline ^ GammaStar) * log
(AgeBaseline))
DerDerQ_W <- sum((AgeEventCensoring ^ GammaStar) * (log
(AgeEventCensoring) ^ 2) - (AgeBaseline ^ GammaStar) * (log
(AgeBaseline) ^ 2))
SecondDerAlphaStar <- -D / AlphaStar ^ 2
# Second partial derivative of the log-likelihood function
wrt AlphaStar/AlphaStar
SecondDerAlphaStarGammaStar <- -DerQ_W
# Second partial derivative of the log-likelihood function
wrt AlphaStar/GammaStar
SecondDerGammaStar <- -1 * (D / GammaStar ^ 2 + AlphaStar *
DerDerQ_W)
# Second partial derivative of the log-likelihood function
wrt GammaStar/GammaStar
FisherInformation <- -1 * matrix(c(SecondDerAlphaStar,
SecondDerAlphaStarGammaStar, SecondDerAlphaStarGammaStar,
SecondDerGammaStar), nrow = 2, ncol = 2)
WeibullVarianceMatrix <- solve(FisherInformation, tol =
1e-35)
AlphaStarSE <- sqrt(WeibullVarianceMatrix[1,1])
GammaStarSE <- sqrt(WeibullVarianceMatrix[2,2])
```

```
AlphaStarCI <- c(AlphaStar - 1.96 * AlphaStarSE, AlphaStar +
1.96 * AlphaStarSE)
GammaStarCI <- c(GammaStar - 1.96 * GammaStarSE, GammaStar +
1.96 * GammaStarSE)

# Fitted event rates
WeibullFittedEventRate <- AlphaStar * GammaStar * (Age[1:10]
- 10) ^ (GammaStar - 1)
WeibullFittedLogEventRate <- log(WeibullFittedEventRate)

# Output for Weibull model
summary(WeibullLeastSquares)
list(AlphaStarLeastSquares = AlphaStarLeastSquares,
GammaStarLeastSquares = GammaStarLeastSquares)
colnames(WeibullNewtonMethod) <- c("i", "GammaStar",
"GammaStar change", "Estimating equation",
"Log likelihood")
print(WeibullNewtonMethod, digits = 10)
print(WeibullLogLikelihood, digits = 15)
WeibullVarianceMatrix
descriptive4 <- matrix(c(AlphaStar, AlphaStarSE,
AlphaStarCI, GammaStar, GammaStarSE, GammaStarCI), nrow = 2,
byrow = TRUE)
colnames(descriptive4) <- c("Parameter estimate", "Standard
error", "95% Confidence interval", " ")
rownames(descriptive4) <- c("AlphaStar", "GammaStar")
descriptive4
descriptive5 <- cbind(Age[1:10], EventRate[1:10],
WeibullFittedEventRate, LogEventRate[1:10],
WeibullFittedLogEventRate)
colnames(descriptive5) <- c("Age", "Event rate", "Weibull
fitted", "Log event rate", "Weibull fitted")
descriptive5


#### Likelihood ratio for the Gompertz model versus the
Weibull model ####

GompertzLogLikelihood <- GompertzLogLik(LambdaStar,
ThetaStar)
WeibullLogLikelihood <- WeibullLogLik(AlphaStar,
GammaStar)
LogLR <- GompertzLogLikelihood - WeibullLogLikelihood
LR <- exp(LogLR)
```

```
list(GompertzLogLikelihood = GompertzLogLikelihood,
WeibullLogLikelihood = WeibullLogLikelihood, LogLR = LogLR,
LR = LR)



############## 5-parameter mixture model ##############

f <- function(X, Mu, Theta, Beta, Gamma, Logit) {(exp(Logit) /
(1 + exp(Logit))) * exp(Mu) * exp(Theta * X - (exp(Mu) / Theta) *
(exp(Theta * X) - 1)) + (1 / (1 + exp(Logit))) * exp(Beta) * Gamma
* X ^ (Gamma - 1) * exp(-exp(Beta) * X ^ Gamma)}
fMu <- function(X, Mu, Theta, Logit) {(exp(Logit) / (1 + exp
(Logit))) * exp(Theta * X + Mu - (exp(Mu) / Theta) * (exp(Theta *
X) - 1)) * (1 - (exp(Mu) / Theta) * (exp(Theta * X) - 1))}
fTheta <- function(X, Mu, Theta, Logit) {(exp(Logit) / (1 + exp
(Logit))) * exp(Mu) * exp(Theta * X - (exp(Mu) / Theta) * (exp
(Theta * X) - 1)) * (X - (exp(Mu) / Theta) * (X * exp(Theta * X)
- (exp(Theta * X) - 1) / Theta))}
fBeta <- function(X, Beta, Gamma, Logit) {(1 / (1 + exp
(Logit))) * Gamma * X ^ (Gamma - 1) * exp(Beta - exp(Beta) * X ^
Gamma) * (1 - exp(Beta) * X ^ Gamma)}
fGamma <- function(X, Beta, Gamma, Logit) {(1 / (1 + exp
(Logit))) * exp(Beta) * X ^ (Gamma - 1) * exp(-exp(Beta) * X ^
Gamma) * (1 + Gamma * log(X) * (1 - exp(Beta) * X ^ Gamma))}
fLogit <- function(X, Mu, Theta, Beta, Gamma, Logit) {(exp
(Logit) / (1 + exp(Logit)) ^ 2) * (exp(Mu) * exp(Theta * X - (exp
(Mu) / Theta) * (exp(Theta * X) - 1)) - exp(Beta) * Gamma * X ^
(Gamma - 1) * exp(-exp(Beta) * X ^ Gamma))}
fMuMu <- function(X, Mu, Theta, Logit) {(exp(Logit) / (1 + exp
(Logit))) * exp(Theta * X + Mu - (exp(Mu) / Theta) * (exp(Theta *
X) - 1)) * ((1 - (exp(Mu) / Theta) * (exp(Theta * X) - 1)) ^ 2 - (exp
(Mu) / Theta) * (exp(Theta * X) - 1))}
fThetaTheta <- function(X, Mu, Theta, Logit) {(exp(Logit) / (1
+ exp(Logit))) * exp(Mu) * exp(Theta * X - (exp(Mu) / Theta) *
(exp(Theta * X) - 1)) * (-(exp(Mu) / Theta) * ((X * exp(Theta * X)
- (exp(Theta * X) - 1) / Theta) * (-(exp(Mu) / Theta) * (X * exp
(Theta * X) - (exp(Theta * X) - 1) / Theta) + 2 * X - 2 / Theta) + X ^ 2
* exp(Theta * X)) + X ^ 2)}
fBetaBeta <- function(X, Beta, Gamma, Logit) {(1 / (1 + exp
(Logit))) * Gamma * X ^ (Gamma - 1) * exp(Beta - exp(Beta) * X ^
Gamma) * ((1 - exp(Beta) * X ^ Gamma) ^ 2 - exp(Beta) * X ^ Gamma)}
fGammaGamma <- function(X, Beta, Gamma, Logit) {(1 / (1 + exp
(Logit))) * exp(Beta) * X ^ (Gamma - 1) * exp(-exp(Beta) * X ^
```

```
Gamma) * (-exp(Beta) * X ^ Gamma * log(X) * (Gamma * log(X) * (3 -
exp(Beta) * X ^ Gamma) + 2) + log(X) * (Gamma * log(X) + 2))}
fLogitLogit <- function(X, Mu, Theta, Beta, Gamma, Logit)
{(exp(Logit) * (1 - exp(Logit)) / (1 + exp(Logit)) ^ 3) * (exp
(Mu) * exp(Theta * X - (exp(Mu) / Theta) * (exp(Theta * X) - 1)) -
exp(Beta) * Gamma * X ^ (Gamma - 1) * exp(-exp(Beta) * X
^ Gamma))}
fMuTheta <- function(X, Mu, Theta, Logit) {(exp(Logit) / (1 +
exp(Logit))) * exp(Theta * X + Mu - (exp(Mu) / Theta) * (exp
(Theta * X) - 1)) * (-(exp(Mu) / Theta) * (X * exp(Theta * X) - (exp
(Theta * X) - 1) / Theta) * (2 - (exp(Mu) / Theta) * (exp(Theta * X)
- 1)) + X * (1 - (exp(Mu) / Theta) * (exp(Theta * X) - 1)))}
fBetaGamma <- function(X, Beta, Gamma, Logit) {(1 / (1 + exp
(Logit))) * X ^ (Gamma - 1) * exp(Beta - exp(Beta) * X ^ Gamma) *
(-exp(Beta) * X ^ Gamma * (Gamma * log(X) * (3 - exp(Beta) * X ^
Gamma) + 1) + Gamma * log(X) + 1)}
fMuLogit <- function(X, Mu, Theta, Logit) {(exp(Logit) / (1 +
exp(Logit)) ^ 2) * exp(Theta * X + Mu - (exp(Mu) / Theta) * (exp
(Theta * X) - 1)) * (1 - (exp(Mu) / Theta) * (exp(Theta * X) - 1))}
fThetaLogit <- function(X, Mu, Theta, Logit) {(exp(Logit) / (1
+ exp(Logit)) ^ 2) * exp(Mu) * exp(Theta * X - (exp(Mu) / Theta) *
(exp(Theta * X) - 1)) * (X - (exp(Mu) / Theta) * (X * exp(Theta * X)
- (exp(Theta * X) - 1) / Theta))}
fBetaLogit <- function(X, Beta, Gamma, Logit) {- (exp(Logit) /
(1 + exp(Logit)) ^ 2) * Gamma * X ^ (Gamma - 1) * exp(Beta - exp
(Beta) * X ^ Gamma) * (1 - exp(Beta) * X ^ Gamma)}
fGammaLogit <- function(X, Beta, Gamma, Logit) {- (exp(Logit) /
(1 + exp(Logit)) ^ 2) * exp(Beta) * X ^ (Gamma - 1) * exp(-exp(Beta)
* X ^ Gamma) * (1 + Gamma * log(X) * (1 - exp(Beta) * X ^ Gamma))}


S <- function(X, Mu, Theta, Beta, Gamma, Logit) {(exp(Logit) /
(1 + exp(Logit))) * exp(-(exp(Mu) / Theta) * (exp(Theta * X) -
1)) + (1 / (1 + exp(Logit))) * exp(-exp(Beta) * X ^ Gamma)}
SMu <- function(X, Mu, Theta, Logit) {(exp(Logit) / (1 + exp
(Logit))) * exp(Mu - (exp(Mu) / Theta) * (exp(Theta * X) - 1)) *
(-(exp(Theta * X) - 1) / Theta)}
STheta <- function(X, Mu, Theta, Logit) {(exp(Logit) / (1 + exp
(Logit))) * exp(-(exp(Mu) / Theta) * (exp(Theta * X) - 1)) *
(-(exp(Mu) / Theta) * (X * exp(Theta * X) - (exp(Theta * X) - 1)
/ Theta))}
SBeta <- function(X, Beta, Gamma, Logit) {(1 / (1 + exp(Logit))) *
exp(Beta - exp(Beta) * X ^ Gamma) * (-X ^ Gamma)}
SGamma <- function(X, Beta, Gamma, Logit) {(1 / (1 + exp(Logit)))
* exp(-exp(Beta) * X ^ Gamma) * (-exp(Beta) * X ^ Gamma * log(X))}
```

```r
SLogit <- function(X, Mu, Theta, Beta, Gamma, Logit) {(exp
(Logit) / (1 + exp(Logit)) ^ 2) * (exp(-(exp(Mu) / Theta) * (exp
(Theta * X) - 1)) - exp(-exp(Beta) * X ^ Gamma))}
SMuMu <- function(X, Mu, Theta, Logit) {(exp(Logit) / (1 + exp
(Logit))) * exp(-(exp(Mu) / Theta) * (exp(Theta * X) - 1)) *
((-(exp(Mu) / Theta) * (exp(Theta * X) - 1)) ^ 2 - (exp(Mu) /
Theta) * (exp(Theta * X) - 1))}
SThetaTheta <- function(X, Mu, Theta, Logit) {(exp(Logit) /
(1 + exp(Logit))) * exp(-(exp(Mu) / Theta) * (exp(Theta * X) -
1)) * (-(exp(Mu) / Theta) * ((X * exp(Theta * X) - (exp(Theta *
X) - 1) / Theta) * (-(exp(Mu) / Theta) * (X * exp(Theta * X) -
(exp(Theta * X) - 1) / Theta) - 2 / Theta) + X ^ 2 * exp(Theta
* X)))}
SBetaBeta <- function(X, Beta, Gamma, Logit) {(1 / (1 + exp
(Logit))) * exp(-exp(Beta) * X ^ Gamma) * ((-exp(Beta) * X ^
Gamma) ^ 2 - exp(Beta) * X ^ Gamma)}
SGammaGamma <- function(X, Beta, Gamma, Logit) {(1 / (1 + exp
(Logit))) * exp(-exp(Beta) * X ^ Gamma) * (-exp(Beta) * X ^ Gamma
* log(X) ^ 2) * (1 - exp(Beta) * X ^ Gamma)}
SLogitLogit <- function(X, Mu, Theta, Beta, Gamma, Logit)
{(exp(Logit) * (1 - exp(Logit)) / (1 + exp(Logit)) ^ 3) * (exp
(-(exp(Mu) / Theta) * (exp(Theta * X) - 1)) - exp(-exp(Beta) * X
^ Gamma))}
SMuTheta <- function(X, Mu, Theta, Logit) {(exp(Logit) / (1 +
exp(Logit))) * exp(Mu - (exp(Mu) / Theta) * (exp(Theta * X) -
1)) * (-1 / Theta) * (X * exp(Theta * X) - (exp(Theta * X) - 1) /
Theta) * (1 - (exp(Mu) / Theta) * (exp(Theta * X) - 1))}
SBetaGamma <- function(X, Beta, Gamma, Logit) {(1 / (1 + exp
(Logit))) * exp(Beta - exp(Beta) * X ^ Gamma) * (-X ^ Gamma * log
(X)) * (1 - exp(Beta) * X ^ Gamma)}
SMuLogit <- function(X, Mu, Theta, Logit) {(exp(Logit) / (1 +
exp(Logit)) ^ 2) * exp(Mu - (exp(Mu) / Theta) * (exp(Theta * X) -
1)) * (-(exp(Theta * X) - 1) / Theta)}
SThetaLogit <- function(X, Mu, Theta, Logit) {(exp(Logit) /
(1 + exp(Logit)) ^ 2) * exp(-(exp(Mu) / Theta) * (exp(Theta * X) -
1)) * (-(exp(Mu) / Theta) * (X * exp(Theta * X) - (exp(Theta * X)
- 1) / Theta))}
SBetaLogit <- function(X, Beta, Gamma, Logit) {(exp(Logit) /
(1 + exp(Logit)) ^ 2) * exp(Beta - exp(Beta) * X ^ Gamma) * X
^ Gamma}
SGammaLogit <- function(X, Beta, Gamma, Logit) {(exp(Logit) /
(1 + exp(Logit)) ^ 2) * exp(-exp(Beta) * X ^ Gamma) * exp(Beta) *
X ^ Gamma * log(X)}

# Function to compute log-likelihood function
MixtureLogLik <- function(Mu, Theta, Beta, Gamma, Logit) {
```

```
  MixtureLogLikValue <- sum(Event * log(f
(AgeEventCensoring, Mu, Theta, Beta, Gamma, Logit)) + (1 -
Event) * log(S(AgeEventCensoring, Mu, Theta, Beta, Gamma,
Logit)) - log(S(AgeBaseline, Mu, Theta, Beta, Gamma, Logit)))
  return(MixtureLogLikValue)
}

# Function to compute estimating equations (gradient vector)
MixtureEquation <- function(Mu, Theta, Beta, Gamma,
Logit) {
  MixtureLogLikMu <- sum(Event * fMu(AgeEventCensoring, Mu,
Theta, Logit) / f(AgeEventCensoring, Mu, Theta, Beta, Gamma,
Logit) + (1 - Event) * SMu(AgeEventCensoring, Mu, Theta,
Logit) / S(AgeEventCensoring, Mu, Theta, Beta, Gamma, Logit) -
SMu(AgeBaseline, Mu, Theta, Logit) / S(AgeBaseline, Mu,
Theta, Beta, Gamma, Logit))
  MixtureLogLikTheta <- sum(Event * fTheta
(AgeEventCensoring, Mu, Theta, Logit) / f(AgeEventCensoring,
Mu, Theta, Beta, Gamma, Logit) + (1 - Event) * STheta
(AgeEventCensoring, Mu, Theta, Logit) / S(AgeEventCensoring,
Mu, Theta, Beta, Gamma, Logit) - STheta(AgeBaseline, Mu,
Theta, Logit) / S(AgeBaseline, Mu, Theta, Beta, Gamma, Logit))
  MixtureLogLikBeta <- sum(Event * fBeta(AgeEventCensoring,
Beta, Gamma, Logit) / f(AgeEventCensoring, Mu, Theta, Beta,
Gamma, Logit) + (1 - Event) * SBeta(AgeEventCensoring, Beta,
Gamma, Logit) / S(AgeEventCensoring, Mu, Theta, Beta, Gamma,
Logit) - SBeta(AgeBaseline, Beta, Gamma, Logit) /
S(AgeBaseline, Mu, Theta, Beta, Gamma, Logit))
  MixtureLogLikGamma <- sum(Event * fGamma
(AgeEventCensoring, Beta, Gamma, Logit) /
f(AgeEventCensoring, Mu, Theta, Beta, Gamma, Logit) + (1 -
Event) * SGamma(AgeEventCensoring, Beta, Gamma, Logit) /
S(AgeEventCensoring, Mu, Theta, Beta, Gamma, Logit) - SGamma
(AgeBaseline, Beta, Gamma, Logit) / S(AgeBaseline, Mu, Theta,
Beta, Gamma, Logit))
  MixtureLogLikLogit <- sum(Event * fLogit
(AgeEventCensoring, Mu, Theta, Beta, Gamma, Logit) /
f(AgeEventCensoring, Mu, Theta, Beta, Gamma, Logit) + (1 -
Event) * SLogit(AgeEventCensoring, Mu, Theta, Beta, Gamma,
Logit) / S(AgeEventCensoring, Mu, Theta, Beta, Gamma, Logit) -
SLogit(AgeBaseline, Mu, Theta, Beta, Gamma, Logit) /
S(AgeBaseline, Mu, Theta, Beta, Gamma, Logit))
  Gradient <- c(MixtureLogLikMu, MixtureLogLikTheta,
MixtureLogLikBeta, MixtureLogLikGamma, MixtureLogLikLogit)
  return(Gradient)
}
```

```
# Function to compute derivatives of estimating equations
(Hessian matrix)
  MixtureDerEquation <- function(Mu, Theta, Beta, Gamma,
Logit) {
  MixtureLogLikMuMu <- sum(Event * (fMuMu
(AgeEventCensoring, Mu, Theta, Logit) / f(AgeEventCensoring,
Mu, Theta, Beta, Gamma, Logit) - (fMu(AgeEventCensoring, Mu,
Theta, Logit) / f(AgeEventCensoring, Mu, Theta, Beta, Gamma,
Logit)) ^ 2) + (1 - Event) * (SMuMu(AgeEventCensoring, Mu,
Theta, Logit) / S(AgeEventCensoring, Mu, Theta, Beta, Gamma,
Logit) - (SMu(AgeEventCensoring, Mu, Theta, Logit) /
S(AgeEventCensoring, Mu, Theta, Beta, Gamma, Logit)) ^ 2) -
(SMuMu(AgeBaseline, Mu, Theta, Logit) / S(AgeBaseline, Mu,
Theta, Beta, Gamma, Logit) - (SMu(AgeBaseline, Mu, Theta,
Logit) / S(AgeBaseline, Mu, Theta, Beta, Gamma, Logit)) ^ 2))
  MixtureLogLikThetaTheta <- sum(Event * (fThetaTheta
(AgeEventCensoring, Mu, Theta, Logit) / f(AgeEventCensoring,
Mu, Theta, Beta, Gamma, Logit) - (fTheta(AgeEventCensoring,
Mu, Theta, Logit) / f(AgeEventCensoring, Mu, Theta, Beta,
Gamma, Logit)) ^ 2) + (1 - Event) * (SThetaTheta
(AgeEventCensoring, Mu, Theta, Logit) / S(AgeEventCensoring,
Mu, Theta, Beta, Gamma, Logit) - (STheta(AgeEventCensoring,
Mu, Theta, Logit) / S(AgeEventCensoring, Mu, Theta, Beta,
Gamma, Logit)) ^ 2) - (SThetaTheta(AgeBaseline, Mu, Theta,
Logit) / S(AgeBaseline, Mu, Theta, Beta, Gamma, Logit) -
(STheta(AgeBaseline, Mu, Theta, Logit) / S(AgeBaseline, Mu,
Theta, Beta, Gamma, Logit)) ^ 2))
  MixtureLogLikBetaBeta <- sum(Event * (fBetaBeta
(AgeEventCensoring, Beta, Gamma, Logit) /
f(AgeEventCensoring, Mu, Theta, Beta, Gamma, Logit) - (fBeta
(AgeEventCensoring, Beta, Gamma, Logit) /
f(AgeEventCensoring, Mu, Theta, Beta, Gamma, Logit)) ^ 2) + (1
- Event) * (SBetaBeta(AgeEventCensoring, Beta, Gamma, Logit)
/ S(AgeEventCensoring, Mu, Theta, Beta, Gamma, Logit) - (SBeta
(AgeEventCensoring, Beta, Gamma, Logit) /
S(AgeEventCensoring, Mu, Theta, Beta, Gamma, Logit)) ^ 2) -
(SBetaBeta(AgeBaseline, Beta, Gamma, Logit) / S(AgeBaseline,
Mu, Theta, Beta, Gamma, Logit) - (SBeta(AgeBaseline, Beta,
Gamma, Logit) / S(AgeBaseline, Mu, Theta, Beta, Gamma,
Logit)) ^ 2))
  MixtureLogLikGammaGamma <- sum(Event * (fGammaGamma
(AgeEventCensoring, Beta, Gamma, Logit) /
f(AgeEventCensoring, Mu, Theta, Beta, Gamma, Logit) - (fGamma
(AgeEventCensoring, Beta, Gamma, Logit) /
```

```
f(AgeEventCensoring, Mu, Theta, Beta, Gamma, Logit)) ^ 2) + (1
- Event) * (SGammaGamma(AgeEventCensoring, Beta, Gamma,
Logit) / S(AgeEventCensoring, Mu, Theta, Beta, Gamma, Logit) -
(SGamma(AgeEventCensoring, Beta, Gamma, Logit) /
S(AgeEventCensoring, Mu, Theta, Beta, Gamma, Logit)) ^ 2) -
(SGammaGamma(AgeBaseline, Beta, Gamma, Logit) /
S(AgeBaseline, Mu, Theta, Beta, Gamma, Logit) - (SGamma
(AgeBaseline, Beta, Gamma, Logit) / S(AgeBaseline, Mu, Theta,
Beta, Gamma, Logit)) ^ 2))
   MixtureLogLikLogitLogit <- sum(Event * (fLogitLogit
(AgeEventCensoring, Mu, Theta, Beta, Gamma, Logit) /
f(AgeEventCensoring, Mu, Theta, Beta, Gamma, Logit) - (fLogit
(AgeEventCensoring, Mu, Theta, Beta, Gamma, Logit) /
f(AgeEventCensoring, Mu, Theta, Beta, Gamma, Logit)) ^ 2) + (1
- Event) * (SLogitLogit(AgeEventCensoring, Mu, Theta, Beta,
Gamma, Logit) / S(AgeEventCensoring, Mu, Theta, Beta, Gamma,
Logit) - (SLogit(AgeEventCensoring, Mu, Theta, Beta, Gamma,
Logit) / S(AgeEventCensoring, Mu, Theta, Beta, Gamma, Logit))
^ 2) - (SLogitLogit(AgeBaseline, Mu, Theta, Beta, Gamma,
Logit) / S(AgeBaseline, Mu, Theta, Beta, Gamma, Logit) -
(SLogit(AgeBaseline, Mu, Theta, Beta, Gamma, Logit) /
S(AgeBaseline, Mu, Theta, Beta, Gamma, Logit)) ^ 2))
   MixtureLogLikMuTheta <- sum(Event * (fMuTheta
(AgeEventCensoring, Mu, Theta, Logit) / f(AgeEventCensoring,
Mu, Theta, Beta, Gamma, Logit) - fMu(AgeEventCensoring, Mu,
Theta, Logit) * fTheta(AgeEventCensoring, Mu, Theta, Logit) /
f(AgeEventCensoring, Mu, Theta, Beta, Gamma, Logit) ^ 2) + (1 -
Event) * (SMuTheta(AgeEventCensoring, Mu, Theta, Logit) /
S(AgeEventCensoring, Mu, Theta, Beta, Gamma, Logit) - SMu
(AgeEventCensoring, Mu, Theta, Logit) * STheta
(AgeEventCensoring, Mu, Theta, Logit) / S(AgeEventCensoring,
Mu, Theta, Beta, Gamma, Logit) ^ 2) - (SMuTheta(AgeBaseline,
Mu, Theta, Logit) / S(AgeBaseline, Mu, Theta, Beta, Gamma,
Logit) - SMu(AgeBaseline, Mu, Theta, Logit) * STheta
(AgeBaseline, Mu, Theta, Logit) / S(AgeBaseline, Mu, Theta,
Beta, Gamma, Logit) ^ 2))
   MixtureLogLikBetaGamma <- sum(Event * (fBetaGamma
(AgeEventCensoring, Beta, Gamma, Logit) /
f(AgeEventCensoring, Mu, Theta, Beta, Gamma, Logit) - fBeta
(AgeEventCensoring, Beta, Gamma, Logit) * fGamma
(AgeEventCensoring, Beta, Gamma, Logit) /
f(AgeEventCensoring, Mu, Theta, Beta, Gamma, Logit) ^ 2) + (1 -
Event) * (SBetaGamma(AgeEventCensoring, Beta, Gamma, Logit)
/ S(AgeEventCensoring, Mu, Theta, Beta, Gamma, Logit) - SBeta
```

```
(AgeEventCensoring, Beta, Gamma, Logit) * SGamma
(AgeEventCensoring, Beta, Gamma, Logit) /
S(AgeEventCensoring, Mu, Theta, Beta, Gamma, Logit) ^ 2) -
(SBetaGamma(AgeBaseline, Beta, Gamma, Logit) /
S(AgeBaseline, Mu, Theta, Beta, Gamma, Logit) - SBeta
(AgeBaseline, Beta, Gamma, Logit) * SGamma(AgeBaseline, Beta,
Gamma, Logit) / S(AgeBaseline, Mu, Theta, Beta, Gamma, Logit)
^ 2))
    MixtureLogLikMuLogit <- sum(Event * (fMuLogit
(AgeEventCensoring, Mu, Theta, Logit) / f(AgeEventCensoring,
Mu, Theta, Beta, Gamma, Logit) - fMu(AgeEventCensoring, Mu,
Theta, Logit) * fLogit(AgeEventCensoring, Mu, Theta, Beta,
Gamma, Logit) / f(AgeEventCensoring, Mu, Theta, Beta, Gamma,
Logit) ^ 2) + (1 - Event) * (SMuLogit(AgeEventCensoring, Mu,
Theta, Logit) / S(AgeEventCensoring, Mu, Theta, Beta, Gamma,
Logit) - SMu(AgeEventCensoring, Mu, Theta, Logit) * SLogit
(AgeEventCensoring, Mu, Theta, Beta, Gamma, Logit) /
S(AgeEventCensoring, Mu, Theta, Beta, Gamma, Logit) ^ 2) -
(SMuLogit(AgeBaseline, Mu, Theta, Logit) / S(AgeBaseline, Mu,
Theta, Beta, Gamma, Logit) - SMu(AgeBaseline, Mu, Theta,
Logit) * SLogit(AgeBaseline, Mu, Theta, Beta, Gamma, Logit) /
S(AgeBaseline, Mu, Theta, Beta, Gamma, Logit) ^ 2))
    MixtureLogLikThetaLogit <- sum(Event * (fThetaLogit
(AgeEventCensoring, Mu, Theta, Logit) / f(AgeEventCensoring,
Mu, Theta, Beta, Gamma, Logit) - fTheta(AgeEventCensoring,
Mu, Theta, Logit) * fLogit(AgeEventCensoring, Mu, Theta,
Beta, Gamma, Logit) / f(AgeEventCensoring, Mu, Theta, Beta,
Gamma, Logit) ^ 2) + (1 - Event) * (SThetaLogit
(AgeEventCensoring, Mu, Theta, Logit) / S(AgeEventCensoring,
Mu, Theta, Beta, Gamma, Logit) - STheta(AgeEventCensoring,
Mu, Theta, Logit) * SLogit(AgeEventCensoring, Mu, Theta,
Beta, Gamma, Logit) / S(AgeEventCensoring, Mu, Theta, Beta,
Gamma, Logit) ^ 2) - (SThetaLogit(AgeBaseline, Mu, Theta,
Logit) / S(AgeBaseline, Mu, Theta, Beta, Gamma, Logit) -
STheta(AgeBaseline, Mu, Theta, Logit) * SLogit(AgeBaseline,
Mu, Theta, Beta, Gamma, Logit) / S(AgeBaseline, Mu, Theta,
Beta, Gamma, Logit) ^ 2))
    MixtureLogLikBetaLogit <- sum(Event * (fBetaLogit
(AgeEventCensoring, Beta, Gamma, Logit) /
f(AgeEventCensoring, Mu, Theta, Beta, Gamma, Logit) - fBeta
(AgeEventCensoring, Beta, Gamma, Logit) * fLogit
(AgeEventCensoring, Mu, Theta, Beta, Gamma, Logit) /
f(AgeEventCensoring, Mu, Theta, Beta, Gamma, Logit) ^ 2) + (1 -
Event) * (SBetaLogit(AgeEventCensoring, Beta, Gamma, Logit)
/ S(AgeEventCensoring, Mu, Theta, Beta, Gamma, Logit) - SBeta
```

```
(AgeEventCensoring, Beta, Gamma, Logit) * SLogit
(AgeEventCensoring, Mu, Theta, Beta, Gamma, Logit) /
S(AgeEventCensoring, Mu, Theta, Beta, Gamma, Logit) ^ 2) -
(SBetaLogit(AgeBaseline, Beta, Gamma, Logit) /
S(AgeBaseline, Mu, Theta, Beta, Gamma, Logit) - SBeta
(AgeBaseline, Beta, Gamma, Logit) * SLogit(AgeBaseline, Mu,
Theta, Beta, Gamma, Logit) / S(AgeBaseline, Mu, Theta, Beta,
Gamma, Logit) ^ 2))
  MixtureLogLikGammaLogit <- sum(Event * (fGammaLogit
(AgeEventCensoring, Beta, Gamma, Logit) /
f(AgeEventCensoring, Mu, Theta, Beta, Gamma, Logit) - fGamma
(AgeEventCensoring, Beta, Gamma, Logit) * fLogit
(AgeEventCensoring, Mu, Theta, Beta, Gamma, Logit) /
f(AgeEventCensoring, Mu, Theta, Beta, Gamma, Logit) ^ 2) + (1 -
Event) * (SGammaLogit(AgeEventCensoring, Beta, Gamma, Logit)
/ S(AgeEventCensoring, Mu, Theta, Beta, Gamma, Logit) - SGamma
(AgeEventCensoring, Beta, Gamma, Logit) * SLogit
(AgeEventCensoring, Mu, Theta, Beta, Gamma, Logit) /
S(AgeEventCensoring, Mu, Theta, Beta, Gamma, Logit) ^ 2) -
(SGammaLogit(AgeBaseline, Beta, Gamma, Logit) /
S(AgeBaseline, Mu, Theta, Beta, Gamma, Logit) - SGamma
(AgeBaseline, Beta, Gamma, Logit) * SLogit(AgeBaseline, Mu,
Theta, Beta, Gamma, Logit) / S(AgeBaseline, Mu, Theta, Beta,
Gamma, Logit) ^ 2))
  MixtureLogLikMuBeta <- sum(-Event * fMu
(AgeEventCensoring, Mu, Theta, Logit) * fBeta
(AgeEventCensoring, Beta, Gamma, Logit) /
f(AgeEventCensoring, Mu, Theta, Beta, Gamma, Logit) ^ 2 - (1 -
Event) * SMu(AgeEventCensoring, Mu, Theta, Logit) * SBeta
(AgeEventCensoring, Beta, Gamma, Logit) /
S(AgeEventCensoring, Mu, Theta, Beta, Gamma, Logit) ^ 2 + SMu
(AgeBaseline, Mu, Theta, Logit) * SBeta(AgeBaseline, Beta,
Gamma, Logit) / S(AgeBaseline, Mu, Theta, Beta, Gamma,
Logit) ^ 2)
  MixtureLogLikMuGamma <- sum(-Event * fMu(AgeEventCensoring,
Mu, Theta, Logit) * fGamma(AgeEventCensoring, Beta, Gamma,
Logit) / f(AgeEventCensoring, Mu, Theta, Beta, Gamma, Logit) ^ 2 -
(1 - Event) * SMu(AgeEventCensoring, Mu, Theta, Logit) * SGamma
(AgeEventCensoring, Beta, Gamma, Logit) / S(AgeEventCensoring,
Mu, Theta, Beta, Gamma, Logit) ^ 2 + SMu(AgeBaseline, Mu, Theta,
Logit) * SGamma(AgeBaseline, Beta, Gamma, Logit) /
S(AgeBaseline, Mu, Theta, Beta, Gamma, Logit) ^ 2)
  MixtureLogLikThetaBeta <- sum(-Event * fTheta
(AgeEventCensoring, Mu, Theta, Logit) * fBeta
(AgeEventCensoring, Beta, Gamma, Logit) / f(AgeEventCensoring,
```

```
Mu, Theta, Beta, Gamma, Logit) ^ 2 - (1 - Event) * STheta
(AgeEventCensoring, Mu, Theta, Logit) * SBeta
(AgeEventCensoring, Beta, Gamma, Logit) / S (AgeEventCensoring,
Mu, Theta, Beta, Gamma, Logit) ^ 2 + STheta (AgeBaseline, Mu,
Theta, Logit) * SBeta (AgeBaseline, Beta, Gamma, Logit) /
S (AgeBaseline, Mu, Theta, Beta, Gamma, Logit) ^ 2)
  MixtureLogLikThetaGamma <- sum (-Event * fTheta
(AgeEventCensoring, Mu, Theta, Logit) * fGamma
(AgeEventCensoring, Beta, Gamma, Logit) /
f (AgeEventCensoring, Mu, Theta, Beta, Gamma, Logit) ^ 2 - (1 -
Event) * STheta (AgeEventCensoring, Mu, Theta, Logit) * SGamma
(AgeEventCensoring, Beta, Gamma, Logit) /
S (AgeEventCensoring, Mu, Theta, Beta, Gamma, Logit) ^ 2 + STheta
(AgeBaseline, Mu, Theta, Logit) * SGamma (AgeBaseline, Beta,
Gamma, Logit) / S (AgeBaseline, Mu, Theta, Beta, Gamma, Logit)
^ 2)
  Hessian <- matrix (rep (NA, 25), ncol = 5)
  Hessian [1,1] <- MixtureLogLikMuMu
  Hessian [2,2] <- MixtureLogLikThetaTheta
  Hessian [3,3] <- MixtureLogLikBetaBeta
  Hessian [4,4] <- MixtureLogLikGammaGamma
  Hessian [5,5] <- MixtureLogLikLogitLogit
  Hessian [1,2] <- Hessian [2,1] <- MixtureLogLikMuTheta
  Hessian [1,3] <- Hessian [3,1] <- MixtureLogLikMuBeta
  Hessian [1,4] <- Hessian [4,1] <- MixtureLogLikMuGamma
  Hessian [1,5] <- Hessian [5,1] <- MixtureLogLikMuLogit
  Hessian [2,3] <- Hessian [3,2] <- MixtureLogLikThetaBeta
  Hessian [2,4] <- Hessian [4,2] <- MixtureLogLikThetaGamma
  Hessian [2,5] <- Hessian [5,2] <- MixtureLogLikThetaLogit
  Hessian [3,4] <- Hessian [4,3] <- MixtureLogLikBetaGamma
  Hessian [3,5] <- Hessian [5,3] <- MixtureLogLikBetaLogit
  Hessian [4,5] <- Hessian [5,4] <- MixtureLogLikGammaLogit
  return (Hessian)
}


# E-M algorithm
f_G <- function (X, Lambda, Theta) {Lambda * exp (Theta * X) * exp
(-(Lambda / Theta) * (exp (Theta * X) - 1))}
f_W <- function (X, Alpha, Gamma) {Alpha * Gamma * X ^ (Gamma - 1)
* exp (-Alpha * X ^ Gamma)}
S_G <- function (X, Lambda, Theta) {exp (-(Lambda / Theta) *
(exp (Theta * X) - 1))}
S_W <- function (X, Alpha, Gamma) {exp (-Alpha * X ^ Gamma)}
```

```
# Functions to compute Theta estimating equation and
derivative of estimating equation from complete-data
likelihood (E-M algorithm)
GompertzEquation_EM <- function(Theta) {
  Q_G_EM <- sum(Y_x * (exp(Theta * AgeEventCensoring) - 1) -
Y_a * (exp(Theta * AgeBaseline) - 1))
  DerQ_G_EM <- sum(Y_x * AgeEventCensoring * exp(Theta *
AgeEventCensoring) - Y_a * AgeBaseline * exp(Theta *
AgeBaseline))
  GompertzEquationValue_EM <- T_G_EM + D_G_EM / Theta - D_G_EM
* DerQ_G_EM / Q_G_EM
  return(GompertzEquationValue_EM)
}
GompertzDerEquation_EM <- function(Theta) {
  Q_G_EM <- sum(Y_x * (exp(Theta * AgeEventCensoring) - 1) -
Y_a * (exp(Theta * AgeBaseline) - 1))
  DerQ_G_EM <- sum(Y_x * AgeEventCensoring * exp(Theta *
AgeEventCensoring) - Y_a * AgeBaseline * exp(Theta *
AgeBaseline))
  DerDerQ_G_EM <- sum(Y_x * AgeEventCensoring ^ 2 * exp(Theta *
AgeEventCensoring) - Y_a * AgeBaseline ^ 2 * exp(Theta *
AgeBaseline))
  GompertzDerEquationValue_EM <- D_G_EM * ((DerQ_G_EM /
Q_G_EM) ^ 2 - DerDerQ_G_EM / Q_G_EM - Theta ^ -2)
  return(GompertzDerEquationValue_EM)
}

# Functions to compute Gamma estimating equation and
derivative of estimating equation from complete-data
likelihood (E-M algorithm)
WeibullEquation_EM <- function(Gamma) {
  Q_W_EM <- sum((1 - Y_x) * AgeEventCensoring ^ Gamma - (1 - Y_a)
* AgeBaseline ^ Gamma)
  DerQ_W_EM <- sum((1 - Y_x) * AgeEventCensoring ^ Gamma * log
(AgeEventCensoring) - (1 - Y_a) * AgeBaseline ^ Gamma * log
(AgeBaseline))
  WeibullEquationValue_EM <- T_W_EM + D_W_EM / Gamma - D_W_EM *
DerQ_W_EM / Q_W_EM
  return(WeibullEquationValue_EM)
}
WeibullDerEquation_EM <- function(Gamma) {
  Q_W_EM <- sum((1 - Y_x) * AgeEventCensoring ^ Gamma - (1 - Y_a)
* AgeBaseline ^ Gamma)
```

```
  DerQ_W_EM <- sum((1 - Y_x) * AgeEventCensoring ^ Gamma * log
(AgeEventCensoring) - (1 - Y_a) * AgeBaseline ^ Gamma * log
(AgeBaseline))
  DerDerQ_W_EM <- sum((1 - Y_x) * AgeEventCensoring ^ Gamma *
log(AgeEventCensoring) ^ 2 - (1 - Y_a) * AgeBaseline ^ Gamma *
log(AgeBaseline) ^ 2)
  WeibullDerEquationValue_EM <- D_W_EM * ((DerQ_W_EM /
Q_W_EM) ^ 2 - DerDerQ_W_EM / Q_W_EM - Gamma ^ -2)
  return(WeibullDerEquationValue_EM)
}


# Initial values for E-M algorithm
LambdaInitial <- LambdaStar
ThetaInitial <- ThetaStar
AlphaInitial <- AlphaStar
GammaInitial <- GammaStar
PiInitial <- 0.5


# Iterative procedure (EM algorithm) to estimate the 5
parameters
i <- 0
MixtureEM <- c(i, LambdaInitial, NA, ThetaInitial, NA,
AlphaInitial, NA, GammaInitial, NA, PiInitial, NA,
MixtureLogLik(log(LambdaInitial), ThetaInitial, log
(AlphaInitial), GammaInitial, log(PiInitial / (1 -
PiInitial)))))
LambdaCurrent <- LambdaInitial
ThetaCurrent <- ThetaInitial
AlphaCurrent <- AlphaInitial
GammaCurrent <- GammaInitial
PiCurrent <- PiInitial
LambdaPrevious_EM <- ThetaPrevious_EM <- AlphaPrevious_EM <-
GammaPrevious_EM <- PiPrevious_EM <- -1e-100
# To make sure it iterates
while (i < 100000 && (abs((LambdaCurrent - LambdaPrevious_EM) /
LambdaPrevious_EM) > 1e-5 || abs((ThetaCurrent -
ThetaPrevious_EM) / ThetaPrevious_EM) > 1e-5 || abs
((AlphaCurrent - AlphaPrevious_EM) / AlphaPrevious_EM) > 1e-5 ||
abs((GammaCurrent - GammaPrevious_EM) / GammaPrevious_EM) > 1e-
5 || abs((PiCurrent - PiPrevious_EM) / PiPrevious_EM) > 1e-5)) {
  LambdaPrevious_EM <- LambdaCurrent
  ThetaPrevious_EM <- ThetaCurrent
  AlphaPrevious_EM <- AlphaCurrent
  GammaPrevious_EM <- GammaCurrent
  PiPrevious_EM <- PiCurrent
```

```
  # Expectation step to calculate expected value of "random
variable" Y
  Y_x <- Event * PiCurrent * f_G(AgeEventCensoring,
LambdaCurrent, ThetaCurrent) / f(AgeEventCensoring, log
(LambdaCurrent), ThetaCurrent, log(AlphaCurrent),
GammaCurrent, log(PiCurrent / (1 - PiCurrent))) + (1 - Event) *
PiCurrent * S_G(AgeEventCensoring, LambdaCurrent,
ThetaCurrent) / S(AgeEventCensoring, log(LambdaCurrent),
ThetaCurrent, log(AlphaCurrent), GammaCurrent, log
(PiCurrent / (1 - PiCurrent)))
  # Maximization sub-step to calculate Y_a for given Lambda,
Theta, Alpha, Gamma, and Pi
  Y_a <- PiCurrent * S_G(AgeBaseline, LambdaCurrent,
ThetaCurrent) / S(AgeBaseline, log(LambdaCurrent),
ThetaCurrent, log(AlphaCurrent), GammaCurrent, log
(PiCurrent / (1 - PiCurrent)))
  # Maximization sub-step to calculate Theta (using Newton
method) and Lambda for given Y_a
  j <- 0
  D_G_EM <- sum(Y_x * Event)
  T_G_EM <- sum(Y_x * Event * AgeEventCensoring)
  ThetaPrevious <- -Inf                # To make sure it iterates
  while (abs(ThetaCurrent - ThetaPrevious) > 1e-10) {
    ThetaPrevious <- ThetaCurrent
    ThetaCurrent <- ThetaPrevious - GompertzEquation_EM
(ThetaPrevious) / GompertzDerEquation_EM
(ThetaPrevious)
    j <- j + 1
  }
  Q_G_EM <- sum(Y_x * (exp(ThetaCurrent * AgeEventCensoring)
- 1) - Y_a * (exp(ThetaCurrent * AgeBaseline) - 1))
  LambdaCurrent <- D_G_EM * ThetaCurrent / Q_G_EM
  # Maximization sub-step to calculate Gamma (using Newton
method) and Alpha for given Y_a
  k <- 0
  D_W_EM <- sum((1 - Y_x) * Event)
  T_W_EM <- sum((1 - Y_x) * Event * log(AgeEventCensoring))
  GammaPrevious <- -Inf                # To make sure it iterates
  while (abs(GammaCurrent - GammaPrevious) > 1e-10) {
    GammaPrevious <- GammaCurrent
    GammaCurrent <- GammaPrevious - WeibullEquation_EM
(GammaPrevious) / WeibullDerEquation_EM(GammaPrevious)
    k <- k + 1
  }
```

```
  Q_W_EM <- sum((1 - Y_x) * AgeEventCensoring ^ GammaCurrent -
(1 - Y_a) * AgeBaseline ^ GammaCurrent)
  AlphaCurrent <- D_W_EM / Q_W_EM
  # Maximization sub-step to calculate Pi using logistic
regression for given Alpha, Gamma, Lambda, and Theta
  LogisticOffset <- log(S_G(AgeBaseline, LambdaCurrent,
ThetaCurrent) / S_W(AgeBaseline, AlphaCurrent,
GammaCurrent))
  Logistic <- glm(Y_x ~ offset(LogisticOffset), family =
binomial(link = "logit"))
  Intercept <- as.numeric(coef(Logistic))
  PiCurrent <- exp(Intercept) / (1 + exp(Intercept))
  i <- i + 1
  MixtureEM <- rbind(MixtureEM, c(i, LambdaCurrent,
(LambdaCurrent - LambdaPrevious_EM) / LambdaPrevious_EM,
ThetaCurrent, (ThetaCurrent - ThetaPrevious_EM) /
ThetaPrevious_EM, AlphaCurrent, (AlphaCurrent -
AlphaPrevious_EM) / AlphaPrevious_EM, GammaCurrent,
(GammaCurrent - GammaPrevious_EM) / GammaPrevious_EM,
PiCurrent, (PiCurrent - PiPrevious_EM) / PiPrevious_EM,
MixtureLogLik(log(LambdaCurrent), ThetaCurrent, log
(AlphaCurrent), GammaCurrent, log(PiCurrent / (1 -
PiCurrent)))))
  colnames(MixtureEM) <- c("i", "Lambda", "Relative change",
"Theta", "Relative change", "Alpha", "Relative change",
"Gamma", "Relative change", "Pi", "Relative change",
"Mixture log lik")
  print(MixtureEM[dim(MixtureEM)[1],], digits = 10)
}
LambdaEM <- LambdaCurrent
ThetaEM <- ThetaCurrent
AlphaEM <- AlphaCurrent
GammaEM <- GammaCurrent
PiEM <- PiCurrent
MixtureLogLikelihoodEM <- MixtureLogLik(log
(LambdaEM), ThetaEM, log(AlphaEM), GammaEM, log(PiEM / (1
- PiEM)))

# Output for E-M algorithm
colnames(MixtureEM) <- c("i", "Lambda", "Relative change",
"Theta", "Relative change", "Alpha", "Relative change",
"Gamma", "Relative change", "Pi", "Relative change",
"Mixture log lik")
# print(MixtureEM, digits = 10)
max.col(t(MixtureEM[,12]), "first")
```

```
max.col(t(MixtureEM[,12]), "last")
print(MixtureLogLikelihoodEM, digits = 15)

# Initial values for N-R algorithm from E-M algorithm
MuInitial <- log(LambdaEM)
ThetaInitial <- ThetaEM
BetaInitial <- log(AlphaEM)
GammaInitial <- GammaEM
LogitInitial <- log(PiEM / (1 - PiEM))

# Iterative procedure (Newton–Raphson method) to estimate
the 5 parameters
i <- 0
MixtureNR <- c(i, MuInitial, NA, ThetaInitial, NA,
BetaInitial, NA, GammaInitial, NA, LogitInitial, NA,
MixtureEquation(MuInitial, ThetaInitial, BetaInitial,
GammaInitial, LogitInitial), MixtureLogLik(MuInitial,
ThetaInitial, BetaInitial, GammaInitial, LogitInitial))
MuCurrent <- MuInitial
ThetaCurrent <- ThetaInitial
BetaCurrent <- BetaInitial
GammaCurrent <- GammaInitial
LogitCurrent <- LogitInitial
MuPrevious <- ThetaPrevious <- BetaPrevious <-
GammaPrevious <- LogitPrevious <- -1e-100
# To make sure it iterates
while (i < 40 && (abs((MuCurrent - MuPrevious) / MuPrevious) >
1e-10 || abs((ThetaCurrent - ThetaPrevious) / ThetaPrevious)
> 1e-10 || abs((BetaCurrent - BetaPrevious) / BetaPrevious) >
1e-10 || abs((GammaCurrent - GammaPrevious) / GammaPrevious)
> 1e-10 || abs((LogitCurrent - LogitPrevious) /
LogitPrevious) > 1e-10)) {
  MuPrevious <- MuCurrent
  ThetaPrevious <- ThetaCurrent
  BetaPrevious <- BetaCurrent
  GammaPrevious <- GammaCurrent
  LogitPrevious <- LogitCurrent
  ParamVecPrevious <- c(MuPrevious, ThetaPrevious,
BetaPrevious, GammaPrevious, LogitPrevious)
  ParamVecCurrent <- ParamVecPrevious - (solve
(MixtureDerEquation(MuPrevious, ThetaPrevious,
BetaPrevious, GammaPrevious, LogitPrevious), tol = 1e-35) %*
% MixtureEquation(MuPrevious, ThetaPrevious, BetaPrevious,
GammaPrevious, LogitPrevious))
  MuCurrent <- ParamVecCurrent[1]
```

```
  ThetaCurrent <- ParamVecCurrent[2]
  BetaCurrent <- ParamVecCurrent[3]
  GammaCurrent <- ParamVecCurrent[4]
  LogitCurrent <- ParamVecCurrent[5]
  i <- i + 1
  MixtureNR <- rbind(MixtureNR, c(i, MuCurrent, (MuCurrent -
MuPrevious) / MuPrevious, ThetaCurrent, (ThetaCurrent -
ThetaPrevious) / ThetaPrevious, BetaCurrent, (BetaCurrent -
BetaPrevious) / BetaPrevious, GammaCurrent, (GammaCurrent -
GammaPrevious) / GammaPrevious, LogitCurrent, (LogitCurrent
- LogitPrevious) / LogitPrevious, MixtureEquation
(MuCurrent, ThetaCurrent, BetaCurrent, GammaCurrent,
LogitCurrent), MixtureLogLik(MuCurrent, ThetaCurrent,
BetaCurrent, GammaCurrent, LogitCurrent)))
}
Mu <- MuCurrent
Theta <- ThetaCurrent
Beta <- BetaCurrent
Gamma <- GammaCurrent
Logit <- LogitCurrent
Lambda <- exp(Mu)
Alpha <- exp(Beta)
Pi <- exp(Logit) / (1 + exp(Logit))
MixtureLogLikelihoodNR <- MixtureLogLik(Mu, Theta, Beta,
Gamma, Logit)

# Output for N-R algorithm
colnames(MixtureNR) <- c("i", "Mu", "Relative change",
"Theta", "Relative change", "Beta", "Relative change",
"Gamma", "Relative change", "Logit", "Relative change",
"Estimating equations", " ", " ", " ", " ", "Log likelihood")
print(MixtureNR, digits = 10)
max.col(t(MixtureNR[,17]), "first")
max.col(t(MixtureNR[,17]), "last")
print(MixtureLogLikelihoodNR, digits = 15)

# Standard errors and 95% CIs
FisherInformation <- -1 * MixtureDerEquation(Mu, Theta,
Beta, Gamma, Logit)
MixtureVarianceMatrix <- solve(FisherInformation, tol = 1e-35)
MuSE <- sqrt(MixtureVarianceMatrix[1,1])
ThetaSE <- sqrt(MixtureVarianceMatrix[2,2])
BetaSE <- sqrt(MixtureVarianceMatrix[3,3])
GammaSE <- sqrt(MixtureVarianceMatrix[4,4])
LogitSE <- sqrt(MixtureVarianceMatrix[5,5])
```

```
MuCI <- c(Mu - 1.96 * MuSE, Mu + 1.96 * MuSE)
ThetaCI <- c(Theta - 1.96 * ThetaSE, Theta + 1.96 * ThetaSE)
BetaCI <- c(Beta - 1.96 * BetaSE, Beta + 1.96 * BetaSE)
GammaCI <- c(Gamma - 1.96 * GammaSE, Gamma + 1.96 * GammaSE)
LogitCI <- c(Logit - 1.96 * LogitSE, Logit + 1.96 * LogitSE)
LambdaCI <- exp(MuCI)
AlphaCI <- exp(BetaCI)
PiCI <- exp(LogitCI) / (1 + exp(LogitCI))

# Fitted event rates
MixtureFittedEventRate <- f(Age[1:10] - 10, Mu, Theta, Beta,
Gamma, Logit) / S(Age[1:10] - 10, Mu, Theta, Beta, Gamma, Logit)
MixtureFittedLogEventRate <- log(MixtureFittedEventRate)

# Final output
FisherInformation
MixtureVarianceMatrix
descriptive6 <- matrix(c(Mu, MuSE, MuCI, Theta, ThetaSE,
ThetaCI, Beta, BetaSE, BetaCI, Gamma, GammaSE, GammaCI,
Logit, LogitSE, LogitCI), nrow = 5, byrow = TRUE)
colnames(descriptive6) <- c("Parameter estimate", "Standard
error", "95% Confidence interval", " ")
rownames(descriptive6) <- c("Mu", "Theta", "Beta",
"Gamma", "Logit")
descriptive6
print(Lambda, digits = 10)
print(LambdaCI, digits = 10)
print(Alpha, digits = 10)
print(AlphaCI, digits = 10)
print(Pi, digits = 10)
print(PiCI, digits = 10)
descriptive7 <- cbind(Age[1:10], EventRate[1:10],
MixtureFittedEventRate, LogEventRate[1:10],
MixtureFittedLogEventRate)
colnames(descriptive7) <- c("Age", "Event rate", "Mixture
fitted", "Log event rate", "Mixture fitted")
descriptive7


#### Likelihood ratio (Gompertz versus Weibull) using
parameter estimates from the mixture model ####

GompertzLogLikelihood_mixture <- GompertzLogLik
(Lambda, Theta)
WeibullLogLikelihood_mixture <- WeibullLogLik(Alpha, Gamma)
```

```
LogLR_mixture <- GompertzLogLikelihood_mixture -
WeibullLogLikelihood_mixture
LR_mixture <- exp(LogLR_mixture)
list(GompertzLogLikelihood = GompertzLogLikelihood_mixture,
WeibullLogLikelihood = WeibullLogLikelihood_mixture, LogLR =
LogLR_mixture, LR = LR_mixture)



################## Producing plots ####################

setEPS(horizontal = FALSE, onefile = FALSE, paper = "special")
# Plot of log h(x) versus age with fitted curves for separate
Gompertz and Weibull models
postscript(file = "MortalityIntrinsic1.eps", horizontal = F,
height = 5, width = 5)
plot(Age[1:10], LogEventRate[1:10], type = "n", xlab = "Age",
ylab = "Log h(x)", xlim = c(39, 91), xaxp = c(40, 90, 10), ylim = c
(-8, -1))
points(Age[1:10], LogEventRate[1:10], pch = 19, cex = 2 *
(Events[1:10] / max(Events[1:10])))
curve(log(LambdaStar) + ThetaStar * (x - 10), 40, 90, lty = 1,
n = 20000, add = TRUE)
curve(log(AlphaStar * GammaStar) + (GammaStar - 1) * log(x -
10), 40, 90, lty = 1, n = 20000, add = TRUE)
graphics.off()

# Plot of log h(x) versus age with fitted curves for mixture
model only
postscript(file = "MortalityIntrinsic2.eps", horizontal = F,
height = 5, width = 5)
plot(Age[1:10], LogEventRate[1:10], type = "n", xlab = "Age",
ylab = "Log h(x)", xlim = c(39, 91), xaxp = c(40, 90, 10), ylim =
c(-8, -1))
points(Age[1:10], LogEventRate[1:10], pch = 19, cex = 2 *
(Events[1:10] / max(Events[1:10])))
curve(log(f(x - 10, Mu, Theta, Beta, Gamma, Logit) / S(x - 10, Mu,
Theta, Beta, Gamma, Logit)), 40, 90, lty = 1, n = 20000, add = TRUE)
graphics.off()

# Plot of log h(x) versus age with fitted curves for mixture
model and for mixture model with Pi = 0 and Pi = 1
postscript(file = "MortalityIntrinsic3.eps", horizontal = F,
height = 5, width = 5)
plot(Age[1:10], LogEventRate[1:10], type = "n", xlab = "Age",
ylab = "Log h(x)", xlim = c(39, 91), xaxp = c(40, 90, 10), ylim =
c(-8, -1))
```

```
points(Age[1:10], LogEventRate[1:10], pch = 19, cex = 2 *
(Events[1:10] / max(Events[1:10])))
curve(log(f(x - 10, Mu, Theta, Beta, Gamma, Logit) / S(x - 10,
Mu, Theta, Beta, Gamma, Logit)), 40, 90, lty = 1, n = 20000, add
= TRUE)
curve(log(f_W(x - 10, Alpha, Gamma) / S_W(x - 10, Alpha,
Gamma)), 40, 90, lty = 5, n = 20000, add = TRUE)
curve(log(f_G(x - 10, Lambda, Theta) / S_G(x - 10, Lambda,
Theta)), 40, 90, lty = 5, n = 20000, add = TRUE)
graphics.off()

# Plot of Pi(age) versus age
postscript(file = "MortalityIntrinsic4.eps", horizontal = F,
height = 5, width = 5)
x <- seq(40, 90, by = 1)
y1 <- rep(NA, 51)
y2 <- rep(NA, 51)
for (i in 1:51) {
  y1[i] <- Pi * f_G(x[i] - 10, Lambda, Theta) / f(x[i] - 10, Mu,
Theta, Beta, Gamma, Logit)
  y2[i] <- Pi * S_G(x[i] - 10, Lambda, Theta) / S(x[i] - 10, Mu,
Theta, Beta, Gamma, Logit)
}
y <- cbind(y1, y2)
matplot(x, y, type = "l", xlab = "Age", ylab = "Pi (age)", ylim =
c(0, 1), yaxp = c(0, 1, 10))
abline(h = Pi, lty = 5)
graphics.off()

# Plot of log h(x) versus age with fitted curves for separate
Gompertz and Weibull models and mixture model
postscript(file = "MortalityIntrinsic5.eps", horizontal = F,
height = 5, width = 5)
plot(Age[1:10], LogEventRate[1:10], type = "n", xlab = "Age",
ylab = "Log h(x)", xlim = c(39, 91), xaxp = c(40, 90, 10), ylim =
c(-8, -1))
points(Age[1:10], LogEventRate[1:10], pch = 19, cex = 2 *
(Events[1:10] / max(Events[1:10])))
curve(log(LambdaStar) + ThetaStar * (x - 10), 40, 90, lty = 5, n
= 20000, add = TRUE)
curve(log(AlphaStar * GammaStar) + (GammaStar - 1) * log(x -
10), 40, 90, lty = 5, n = 20000, add = TRUE)
curve(log(f(x - 10, Mu, Theta, Beta, Gamma, Logit) / S(x - 10, Mu,
Theta, Beta, Gamma, Logit)), 40, 90, lty = 1, n = 20000, add = TRUE)
graphics.off()
```

```
# Plot of log-likelihood function versus iteration in EM
algorithm
postscript(file = "MortalityIntrinsic6.eps", horizontal = F,
height = 5, width = 5)
plot(MixtureEM[,1], MixtureEM[,12], type = "l", xlab =
"Iteration", ylab = "Log likelihood")
# abline(h = MixtureLogLikelihoodEM, lty = 5)
abline(h = MixtureLogLikelihoodNR, lty = 5)
graphics.off()

# Plot of Pi versus iteration in EM algorithm
postscript(file = "MortalityIntrinsic7.eps", horizontal = F,
height = 5, width = 5)
plot(MixtureEM[,1], MixtureEM[,10], type = "l", xlab =
"Iteration", ylab = "Pi")
abline(h = Pi, lty = 5)
graphics.off()


########## Nelson-Aalen estimate of cumulative hazard
function ##########

AgeEventCensoringNA <- AgeEventCensoring + 10
AgeBaselineNA <- AgeBaseline + 10
AtRiskNA <- rep(0, n)
for (i in 1:n) {
  for (j in 1:n) {
    if (AgeEventCensoringNA[i] >= AgeBaselineNA[j] &&
AgeEventCensoringNA[i] <= AgeEventCensoringNA[j])
      AtRiskNA[i] <- AtRiskNA[i] + 1
  }
}
EventRiskNA <- Event / AtRiskNA
o <- order(AgeEventCensoringNA)
NelsonAalenMatrix <- cbind(AgeEventCensoringNA[o],
Event[o], AtRiskNA[o], EventRiskNA[o], rep(NA, n))
for (i in 1:n)
  NelsonAalenMatrix[i,5] <- sum(NelsonAalenMatrix[1:i,4])
colnames(NelsonAalenMatrix) <- c("Age", "Event", "At risk",
"Event risk", "Cumulative hazard")
NelsonAalenMatrix <- rbind(c(40, NA, NA, NA, 0),
NelsonAalenMatrix)
NelsonAalenMatrix[1:100,]

setEPS(horizontal = FALSE, onefile = FALSE, paper = "special")
```

```
# Plot of Nelson-Aalen estimate of cumulative hazard function
and mixture model cumulative hazard function
postscript(file =
"MortalityIntrinsicGoodnessOfFit_Mixture.eps", horizontal
= F, height = 5, width = 5)
plot(NelsonAalenMatrix[,1], NelsonAalenMatrix[,5], type =
"s", xlab = "Age", ylab = "Cumulative hazard function", xlim = c
(39, 91), xaxp = c(40, 90, 10))
curve(-log(S(x - 10, Mu, Theta, Beta, Gamma, Logit)) + log(S
(30, Mu, Theta, Beta, Gamma, Logit)), 40, 90, lty = 1, col =
"red", n = 20000, add = TRUE)
graphics.off()

# Plot of Nelson-Aalen estimate of cumulative hazard function
and Gompertz model cumulative hazard function
postscript(file =
"MortalityIntrinsicGoodnessOfFit_Gompertz.eps",
horizontal = F, height = 5, width = 5)
plot(NelsonAalenMatrix[,1], NelsonAalenMatrix[,5], type =
"s", xlab = "Age", ylab = "Cumulative hazard function", xlim = c
(39, 91), xaxp = c(40, 90, 10))
curve(-log(S_G(x - 10, LambdaStar, ThetaStar)) + log(S_G(30,
LambdaStar, ThetaStar)), 40, 90, lty = 1, col = "red",
n = 20000, add = TRUE)
graphics.off()

# Plot of Nelson-Aalen estimate of cumulative hazard function
and Weibull model cumulative hazard function
postscript(file =
"MortalityIntrinsicGoodnessOfFit_Weibull.eps", horizontal
= F, height = 5, width = 5)
plot(NelsonAalenMatrix[,1], NelsonAalenMatrix[,5], type =
"s", xlab = "Age", ylab = "Cumulative hazard function", xlim = c
(39, 91), xaxp = c(40, 90, 10))
curve(-log(S_W(x - 10, AlphaStar, GammaStar)) + log(S_W(30,
AlphaStar, GammaStar)), 40, 90, lty = 1, col = "red", n = 20000,
add = TRUE)
graphics.off()


################### Goodness-of-fit chi-squared test for
intrinsic mortality (5 age intervals) ###################

Observed40to50 <- Observed50to60 <- Observed60to70 <-
Observed70to80 <- Observed80to90 <- 0
```

```
ExpectedGompertz40to50 <- ExpectedGompertz50to60 <-
ExpectedGompertz60to70 <- ExpectedGompertz70to80 <-
ExpectedGompertz80to90 <- 0
ExpectedWeibull40to50 <- ExpectedWeibull50to60 <-
ExpectedWeibull60to70 <- ExpectedWeibull70to80 <-
ExpectedWeibull80to90 <- 0
ExpectedMixture40to50 <- ExpectedMixture50to60 <-
ExpectedMixture60to70 <- ExpectedMixture70to80 <-
ExpectedMixture80to90 <- 0
for (i in 1:n) {
  if (NelsonAalenMatrix[i,1] > 40 && NelsonAalenMatrix[i,1]
<= 50)
    Observed40to50 <- Observed40to50 + NelsonAalenMatrix[i,2]
  if (NelsonAalenMatrix[i,1] > 50 && NelsonAalenMatrix[i,1]
<= 60)
    Observed50to60 <- Observed50to60 + NelsonAalenMatrix[i,2]
  if (NelsonAalenMatrix[i,1] > 60 && NelsonAalenMatrix[i,1]
<= 70)
    Observed60to70 <- Observed60to70 + NelsonAalenMatrix[i,2]
  if (NelsonAalenMatrix[i,1] > 70 && NelsonAalenMatrix[i,1]
<= 80)
    Observed70to80 <- Observed70to80 + NelsonAalenMatrix[i,2]
  if (NelsonAalenMatrix[i,1] > 80 && NelsonAalenMatrix[i,1]
<= 90)
    Observed80to90 <- Observed80to90 + NelsonAalenMatrix[i,2]
}

AgeY <- sort(c(AgeBaselineNA, AgeEventCensoringNA))
AtRiskY <- rep(0, 2*n)
for (i in 1:(2*n)) {
  for (j in 1:n) {
    if (AgeY[i] >= AgeBaselineNA[j] && AgeY[i] <=
AgeEventCensoringNA[j])
      AtRiskY[i] <- AtRiskY[i] + 1
  }
}
AtRiskY <- c(0, AtRiskY)

Y <- stepfun(AgeY, AtRiskY, f = 0, right = FALSE)
GompertzHazard <- function(x) {LambdaStar * exp(ThetaStar
* x)}
WeibullHazard <- function(x) {AlphaStar * GammaStar * x ^
(GammaStar - 1)}
MixtureHazard <- function(x) {f(x, Mu, Theta, Beta, Gamma,
Logit) / S(x, Mu, Theta, Beta, Gamma, Logit)}
```

```
setEPS(horizontal = FALSE, onefile = FALSE, paper = "special")
postscript(file =
"MortalityIntrinsicGoodnessOfFit_AtRisk.eps", horizontal
= F, height = 5, width = 5)
plot(Y)
graphics.off()


YGompertz <- function(x) {Y(x) * GompertzHazard(x -10)}
ExpectedGompertz40to50 <- integrate(YGompertz, 40, 50,
subdivisions = 1000, abs.tol = 1e-10)$value
ExpectedGompertz50to60 <- integrate(YGompertz, 50, 60,
subdivisions = 1000, abs.tol = 1e-10)$value
ExpectedGompertz60to70 <- integrate(YGompertz, 60, 70,
subdivisions = 1000, abs.tol = 1e-10)$value
ExpectedGompertz70to80 <- integrate(YGompertz, 70, 80,
subdivisions = 1000, abs.tol = 1e-10)$value
ExpectedGompertz80to90 <- integrate(YGompertz, 80, 90,
subdivisions = 1000, abs.tol = 1e-10)$value


YWeibull <- function(x) {Y(x) * WeibullHazard(x - 10)}
ExpectedWeibull40to50 <- integrate(YWeibull, 40, 50,
subdivisions = 1000, abs.tol = 1e-10)$value
ExpectedWeibull50to60 <- integrate(YWeibull, 50, 60,
subdivisions = 1000, abs.tol = 1e-10)$value
ExpectedWeibull60to70 <- integrate(YWeibull, 60, 70,
subdivisions = 1000, abs.tol = 1e-10)$value
ExpectedWeibull70to80 <- integrate(YWeibull, 70, 80,
subdivisions = 1000, abs.tol = 1e-10)$value
ExpectedWeibull80to90 <- integrate(YWeibull, 80, 90,
subdivisions = 1000, abs.tol = 1e-10)$value


YMixture <- function(x) {Y(x) * MixtureHazard(x - 10)}
ExpectedMixture40to50 <- integrate(YMixture, 40, 50,
subdivisions = 1000, abs.tol = 1e-10)$value
ExpectedMixture50to60 <- integrate(YMixture, 50, 60,
subdivisions = 1000, abs.tol = 1e-10)$value
ExpectedMixture60to70 <- integrate(YMixture, 60, 70,
subdivisions = 1000, abs.tol = 1e-10)$value
ExpectedMixture70to80 <- integrate(YMixture, 70, 80,
subdivisions = 1000, abs.tol = 1e-10)$value
ExpectedMixture80to90 <- integrate(YMixture, 80, 90,
subdivisions = 1000, abs.tol = 1e-10)$value


Observed <- c(Observed40to50, Observed50to60,
Observed60to70, Observed70to80, Observed80to90)
```

```
ExpectedGompertz <- c(ExpectedGompertz40to50,
ExpectedGompertz50to60, ExpectedGompertz60to70,
ExpectedGompertz70to80, ExpectedGompertz80to90)
ExpectedWeibull <- c(ExpectedWeibull40to50,
ExpectedWeibull50to60, ExpectedWeibull60to70,
ExpectedWeibull70to80, ExpectedWeibull80to90)
ExpectedMixture <- c(ExpectedMixture40to50,
ExpectedMixture50to60, ExpectedMixture60to70,
ExpectedMixture70to80, ExpectedMixture80to90)
Observed
ExpectedGompertz
ExpectedWeibull
ExpectedMixture

ChiSquaredGompertz <- (Observed - ExpectedGompertz) ^ 2 /
ExpectedGompertz
ChiSquaredGompertzSum <- sum(ChiSquaredGompertz)
ChiSquaredGompertzPvalue <- pchisq(ChiSquaredGompertzSum,
df = 5, lower.tail = FALSE)
ChiSquaredGompertzMatrix <- rbind(Observed,
ExpectedGompertz, ChiSquaredGompertz)
ChiSquaredGompertzMatrix
list(ChiSquaredGompertz = ChiSquaredGompertzSum, df = 5,
ChiSquaredGompertzPvalue = ChiSquaredGompertzPvalue)

ChiSquaredWeibull <- (Observed - ExpectedWeibull) ^ 2 /
ExpectedWeibull
ChiSquaredWeibullSum <- sum(ChiSquaredWeibull)
ChiSquaredWeibullPvalue <- pchisq(ChiSquaredWeibullSum, df
= 5, lower.tail = FALSE)
ChiSquaredWeibullMatrix <- rbind(Observed,
ExpectedWeibull, ChiSquaredWeibull)
ChiSquaredWeibullMatrix
list(ChiSquaredWeibull = ChiSquaredWeibullSum, df = 5,
ChiSquaredWeibullPvalue = ChiSquaredWeibullPvalue)

ChiSquaredMixture <- (Observed - ExpectedMixture) ^ 2 /
ExpectedMixture
ChiSquaredMixtureSum <- sum(ChiSquaredMixture)
ChiSquaredMixturePvalue <- pchisq(ChiSquaredMixtureSum, df
= 5, lower.tail = FALSE)
ChiSquaredMixtureMatrix <- rbind(Observed,
ExpectedMixture, ChiSquaredMixture)
ChiSquaredMixtureMatrix
```

```
list(ChiSquaredMixture = ChiSquaredMixtureSum, df = 5,
ChiSquaredMixturePvalue = ChiSquaredMixturePvalue)


########## Goodness-of-fit likelihood ratio test ##########

ChiSquaredMixtureGompertz <- 2 * (MixtureLogLikelihoodNR -
GompertzLogLikelihood)
ChiSquaredMixtureGompertzPvalue <- pchisq
(ChiSquaredMixtureGompertz, df = 3, lower.tail = FALSE)
list(GompertzLogLikelihood = GompertzLogLikelihood,
MixtureLogLikelihood = MixtureLogLikelihoodNR,
ChiSquaredMixtureGompertz = ChiSquaredMixtureGompertz,
df = 3, ChiSquaredMixtureGompertzPvalue =
ChiSquaredMixtureGompertzPvalue)

ChiSquaredMixtureWeibull <- 2 * (MixtureLogLikelihoodNR -
WeibullLogLikelihood)
ChiSquaredMixtureWeibullPvalue <- pchisq
(ChiSquaredMixtureWeibull, df = 3, lower.tail = FALSE)
list(WeibullLogLikelihood = WeibullLogLikelihood,
MixtureLogLikelihood = MixtureLogLikelihoodNR,
ChiSquaredMixtureWeibull = ChiSquaredMixtureWeibull, df = 3,
ChiSquaredMixtureWeibullPvalue =
ChiSquaredMixtureWeibullPvalue)
```

REFERENCES

Abernethy, J. (1998). Gompertzian mortality originates in the winding-down of the mitotic clock. *Journal of Theoretical Biology*, **192**, 419–435.

Abernethy, J. D. (1979). The exponential increase in mortality rate with age attributed to wearing-out of biological components. *Journal of Theoretical Biology*, **80**, 333–354.

Abramowitz, M. and Stegun, I. A. (1972). *Handbook of Mathematical Functions with Formulas, Graphs, and Mathematical Tables*. Applied Mathematics Series 55. Washington, DC: National Bureau of Standards.

Abrams, P. A. and Ludwig, D. (1995). Optimality theory, Gompertz' law, and the disposable soma theory of senescence. *Evolution*, **49**, 1055–1066.

Ackermann, M. and Pletcher, S. D. (2008). Evolutionary biology as a foundation for studying aging and aging-related disease. In: Stearns, S. C. and Koella, J. C. (Eds.). *Evolution in Health and Disease*, 2nd ed., pp. 241–252. Oxford: Oxford University Press.

Adamovic, D. D. (1966). Sur quelques propriétés des fonctions à croissance lente de Karamata I. *Matematicki Vesnik*, **3**, 123–136.

Adelman, R. C. (1980). Definition of biological aging. In: Haynes, S. G. and Feinleib, M. (Eds.). *Second Conference on the Epidemiology of Aging*, pp. 9–13. Bethesda, MD: DHHS, NIH Pub. No. 80-969.

Adelman, R. C. (1987). Biomarkers of aging. *Experimental Gerontology*, **22**, 227–229.

Aguilera, O., Fernández, A. F., Muñoz, A., and Fraga, M. F. (2010). Epigenetics and environment: A complex relationship. *Journal of Applied Physiology*, **109**, 243–251.

The Biostatistics of Aging: From Gompertzian Mortality to an Index of Aging-Relatedness,
First Edition. Gilberto Levy and Bruce Levin.
© 2014 John Wiley & Sons, Inc. Published 2014 by John Wiley & Sons, Inc.

Aickin, M. (2002). *Causal Analysis in Biomedicine and Epidemiology: Based on Minimal Sufficient Causation*. New York: Marcel Dekker.

Al-Samarrai, T., Madsen, A., Zimmerman, R., Maduro, G., Li, W., Greene, C., et al. (2013). Impact of a hospital-level intervention to reduce heart disease overreporting on leading causes of death. *Preventing Chronic Disease*, **10**, 120210.

Albin, R. L. (1993). Antagonistic pleiotropy, mutation accumulation, and human genetic disease. *Genetica*, **91**, 279–286.

Andersen, P. K., Borgan, Ø., Gill, R. D., and Keiding, N. (1993). *Statistical Models Based on Counting Processes*. New York: Springer Verlag.

Austad, S. N. (1994). Menopause: An evolutionary perspective. *Experimental Gerontology*, **29**, 255–263.

Austad, S. N. (2001). Concepts and theories of aging. In: Masoro, E. J. and Austad, S. N. (Eds.). *Handbook of the Biology of Aging*, 5th ed., pp. 3–22. San Diego, CA: Academic Press.

Austad, S. N. (2006). Why women live longer than men: Sex differences in longevity. *Gender Medicine*, **3**, 79–92.

Bailey, R. C. (1997). Hereditarian scientific fallacies. *Genetica*, **99**, 125–133.

Baker III, G. T. and Sprott, R. L. (1988). Biomarkers of aging. *Experimental Gerontology*, **23**, 223–239.

Barker, D. J. (1993). Fetal origins of coronary heart disease. *British Heart Journal*, **69**, 195–196.

Barker, D. J. (1995a). Fetal origins of coronary heart disease. *British Medical Journal*, **311**, 171–174.

Barker, D. J. P. (1995b). The Wellcome Foundation Lecture, 1994. The fetal origins of adult disease. *Proceedings of the Royal Society of London. Series B: Biological Sciences*, **262**, 37–43.

Barker, D. J. P. (2004). The developmental origins of adult disease. *Journal of the American College of Nutrition*, **23**, 588S–595S.

Barker, D. J. P., Eriksson, J. G., Forsen, T., and Osmond, C. (2002). Fetal origins of adult disease: Strength of effects and biological basis. *International Journal of Epidemiology*, **31**, 1235–1239.

Barlow, R. E. and Proschan, F. (1981). *Statistical Theory of Reliability and Life Testing: Probability Models*. Silver Spring, MD: To Begin With.

Barrès, R., Yan, J., Egan, B., Treebak, J. T., Rasmussen, M., Fritz, T., et al. (2012). Acute exercise remodels promoter methylation in human skeletal muscle. *Cell Metabolism*, **15**, 405–411.

Baudisch, A. (2005). Hamilton's indicators of the force of selection. *Proceedings of the National Academy of Sciences of the United States of America*, **102**, 8263–8268.

Beard, R. E. (1959). Note on some mathematical mortality models. In: Wolstenholme, G. E. W. and O'Connor, M. (Eds.). *Ciba Foundation Colloquia on Ageing, Volume 5: The Lifespan of Animals*, pp. 302–311. Boston, MA: Little, Brown and Company.

Belinsky, S. A., Palmisano, W. A., Gilliland, F. D., Crooks, L. A., Divine, K. K., Winters, S. A., et al. (2002). Aberrant promoter methylation in bronchial epithelium and sputum from current and former smokers. *Cancer Research*, **62**, 2370–2377.

Bell, J. T., Tsai, P., Yang, T., Pidsley, R., Nisbet, J., Glass, D., et al. (2012). Epigenome-wide scans identify differentially methylated regions for age and age-related phenotypes in a healthy ageing population. *PLoS Genetics*, **8**, e1002629.

Ben-Shlomo, Y. and Kuh, D. (2002). A life course approach to chronic disease epidemiology: Conceptual models, empirical challenges and interdisciplinary perspectives. *International Journal of Epidemiology*, **31**, 285–293.

Bergman, R. A. M. (1948). Who is old? Death rate in a Japanese concentration camp as a criterion of age. *Journal of Gerontology*, **3**, 14–17.

Bertram, L. and Tanzi, R. E. (2005). The genetic epidemiology of neurodegenerative disease. *Journal of Clinical Investigation*, **115**, 1449–1457.

Bird, A. (2007). Perceptions of epigenetics. *Nature*, **447**, 396–398.

Bjornsson, H. T., Fallin, M. D., and Feinberg, A. P. (2004). An integrated epigenetic and genetic approach to common human disease. *Trends in Genetics*, **20**, 350–358.

Bjornsson, H. T., Sigurdsson, M. I., Fallin, M. D., Irizarry, R. A., Aspelund, T., Cui, H., et al. (2008). Intra-individual change over time in DNA methylation with familial clustering. *Journal of the American Medical Association*, **299**, 2877–2883.

Blumenthal, H. T. (2003). The aging–disease dichotomy: True or false? *The Journals of Gerontology Series A: Biological Sciences and Medical Sciences*, **58**, M138–M145.

Bodmer, W. and Bonilla, C. (2008). Common and rare variants in multifactorial susceptibility to common diseases. *Nature Genetics*, **40**, 695–701.

Boks, M. P., Derks, E. M., Weisenberger, D. J., Strengman, E., Janson, E., Sommer, I. E., et al. (2009). The relationship of DNA methylation with age, gender and genotype in twins and healthy controls. *PLoS One*, **4**, e6767.

Bonneux, L., Barendregt, J. J., and Van der Maas, P. J. (1998). The expiry date of man: A synthesis of evolutionary biology and public health. *Journal of Epidemiology and Community Health*, **52**, 619–623.

Bors, D. A. (1994). Is the nature-nurture debate on the verge of extinction? *Canadian Psychology*, **35**, 231–243.

Bourgeois-Pichat, J. (1952). Essai sur la mortalité "biologique" de l'homme. *Population (French Edition)*, **7**, 381–394.

Boyd Eaton, S., Cordain, L., and Lindeberg, S. (2002a). Evolutionary health promotion: A consideration of common counterarguments. *Preventive Medicine*, **34**, 119–123.

Boyd Eaton, S. and Konner, M. (1985). Paleolithic nutrition. A consideration of its nature and current implications. *New England Journal of Medicine*, **312**, 283–289.

Boyd Eaton, S., Konner, M., and Shostak, M. (1988). Stone agers in the fast lane: Chronic degenerative diseases in evolutionary perspective. *The American Journal of Medicine*, **84**, 739–749.

Boyd Eaton, S., Strassman, B. I., Nesse, R. M., Neel, J. V., Ewald, P. W., Williams, G. C., et al. (2002b). Evolutionary health promotion. *Preventive Medicine*, **34**, 109–118.

Britton, A., Shipley, M., Singh-Manoux, A., and Marmot, M. G. (2008). Successful aging: The contribution of early-life and midlife risk factors. *Journal of the American Geriatrics Society*, **56**, 1098–1105.

Brody, J. A. (1985). Prospects for an ageing population. *Nature*, **315**, 463–466.

Brody, J. A. and Schneider, E. L. (1986). Diseases and disorders of aging: An hypothesis. *Journal of Chronic Diseases*, **39**, 871–876.

Brownlee, J. (1919). Notes on the biology of a life-table. *Journal of the Royal Statistical Society*, **82**, 34–77.

Buchanan, A. V., Weiss, K. M., and Fullerton, S. M. (2006). Dissecting complex disease: The quest for the Philosopher's Stone? *International Journal of Epidemiology*, **35**, 562–571.

Burke, M. K., Dunham, J. P., Shahrestani, P., Thornton, K. R., Rose, M. R., and Long, A. D. (2010). Genome-wide analysis of a long-term evolution experiment with Drosophila. *Nature*, **467**, 587–590.

Callinan, P. A. and Feinberg, A. P. (2006). The emerging science of epigenomics. *Human Molecular Genetics*, **15**, R95–R101.

Calvanese, V., Lara, E., Kahn, A., and Fraga, M. F. (2009). The role of epigenetics in aging and age-related diseases. *Ageing Research Reviews*, **8**, 268–276.

Carey, J. R. (1999). Population study of mortality and longevity with Gompertzian analysis. In: Yu, B. P. (Ed.). *Methods in Aging Research*, 2nd ed., pp. 3–24. Boca Raton, FL: CRC Press.

Carey, J. R. (2003). *Longevity: The Biology and Demography of Life Span*. Princeton, NJ: Princeton University Press.

Carey, J. R., Liedo, P., Orozco, D., and Vaupel, J. W. (1992). Slowing of mortality rates at older ages in large medfly cohorts. *Science*, **258**, 457–461.

Carnes, B. A., Holden, L. R., Olshansky, S. J., Witten, M. T., and Siegel, J. S. (2006). Mortality partitions and their relevance to research on senescence. *Biogerontology*, **7**, 183–198.

Carnes, B. A. and Olshansky, S. J. (1997). A biologically motivated partitioning of mortality. *Experimental Gerontology*, **32**, 615–631.

Carnes, B. A. and Olshansky, S. J. (2001). Heterogeneity and its biodemographic implications for longevity and mortality. *Experimental Gerontology*, **36**, 419–430.

Carnes, B. A., Olshansky, S. J., and Grahn, D. (1996). Continuing the search for a law of mortality. *Population and Development Review*, **22**, 231–264.

Caughley, G. and Birch, L. C. (1971). Rate of increase. *The Journal of Wildlife Management*, **35**, 658–663.

Chakravarti, A. (1999). Population genetics — making sense out of sequence. *Nature Genetics*, **21**, 56–60.

Charlesworth, B. (1973). Selection in populations with overlapping generations. V. Natural selection and life histories. *American Naturalist*, **107**, 303–311.

Charlesworth, B. (1990). Optimization models, quantitative genetics, and mutation. *Evolution*, **44**, 520–538.

Charlesworth, B. (1994). *Evolution in Age-Structured Populations*, 2nd ed. Cambridge: Cambridge University Press.

Charlesworth, B. (2000). Fisher, Medawar, Hamilton and the evolution of aging. *Genetics*, **156**, 927–931.

Charlesworth, B. (2001). Patterns of age-specific means and genetic variances of mortality rates predicted by the mutation-accumulation theory of ageing. *Journal of Theoretical Biology*, **210**, 47–65.

Charlesworth, B. and Partridge, L. (1997). Ageing: Levelling of the grim reaper. *Current Biology*, **7**, R440–R442.

Charlesworth, B. and Williamson, J. A. (1975). The probability of survival of a mutant gene in an age-structured population and implications for the evolution of life-histories. *Genetical Research*, **26**, 1–10.

Christensen, B. C., Houseman, E. A., Marsit, C. J., Zheng, S., Wrensch, M. R., Wiemels, J. L., et al. (2009). Aging and environmental exposures alter tissue-specific DNA methylation dependent upon CpG island context. *PLoS Genetics*, **5**, e1000602.

Coles, S. (2001). *An Introduction to Statistical Modeling of Extreme Values*. London: Springer Verlag.

Collett, D. (2003). *Modelling Survival Data in Medical Research*, 2nd ed. Boca Raton, FL: Chapman & Hall/CRC.

Comfort, A. (1979). *The Biology of Senescence*, 3rd ed. New York: Elsevier.

Cooney, C. A. (1993). Are somatic cells inherently deficient in methylation metabolism? A proposed mechanism for DNA methylation loss, senescence and aging. *Growth, Development, and Aging*, **57**, 261–273.

Cooney, C. A. (2007). Epigenetics — DNA-based mirror of our environment? *Disease Markers*, **23**, 121–137.

Cooney, C. A. (2010). Drugs and supplements that may slow aging of the epigenome. *Drug Discovery Today: Therapeutic Strategies*, **7**, 57–64.

Cordain, L., Boyd Eaton, S., Sebastian, A., Mann, N., Lindeberg, S., Watkins, B. A., et al. (2005). Origins and evolution of the Western diet: Health implications for the 21st century. *The American Journal of Clinical Nutrition*, **81**, 341–354.

Cortopassi, G. A. (2002). Fixation of deleterious alleles, evolution and human aging. *Mechanisms of Ageing and Development*, **123**, 851–855.

Costa Jr, P. T. and McCrae, R. R. (1980). Functional age: A conceptual and empirical critique. In: Haynes, S. G. and Feinleib, M. (Eds.). *Second Conference on the Epidemiology of Aging*, pp. 23–49. Bethesda, MD: DHHS, NIH Pub. No. 80–969.

Costa Jr, P. T. and McCrae, R. R. (1988). Measures and markers of biological aging: "A great clamoring… of fleeting significance". *Archives of Gerontology and Geriatrics*, **7**, 211–214.

Cox, D. R. (1959). The analysis of exponentially distributed life-times with two types of failure. *Journal of the Royal Statistical Society. Series B (Methodological)*, **21**, 411–421.

Crimmins, E. M., Saito, Y., and Ingegneri, D. (1989). Changes in life expectancy and disability-free life expectancy in the United States. *Population and Development Review*, **15**, 235–267.

Crow, J. F. and Kimura, M. (1970). *An Introduction to Population Genetics Theory*. New York: Harper & Row, Publishers.

Curtsinger, J. W., Fukui, H. H., Townsend, D. R., and Vaupel, J. W. (1992). Demography of genotypes: Failure of the limited life-span paradigm in *Drosophila melanogaster*. *Science*, **258**, 461–463.

Danaei, G., Ding, E. L., Mozaffarian, D., Taylor, B., Rehm, J., Murray, C. J. L., et al. (2009). The preventable causes of death in the United States: Comparative risk assessment of dietary, lifestyle, and metabolic risk factors. *PLoS Medicine*, **6**, e1000058.

Davey Smith, G. (2011). Epidemiology, epigenetics and the "Gloomy Prospect": Embracing randomness in population health research and practice. *International Journal of Epidemiology*, **40**, 537–562.

Davey Smith, G. and Kuh, D. (2001). Commentary: William Ogilvy Kermack and the childhood origins of adult health and disease. *International Journal of Epidemiology*, **30**, 696–703.

David, H. A. and Moeschberger, M. L. (1978). *The Theory of Competing Risks*. New York: Macmillan Publishing Co.

David, H. A. and Nagaraja, H. N. (2003). *Order Statistics*, 3rd ed. Hoboken, NJ: John Wiley & Sons.

Daviglus, M. L., Liu, K., Yan, L. L., Pirzada, A., Garside, D. B., Schiffer, L., et al. (2003). Body mass index in middle age and health-related quality of life in older age: The Chicago Heart

Association Detection Project in Industry study. *Archives of Internal Medicine*, **163**, 2448–2455.

de Haan, L. (1970). On regular variation and its application to the weak convergence of sample extremes. *Mathematical Centre Tracts*, **32**, 1–124.

de Haan, L. (1976). Sample extremes: An elementary introduction. *Statistica Neerlandica*, **30**, 161–172.

de Haan, L. and Ferreira, A. (2006). *Extreme Value Theory: An Introduction*. New York: Springer.

Dean, W. and Morgan, R. F. (1988). In defense of the concept of biological aging measurement—current status. *Archives of Gerontology and Geriatrics*, **7**, 191–210.

Deaner, R. O. and Winegard, B. M. (2013). Throwing out the mismatch baby with the paleo-bathwater. *Evolutionary Psychology*, **11**, 263–269.

Dempster, A. P., Laird, N. M., and Rubin, D. B. (1977). Maximum likelihood from incomplete data via the EM algorithm. *Journal of the Royal Statistical Society. Series B (Methodological)*, **39**, 1–38.

Doll, R. and Peto, R. (1998). There is no such thing as ageing. Authors' reply. *British Medical Journal*, **316**, 1532.

Drapeau, M. D., Gass, E. K., Simison, M. D., Mueller, L. D., and Rose, M. R. (2000). Testing the heterogeneity theory of late-life mortality plateaus by using cohorts of *Drosophila melanogaster*. *Experimental Gerontology*, **35**, 71–84.

Economos, A. C. (1982). Rate of aging, rate of dying and the mechanism of mortality. *Archives of Gerontology and Geriatrics*, **1**, 3–27.

Egger, G., Liang, G., Aparicio, A., and Jones, P. A. (2004). Epigenetics in human disease and prospects for epigenetic therapy. *Nature*, **429**, 457–463.

El Shaarawi, A., Prentice, R. L., and Forbes, W. F. (1974). The goodness of fit of certain aging models. *Journal of Chronic Diseases*, **27**, 377–385.

Falconer, D. S. (1965). The inheritance of liability to certain diseases, estimated from the incidence among relatives. *Annals of Human Genetics*, **29**, 51–76.

Feinberg, A. P. (2007). Phenotypic plasticity and the epigenetics of human disease. *Nature*, **447**, 433–440.

Feinberg, A. P. (2008). Epigenetics at the epicenter of modern medicine. *Journal of the American Medical Association*, **299**, 1345–1350.

Feller, W. (1966). *An Introduction to Probability Theory and its Applications, Vol. II*, 1st ed. New York: John Wiley & Sons.

Finch, C. E. (1990). *Longevity, Senescence, and the Genome*. Chicago: The University of Chicago Press.

Finch, C. E., Pike, M. C., and Witten, M. (1990). Slow mortality rate accelerations during aging in some animals approximate that of humans. *Science*, **249**, 902–905.

Fisher, R. A. (1918). The correlation between relatives on the supposition of Mendelian Inheritance. *Transactions of the Royal Society of Edinburgh*, **52**, 399–433.

Fisher, R. A. (1930). *The Genetical Theory of Natural Selection*. London: Oxford University Press.

Fisher, R. A. (1958). *The Genetical Theory of Natural Selection*. New York: Dover Publications.

Fisher, R. A. and Tippett, L. H. C. (1928). Limiting forms of the frequency distribution of the largest or smallest member of a sample. *Mathematical Proceedings of the Cambridge Philosophical Society*, **24**, 180–190.

Flanders, W. D. (2006). On the relationship of sufficient component cause models with potential outcome (counterfactual) models. *European Journal of Epidemiology*, **21**, 847–853.

Fréchet, M. (1927). Sur la loi de probabilité de l'écart maximum. *Annales de la Société Polonaise de Mathématique*, **6**, 93–116.

Freese, J. (2006). Commentary: The analysis of variance and the social complexities of genetic causation. *International Journal of Epidemiology*, **35**, 534–536.

Fried, L. P., Tangen, C. M., Walston, J., Newman, A. B., Hirsch, C., Gottdiener, J., et al. (2001). Frailty in older adults: Evidence for a phenotype. *The Journals of Gerontology Series A: Biological Sciences and Medical Sciences*, **56**, M146–M157.

Fries, J. F. (1980). Aging, natural death, and the compression of morbidity. *New England Journal of Medicine*, **303**, 130–135.

Frontali, M., Sabbadini, G., Novelletto, A., Jodice, C., Naso, F., Spadaro, M., et al. (1996). Genetic fitness in Huntington's Disease and Spinocerebellar Ataxia 1: A population genetics model for CAG repeat expansions. *Annals of Human Genetics*, **60**, 423–435.

Fullerton, S. M., Clark, A. G., Weiss, K. M., Nickerson, D. A., Taylor, S. L., Stengård, J. H., et al. (2000). Apolipoprotein E variation at the sequence haplotype level: Implications for the origin and maintenance of a major human polymorphism. *The American Journal of Human Genetics*, **67**, 881–900.

Galambos, J. (1981). Extreme value theory in applied probability. *The Mathematical Scientist*, **6**, 13–26.

Galambos, J. (1987). *The Asymptotic Theory of Extreme Order Statistics*, 2nd ed. Malabar, FL: Robert E. Krieger Publishing Company.

Galambos, J. and Obretenov, A. (1987). Restricted domains of attraction of $\exp(-\exp(-x))$. *Stochastic Processes and their Applications*, **25**, 265–271.

Galvan, A., Ioannidis, J., and Dragani, T. A. (2010). Beyond genome-wide association studies: Genetic heterogeneity and individual predisposition to cancer. *Trends in Genetics*, **26**, 132–141.

Gandhi, S. and Wood, N. W. (2010). Genome-wide association studies: The key to unlocking neurodegeneration? *Nature Neuroscience*, **13**, 789–794.

Garg, M. L., Rao, B. R., and Redmond, C. K. (1970). Maximum-likelihood estimation of the parameters of the Gompertz survival function. *Applied Statistics*, **19**, 152–159.

Gavrilov, L. A. and Gavrilova, N. S. (1991). *The Biology of Life Span: A Quantitative Approach*. Chur: Harwood Academic Publishers.

Gavrilov, L. A. and Gavrilova, N. S. (2001). The reliability theory of aging and longevity. *Journal of Theoretical Biology*, **213**, 527–545.

Gavrilov, L. A. and Gavrilova, N. S. (2003). The quest for a general theory of aging and longevity. *Science's SAGE KE*, **28**, re5.

Gavrilov, L. A. and Gavrilova, N. S. (2004). The reliability-engineering approach to the problem of biological aging. *Annals of the New York Academy of Sciences*, **1019**, 509–512.

Gavrilov, L. A. and Gavrilova, N. S. (2006). Reliability theory of aging and longevity. In: Masoro, E. J. and Austad, S. N. (Eds.). *Handbook of the Biology of Aging*, 6th ed., pp. 3–42. San Diego, CA: Academic Press.

Gluckman, P. D. and Hanson, M. A. (2006). Evolution, development and timing of puberty. *Trends in Endocrinology & Metabolism*, **17**, 7–12.

Gluckman, P. D., Hanson, M. A., and Beedle, A. S. (2007). Early life events and their consequences for later disease: A life history and evolutionary perspective. *American Journal of Human Biology*, **19**, 1–19.

Gluckman, P. D., Hanson, M. A., and Buklijas, T. (2010). A conceptual framework for the developmental origins of health and disease. *Journal of Developmental Origins of Health and Disease*, **1**, 6–18.

Gluckman, P. D., Hanson, M. A., Spencer, H. G., and Bateson, P. (2005). Environmental influences during development and their later consequences for health and disease: Implications for the interpretation of empirical studies. *Proceedings of the Royal Society B: Biological Sciences*, **272**, 671–677.

Gnedenko, B. (1943). Sur la distribution limite du terme maximum d'une série aleatoire. *The Annals of Mathematics*, **44**, 423–453.

Goldberg, A. D., Allis, C. D., and Bernstein, E. (2007). Epigenetics: A landscape takes shape. *Cell*, **128**, 635–638.

Goldbourt, U., Yaari, S., and Medalie, J. H. (1993). Factors predictive of long-term coronary heart disease mortality among 10,059 male Israeli civil servants and municipal employees. A 23-year mortality follow-up in the Israeli Ischemic Heart Disease Study. *Cardiology*, **82**, 100–121.

Goldstein, D. B. (2009). Common genetic variation and human traits. *New England Journal of Medicine*, **360**, 1696–1698.

Gompertz, B. (1825). On the nature of the function expressive of the law of human mortality, and on a new mode of determining the value of life contingencies. *Philosophical Transactions of the Royal Society of London*, **115**, 513–583.

Gompertz, B. (1871). On one uniform law of mortality from birth to extreme old age, and on the law of sickness. *Journal of the Institute of Actuaries*, **16**, 329–344.

Graham, J. E., Mitnitski, A. B., Mogilner, A. J., and Rockwood, K. (1999). Dynamics of cognitive aging: Distinguishing functional age and disease from chronologic age in a population. *American Journal of Epidemiology*, **150**, 1045–1054.

Greenland, S. (2000). Causal analysis in the health sciences. *Journal of the American Statistical Association*, **95**, 286–289.

Greenland, S. and Brumback, B. (2002). An overview of relations among causal modelling methods. *International Journal of Epidemiology*, **31**, 1030–1037.

Greenwood, M. (1928). "Laws" of mortality from the biological point of view. *The Journal of Hygiene*, **28**, 267–294.

Greenwood, M. and Irwin, J. O. (1939). The biostatistics of senility. *Human Biology*, **11**, 1–23.

Groen, J. J., Medalie, J. H., Neufeld, H. N., Riss, E., Bachrach, C. A., Mount, F. W., et al. (1968). An epidemiologic investigation of hypertension and ischemic heart disease within a defined segment of the adult male population of Israel. *Israel Journal of Medical Sciences*, **4**, 177–194.

Gruenberg, E. M. (1977). The failures of success. *The Milbank Memorial Fund Quarterly. Health and Society*, **55**, 3–24.

Gumbel, E. J. (1954). *Statistical Theory of Extreme Values and some Practical Applications*. Washington, DC: National Bureau of Standards – Applied Mathematics Series 33.

Gumbel, E. J. (1958). *Statistics of Extremes*. New York: Columbia University Press.

Hairston, N. G., Tinkle, D. W., and Wilbur, H. M. (1970). Natural selection and the parameters of population growth. *The Journal of Wildlife Management*, **34**, 681–690.

Haldane, J. B. (1942). *New Paths in Genetics*. New York: Harper & Brothers.

Hamilton, W. D. (1966). The moulding of senescence by natural selection. *Journal of Theoretical Biology*, **12**, 12–45.

Hardy, J. and Singleton, A. (2009). Genomewide association studies and human disease. *New England Journal of Medicine*, **360**, 1759–1768.

Havighurst, R. J. (1961). Successful aging. *The Gerontologist*, **1**, 8–13.

Hawkes, K. (2003). Grandmothers and the evolution of human longevity. *American Journal of Human Biology*, **15**, 380–400.

Hawkes, K. (2004). Human longevity: The grandmother effect. *Nature*, **428**, 128–129.

Hawkes, K., O'Connell, J. F., Jones, N. B., Alvarez, H., and Charnov, E. L. (1998). Grandmothering, menopause, and the evolution of human life histories. *Proceedings of the National Academy of Sciences of the United States of America*, **95**, 1336–1339.

Hayflick, L. (2000). The future of ageing. *Nature*, **408**, 267–269.

Hayflick, L. (2004). The not-so-close relationship between biological aging and age-associated pathologies in humans. *The Journals of Gerontology Series A: Biological Sciences and Medical Sciences*, **59**, B547–B550.

Hernandez, D. G., Nalls, M. A., Gibbs, J. R., Arepalli, S., van der Brug, M., Chong, S., et al. (2011). Distinct DNA methylation changes highly correlated with chronological age in the human brain. *Human Molecular Genetics*, **20**, 1164–1172.

Hill, B. M. (1963). Information for estimating the proportions in mixtures of exponential and normal distributions. *Journal of the American Statistical Association*, **58**, 918–932.

Hirschhorn, J. N. (2009). Genomewide association studies—illuminating biologic pathways. *New England Journal of Medicine*, **360**, 1699–1701.

Hjort, N. L. (1990). Goodness of fit tests in models for life history data based on cumulative hazard rates. *The Annals of Statistics*, **18**, 1221–1258.

Holliday, R. (1987). The inheritance of epigenetic defects. *Science*, **238**, 163–170.

Holliday, R. (2004a). The close relationship between biological aging and age-associated pathologies in humans. *The Journals of Gerontology Series A: Biological Sciences and Medical Sciences*, **59**, B543–B546.

Holliday, R. (2004b). Response to Dr. Hayflick. *The Journals of Gerontology Series A: Biological Sciences and Medical Sciences*, **59**, B551.

Holliday, R. (2005). DNA methylation and epigenotypes. *Biochemistry (Moscow)*, **70**, 500–504.

Hooker, P. F. (1965). Benjamin Gompertz, 1779–1865. *Journal of the Institute of Actuaries*, **91**, 203–212.

Horiuchi, S. and Wilmoth, J. R. (1998). Deceleration in the age pattern of mortality at older ages. *Demography*, **35**, 391–412.

International HapMap Consortium. (2005). A haplotype map of the human genome. *Nature*, **437**, 1299–1320.

Jablonka, E. (2004). Epigenetic epidemiology. *International Journal of Epidemiology*, **33**, 929–935.

Jablonka, E. and Lamb, M. J. (1990). Lamarckism and ageing. *Gerontology*, **36**, 323–332.

Jablonka, E. and Lamb, M. J. (2007). Précis of evolution in four dimensions. *Behavioral and Brain Sciences*, **30**, 353–392.

Jablonka, E. and Raz, G. (2009). Transgenerational epigenetic inheritance: Prevalence, mechanisms, and implications for the study of heredity and evolution. *The Quarterly Review of Biology*, **84**, 131–176.

Jacquard, A. (1983). Heritability: One word, three concepts. *Biometrics*, **39**, 465–477.

Jirtle, R. L. and Skinner, M. K. (2007). Environmental epigenomics and disease susceptibility. *Nature Reviews Genetics*, **8**, 253–262.

Jones, H. B. (1956). A special consideration of the aging process, disease, and life expectancy. In: Lawrence, J. H. and Tobias, C. A. (Eds.). *Advances in Biological and Medical Physics*, pp. 281–337. New York: Academic Press.

Jones, H. B. (1959). The relation of human health to age, place, and time. In: Birren, J. E. (Ed.). *Handbook of Aging and the Individual: Psychological and Biological Aspects*, pp. 336–363. Chicago, IL: The University of Chicago Press.

Juckett, D. A. and Rosenberg, B. (1993). Comparison of the Gompertz and Weibull functions as descriptors for human mortality distributions and their intersections. *Mechanisms of Ageing and Development*, **69**, 1–31.

Juncosa, M. L. (1949). The asymptotic behavior of the minimum in a sequence of random variables. *Duke Mathematical Journal*, **16**, 609–618.

Kaati, G., Bygren, L. O., and Edvinsson, S. (2002). Cardiovascular and diabetes mortality determined by nutrition during parents' and grandparents' slow growth period. *European Journal of Human Genetics*, **10**, 682–688.

Karamata, M. J. (1930). Sur un mode de croissance régulière des fonctions. *Mathematica (Cluj)*, **4**, 38–58.

Karamata, M. J. (1933). Sur un mode de croissance régulière. Théorémes fondamentaux. *Bulletin de la Société Mathématique de France*, **61**, 55–62.

Karasik, D., Demissie, S., Cupples, L. A., and Kiel, D. P. (2005). Disentangling the genetic determinants of human aging: Biological age as an alternative to the use of survival measures. *The Journals of Gerontology Series A: Biological Sciences and Medical Sciences*, **60**, 574–587.

Karasik, D., Hannan, M. T., Cupples, L. A., Felson, D. T., and Kiel, D. P. (2004). Genetic contribution to biological aging: The Framingham Study. *The Journals of Gerontology Series A: Biological Sciences and Medical Sciences*, **59**, B218–B226.

Kempthorne, O. (1978). Logical, epistemological and statistical aspects of nature-nurture data interpretation. *Biometrics*, **34**, 1–23.

Kempthorne, O. (1997). Heritability: Uses and abuses. *Genetica*, **99**, 109–112.

Kermack, W. O., McKendrick, A. G., and McKinlay, P. L. (1934). Death-rates in Great Britain and Sweden. Some general regularities and their significance. *The Lancet*, **223**, 698–703.

Keyfitz, N. (1978). Improving life expectancy: An uphill road ahead. *American Journal of Public Health*, **68**, 954–956.

Keyfitz, N. (1980). What direction of research? *American Journal of Public Health*, **70**, 1201.

Khazaeli, A. A., Pletcher, S. D., and Curtsinger, J. W. (1998). The fractionation experiment: Reducing heterogeneity to investigate age-specific mortality in Drosophila. *Mechanisms of Ageing and Development*, **105**, 301–317.

Khoury, M. J., Beaty, T. H., and Cohen, B. H. (1993). *Fundamentals of Genetic Epidemiology*. New York: Oxford University Press.

Kirkwood, T. (1999). *Time of Our Lives: The Science of Human Aging*. New York: Oxford University Press.

Kirkwood, T. (2010). Why women live longer. *Scientific American*, **303**, 34–35.

Kirkwood, T. B. L. (1985). Comparative and evolutionary aspects of longevity. In: Finch, C. E. and Schneider, E. L. (Eds.). *Handbook of the Biology of Aging*, 2nd ed., pp. 27–44. New York: Van Nostrand Reinhold Company.

Kirkwood, T. B. L. (2008). A systematic look at an old problem. *Nature*, **451**, 644–647.

Kirkwood, T. B. L. and Austad, S. N. (2000). Why do we age? *Nature*, **408**, 233–238.

Kirkwood, T. B. L. and Cremer, T. (1982). Cytogerontology since 1881: A reappraisal of August Weismann and a review of modern progress. *Human Genetics*, **60**, 101–121.

Kirkwood, T. B. L., Martin, G. M., and Partridge, L. (1999). Evolution, senescence, and health in old age. In: Stearns, S. C. (Ed.). *Evolution in Health and Disease*, pp. 219–230. Oxford: Oxford University Press.

Kirkwood, T. B. L. and Rose, M. R. (1991). Evolution of senescence: Late survival sacrificed for reproduction. *Philosophical Transactions of the Royal Society of London. Series B: Biological Sciences*, **332**, 15–24.

Kohn, R. R. (1963). Human aging and disease. *Journal of Chronic Diseases*, **16**, 5–21.

Kohn, R. R. (1982). Cause of death in very old people. *Journal of the American Medical Association*, **247**, 2793–2797.

Konner, M. and Boyd Eaton, S. (2010). Paleolithic nutrition: Twenty-five years later. *Nutrition in Clinical Practice*, **25**, 594–602.

Korevaar, J., Van Aardenne-Ehrenfest, T., and De Bruijn, N. G. (1949). A note on slowly oscillating functions. *Nieuw Archief Voor Wiskunde*, **23**, 77–86.

Korn, E. L., Graubard, B. I., and Midthune, D. (1997). Time-to-event analysis of longitudinal follow-up of a survey: Choice of the time-scale. *American Journal of Epidemiology*, **145**, 72–80.

Kotz, S. and Nadarajah, S. (2000). *Extreme Value Distributions: Theory and Applications*. London: Imperial College Press.

Kowald, A. and Kirkwood, T. B. (1993). Explaining fruit fly longevity. *Science*, **260**, 1664–1665.

Kraft, P. and Hunter, D. J. (2009). Genetic risk prediction: Are we there yet? *New England Journal of Medicine*, **360**, 1701–1703.

Kramer, M. (1980). The rising pandemic of mental disorders and associated chronic diseases and disabilities. *Acta Psychiatrica Scandinavica*, **62**, 382–397.

Kuh, D., Ben-Shlomo, Y., Lynch, J., Hallqvist, J., and Power, C. (2003). Life course epidemiology. *Journal of Epidemiology and Community Health*, **57**, 778–783.

Kuh, D. and Davey Smith, G. (2004). The life course and adult chronic disease: An historical perspective with particular reference to coronary heart disease. In: Kuh, D. and Ben-Shlomo, Y. (Eds.). *A Life Course Approach to Chronic Disease Epidemiology*, 2nd ed., pp. 15–37. New York: Oxford University Press.

Lahdenperä, M., Lummaa, V., Helle, S., Tremblay, M., and Russell, A. F. (2004). Fitness benefits of prolonged post-reproductive lifespan in women. *Nature*, **428**, 178–181.

Lamb, M. J. (1994). Epigenetic inheritance and aging. *Reviews in Clinical Gerontology*, **4**, 97–105.

Lander, E. S. (1996). The new genomics: Global views of biology. *Science*, **274**, 536–539.

Lander, E. S. and Schork, N. J. (1994). Genetic dissection of complex traits. *Science*, **265**, 2037–2048.

Lawless, J. F. (2003). *Statistical Models and Methods for Lifetime Data*, 2nd ed. Hoboken, NJ: John Wiley & Sons.

Le Bourg, E. (1998). Evolutionary theories of aging: Handle with care. *Gerontology*, **44**, 345–348.

Lee, R. D. (2003). Rethinking the evolutionary theory of aging: Transfers, not births, shape senescence in social species. *Proceedings of the National Academy of Sciences of the United States of America*, **100**, 9637–9642.

Levy, G. (2007). The relationship of Parkinson disease with aging. *Archives of Neurology*, **64**, 1242–1246.

Levy, G., Louis, E. D., Cote, L., Perez, M., Mejia-Santana, H., Andrews, H., et al. (2005). Contribution of aging to the severity of different motor signs in Parkinson disease. *Archives of Neurology*, **62**, 467–472.

Levy, G., Schupf, N., Tang, M. X., Cote, L. J., Louis, E. D., Mejia, H., et al. (2002). Combined effect of age and severity on the risk of dementia in Parkinson's disease. *Annals of Neurology*, **51**, 722–729.

Levy, G., Tang, M. X., Cote, L. J., Louis, E. D., Alfaro, B., Mejia, H., et al. (2000). Motor impairment in PD: Relationship to incident dementia and age. *Neurology*, **55**, 539–544.

Lewontin, R. C. (1974). The analysis of variance and the analysis of causes. *American Journal of Human Genetics*, **26**, 400–411.

Lewontin, R. C. (2006). Commentary: Statistical analysis or biological analysis as tools for understanding biological causes. *International Journal of Epidemiology*, **35**, 536–537.

Little, R. J. and Rubin, D. B. (2000). Causal effects in clinical and epidemiological studies via potential outcomes: Concepts and analytical approaches. *Annual Review of Public Health*, **21**, 121–145.

Lotka, A. J. (1907). Relation between birth rates and death rates. *Science*, **26**, 21–22.

Lotka, A. J. (1913). A natural population norm. *Journal of the Washington Academy of Sciences*, **3**, 241–248.

Lotka, A. J. (1922). The stability of the normal age distribution. *Proceedings of the National Academy of Sciences of the United States of America*, **8**, 339–345.

Luckinbill, L. S., Arking, R., Clare, M. J., Cirocco, W. C., and Buck, S. A. (1984). Selection for delayed senescence in Drosophila melanogaster. *Evolution*, **38**, 996–1003.

Lynch, J. and Davey Smith, G. (2005). A life course approach to chronic disease epidemiology. *Annual Review of Public Health*, **26**, 1–35.

Mackie, J. L. (1965). Causes and conditions. *American Philosophical Quarterly*, **2**, 245–264.

Maher, B. (2008). Personal genomes: The case of the missing heritability. *Nature*, **456**, 18–21.

Makeham, W. M. (1860). On the law of mortality and the construction of annuity tables. *Journal of the Institute of Actuaries*, **8**, 301–310.

Makeham, W. M. (1867). On the law of mortality. *Journal of the Institute of Actuaries*, **13**, 325–358.

Mann, D. M. (1997). Molecular biology's impact on our understanding of aging. *British Medical Journal*, **315**, 1078–1081.

Manolio, T. A., Collins, F. S., Cox, N. J., Goldstein, D. B., Hindorff, L. A., Hunter, D. J., et al. (2009). Finding the missing heritability of complex diseases. *Nature*, **461**, 747–753.

Manton, K. G. (1982). Changing concepts of morbidity and mortality in the elderly population. *The Milbank Memorial Fund Quarterly. Health and Society*, **60**, 183–244.

Masoro, E. J. (2006). Are age-associated diseases an integral part of aging? In: Masoro, E. J. and Austad, S. N. (Eds.). *Handbook of the Biology of Aging*, 6th ed., pp. 43–62. San Diego, CA: Academic Press.

Maynard Smith, J. (1962). Review lectures on senescence. I. The causes of ageing. *Proceedings of the Royal Society of London. Series B: Biological Sciences*, **157**, 115–127.

Maynard Smith, J., Barker, D. J., Finch, C. E., Kardia, S. L., Boyd Eaton, S., Kirkwood, T. B., et al. (1999). The evolution of non-infectious and degenerative disease. In: Stearns, S. C. (Ed.). *Evolution in Health and Disease*, pp. 267–272. Oxford: Oxford University Press.

Mayr, E. (1961). Cause and effect in biology. *Science*, **134**, 1501–1506.

McClellan, J. and King, M. (2010). Genetic heterogeneity in human disease. *Cell*, **141**, 210–217.

McKinlay, J. B., McKinlay, S. M., and Beaglehole, R. (1989). A review of the evidence concerning the impact of medical measures on recent mortality and morbidity in the United States. *International Journal of Health Services*, **19**, 181–208.

McLachlan, G. J. and Krishnan, T. (2008). *The EM Algorithm and Extensions*, 2nd ed. Hoboken, NJ: John Wiley & Sons.

McLachlan, G. J. and McGiffin, D. C. (1994). On the role of finite mixture models in survival analysis. *Statistical Methods in Medical Research*, **3**, 211–226.

McLachlan, G. and Peel, D. (2000). *Finite Mixture Models*. New York: John Wiley & Sons.

Medalie, J. H., Kahn, H. A., Neufeld, H. N., Riss, E., Goldbourt, U., Perlstein, T., et al. (1973a). Myocardial infarction over a five-year period—I. Prevalence, incidence and mortality experience. *Journal of Chronic Diseases*, **26**, 63–84.

Medalie, J. H., Snyder, M., Groen, J. J., Neufeld, H. N., Goldbourt, U., and Riss, E. (1973b). Angina pectoris among 10,000 men: 5 year incidence and univariate analysis. *The American Journal of Medicine*, **55**, 583–594.

Medawar, P. B. (1946). Old age and natural death. *Modern Quarterly*, **1**, 30–56.

Medawar, P. B. (1952). *An Unsolved Problem of Biology*. London: H. K. Lewis & Co.

Medawar, P. B. (1955). The definition and measurement of senescence. In: Wolstenholme, G. E. W. and Cameron, M. P. (Eds.). *Ciba Foundation Colloquia on Ageing, Vol. I, General Aspects*, pp. 5–15. Boston, MA: Little, Brown, and Company.

Medawar, P. B. (1985). The future of life expectancy. *Clinical Orthopaedics and Related Research*, **201**, 2–8.

Medvedev, Z. A. (1990). An attempt at a rational classification of theories of ageing. *Biological Reviews*, **65**, 375–398.

Mendenhall, W. and Hader, R. J. (1958). Estimation of parameters of mixed exponentially distributed failure time distributions from censored life test data. *Biometrika*, **45**, 504–520.

Meng, X. and Rubin, D. B. (1993). Maximum likelihood estimation via the ECM algorithm: A general framework. *Biometrika*, **80**, 267–278.

Miller, R. A. (2001). Biomarkers of aging. *Science's SAGE KE*, **1**, pe2.

Mueller, L. D., Drapeau, M. D., Adams, C. S., Hammerle, C. W., Doyal, K. M., Jazayeri, A. J., et al. (2003). Statistical tests of demographic heterogeneity theories. *Experimental Gerontology*, **38**, 373–386.

Mueller, L. D. and Rose, M. R. (1996). Evolutionary theory predicts late-life mortality plateaus. *Proceedings of the National Academy of Sciences of the United States of America*, **93**, 15249–15253.

Nesse, R. M. and Williams, G. C. (1998). Evolution and the origins of disease. *Scientific American*, **279**, 58–65.

Nusbaum, T. J., Graves, J. L., Mueller, L. D., and Rose, M. R. (1993). Fruit fly aging and mortality. *Science*, **260**, 1567.

Nusbaum, T. J., Mueller, L. D., and Rose, M. R. (1996). Evolutionary patterns among measures of aging. *Experimental Gerontology*, **31**, 507–516.

Olshansky, S. J. (1985). Pursuing longevity: Delay vs elimination of degenerative diseases. *American Journal of Public Health*, **75**, 754–757.

Olshansky, S. J. and Ault, A. B. (1986). The fourth stage of the epidemiologic transition: The age of delayed degenerative diseases. *The Milbank Quarterly*, **64**, 355–391.

Olshansky, S. J. and Carnes, B. A. (1997). Ever since gompertz. *Demography*, **34**, 1–15.

Olshansky, S. J., Carnes, B. A., and Cassel, C. (1990). In search of Methuselah: Estimating the upper limits to human longevity. *Science*, **250**, 634–640.

Olshansky, S. J., Carnes, B. A., and Désesquelles, A. (2001). Prospects for human longevity. *Science*, **291**, 1491–1492.

Olshansky, S. J., Hayflick, L., and Carnes, B. A. (2002a). Position statement on human aging. *Journal of Gerontology: Biological Sciences*, **57A**, B292–B297.

Olshansky, S. J., Hayflick, L., and Carnes, B. A. (2002b). No truth to the fountain of youth. *Scientific American*, **286**, 92–95.

Olshansky, S. J., Rudberg, M. A., Carnes, B. A., Cassel, C. K., and Brody, J. A. (1991). Trading off longer life for worsening health: The expansion of morbidity hypothesis. *Journal of Aging and Health*, **3**, 194–216.

Omran, A. R. (1971). The epidemiologic transition: A theory of the epidemiology of population change. *The Milbank Memorial Fund Quarterly*, **49**, 509–538.

Partridge, L. and Barton, N. H. (1993). Optimally, mutation and the evolution of ageing. *Nature*, **362**, 305–311.

Partridge, L. and Barton, N. H. (1996). On measuring the rate of ageing. *Proceedings of the Royal Society of London. Series B: Biological Sciences*, **263**, 1365–1371.

Pearce, N. (2011). Epidemiology in a changing world: Variation, causation and ubiquitous risk factors. *International Journal of Epidemiology*, **40**, 503–512.

Pembrey, M. E. (2002). Time to take epigenetic inheritance seriously. *European Journal of Human Genetics*, **10**, 669–671.

Perks, W. (1932). On some experiments in the graduation of mortality statistics. *Journal of the Institute of Actuaries*, **63**, 12–57.

Peto, R. and Doll, R. (1997). There is no such thing as aging. Old age is associated with disease, but does not cause it. *British Medical Journal*, **315**, 1030–1032.

Petronis, A. (2001). Human morbid genetics revisited: Relevance of epigenetics. *Trends in Genetics*, **17**, 142–146.

Pletcher, S. D. and Curtsinger, J. W. (1998). Mortality plateaus and the evolution of senescence: Why are old-age mortality rates so low? *Evolution*, **52**, 454–464.

Plomin, R. and Daniels, D. (1987). Why are children in the same family so different from one another? *Behavioral and Brain Sciences*, **10**, 1–16.

Polfeldt, T. (1970). Minimum variance order when estimating the location of an irregularity in the density. *The Annals of Mathematical Statistics*, **41**, 673–679.

Poole, C. (2001). Commentary: Positivized epidemiology and the model of sufficient and component causes. *International Journal of Epidemiology*, **30**, 707–709.

Popoviciu, T. (1935). Sur les equations algébriques ayant toutes leurs racines réelles. *Mathematica*, **9**, 129–145.

Powell, D. E. B. (1998). There is no such thing as ageing. Ageing has been defined as to grow or make old. *British Medical Journal*, **316**, 1532.

Prentice, R. L. and El Shaarawi, A. (1973). A model for mortality rates and a test of fit for the Gompertz force of mortality. *Applied Statistics*, **22**, 301–314.

Prentice, R. L., Kalbfleisch, J. D., Peterson Jr, A. V., Flournoy, N., Farewell, V. T., and Breslow, N. E. (1978). The analysis of failure times in the presence of competing risks. *Biometrics*, **34**, 541–554.

Pritchard, J. K. (2001). Are rare variants responsible for susceptibility to complex diseases? *The American Journal of Human Genetics*, **69**, 124–137.

Pritchard, J. K. and Cox, N. J. (2002). The allelic architecture of human disease genes: Common disease–common variant… or not? *Human Molecular Genetics*, **11**, 2417–2423.

Pritchard, J. K., Pickrell, J. K., and Coop, G. (2010). The genetics of human adaptation: Hard sweeps, soft sweeps, and polygenic adaptation. *Current Biology*, **20**, R208–R215.

Promislow, D. E. L., Fedorka, K. M., and Burger, J. M. S. (2006). Evolutionary biology of aging: Future directions. In: Masoro, E. J. and Austad, S. N. (Eds.). *Handbook of the Biology of Aging*, 6th ed., pp. 217–242. San Diego, CA: Academic Press.

Qualls, C. and Watanabe, H. (1972). Asymptotic properties of Gaussian processes. *The Annals of Mathematical Statistics*, **43**, 580–596.

Qureshi, I. A. and Mehler, M. F. (2011). Advances in epigenetics and epigenomics for neuro-degenerative diseases. *Current Neurology and Neuroscience Reports*, **11**, 464–473.

R Development Core Team. (2010). *R: A Language and Environment for Statistical Computing*. Vienna: R Foundation for Statistical Computing.

Rakyan, V. K., Down, T. A., Maslau, S., Andrew, T., Yang, T., Beyan, H., et al. (2010). Human aging-associated DNA hypermethylation occurs preferentially at bivalent chromatin domains. *Genome Research*, **20**, 434–439.

Rando, O. J. and Verstrepen, K. J. (2007). Timescales of genetic and epigenetic inheritance. *Cell*, **128**, 655–668.

Rausand, M. and Høyland, A. (2004). *System Reliability Theory: Models, Statistical Methods, and Applications*, 2nd ed. Hoboken, NJ: John Wiley & Sons.

Rauser, C. L., Mueller, L. D., and Rose, M. R. (2006). The evolution of late life. *Ageing Research Reviews*, **5**, 14–32.

Redner, R. A. and Walker, H. F. (1984). Mixture densities, maximum likelihood and the EM algorithm. *SIAM Review*, **26**, 195–239.

Reich, D. E. and Lander, E. S. (2001). On the allelic spectrum of human disease. *Trends in Genetics*, **17**, 502–510.

Rice, T. K. and Borecki, I. B. (2001). Familial resemblance and heritability. *Advances in Genetics*, **42**, 35–44.

Ries, W. and Pöthig, D. (1984). Chronological and biological age. *Experimental Gerontology*, **19**, 211–216.

Risch, N. and Merikangas, K. (1996). The future of genetic studies of complex human diseases. *Science*, **273**, 1516–1517.

Risch, N. J. (2000). Searching for genetic determinants in the new millennium. *Nature*, **405**, 847–856.

Ritchie, K. and Kildea, D. (1995). Is senile dementia "age-related" or "ageing-related"?— evidence from meta-analysis of dementia prevalence in the oldest old. *The Lancet*, **346**, 931–934.

Robine, J. and Michel, J. (2004). Looking forward to a general theory on population aging. *The Journals of Gerontology Series A: Biological Sciences and Medical Sciences*, **59**, M590–M597.

Robine, J. M. and Ritchie, K. (1993). Explaining fruit fly longevity. *Science*, **260**, 1665.

Rockwood, K., Andrew, M., and Mitnitski, A. (2007). A comparison of two approaches to measuring frailty in elderly people. *The Journals of Gerontology Series A: Biological Sciences and Medical Sciences*, **62**, 738–743.

Roff, D. A. (2002). *Life History Evolution*. Sunderland, MA: Sinauer Associates.

Roff, D. A. (2008). Defining fitness in evolutionary models. *Journal of Genetics*, **87**, 339–348.

Rogers, A. R. (2003). Economics and the evolution of life histories. *Proceedings of the National Academy of Sciences of the United States of America*, **100**, 9114–9115.

Rönn, T., Volkov, P., Davegårdh, C., Dayeh, T., Hall, E., Olsson, A. H., et al. (2013). A six months exercise intervention influences the genome-wide DNA methylation pattern in human adipose tissue. *PLoS Genetics*, **9**, e1003572.

Rose, G. (1985). Sick individuals and sick populations. *International Journal of Epidemiology*, **14**, 32–38.

Rose, M. (2004). Will human aging be postponed? *Scientific American*, **14**, 24–29.

Rose, M. and Charlesworth, B. (1980). A test of evolutionary theories of senescence. *Nature*, **287**, 141–142.

Rose, M. R. (1991). *Evolutionary Biology of Aging*. New York: Oxford University Press.

Rose, M. R. (2009). Adaptation, aging, and genomic information. *Aging*, **1**, 444–451.

Rose, M. R. and Archer, M. A. (1996). Genetic analysis of mechanisms of aging. *Current Opinion in Genetics & Development*, **6**, 366–370.

Rose, M. R. and Burke, M. K. (2011). Genomic Croesus: Experimental evolutionary genetics of Drosophila aging. *Experimental Gerontology*, **46**, 397–403.

Rose, M. R., Burke, M. K., Shahrestani, P., and Mueller, L. D. (2008). Evolution of ageing since Darwin. *Journal of Genetics*, **87**, 363–371.

Rose, M. R. and Charlesworth, B. (1981). Genetics of life history in Drosophila melanogaster. II. Exploratory selection experiments. *Genetics*, **97**, 187–196.

Rose, M. R., Drapeau, M. D., Yazdi, P. G., Shah, K. H., Moise, D. B., Thakar, R. R., et al. (2002). Evolution of late-life mortality in Drosophila melanogaster. *Evolution*, **56**, 1982–1991.

Rose, M. R., Flatt, T., Graves, J. L., Greer, L. F., Martinez, D. E., Matos, M., et al. (2012). What is aging? *Frontiers in Genetics*, **3**, 1–3.

Rose, M. R. and Graves Jr, J. L. (1989). What evolutionary biology can do for gerontology. *Journal of Gerontology*, **44**, B27–B29.

Rose, M. R. and Long, A. D. (2002). Ageing: The many-headed monster. *Current Biology*, **12**, R311–R312.

Rose, M. R. and Mueller, L. D. (1998). Evolution of human lifespan: Past, future, and present. *American Journal of Human Biology*, **10**, 409–420.

Rose, M. R. and Mueller, L. D. (2000). Ageing and immortality. *Philosophical Transactions of the Royal Society of London. Series B: Biological Sciences*, **355**, 1657–1662.

Rose, M. R., Rauser, C. L., Benford, G., Matos, M., and Mueller, L. D. (2007). Hamilton's forces of natural selection after forty years. *Evolution*, **61**, 1265–1276.

Rose, M. R., Rauser, C. L., and Mueller, L. D. (2005). Late life: A new frontier for physiology. *Physiological and Biochemical Zoology*, **78**, 869–878.

Rose, M. R., Rauser, C. L., Mueller, L. D., and Benford, G. (2006). A revolution for aging research. *Biogerontology*, **7**, 269–277.

Rose, S. P. (2006). Commentary: Heritability estimates—long past their sell-by date. *International Journal of Epidemiology*, **35**, 525–527.

Rowe, J. W. and Kahn, R. L. (1987). Human aging: Usual and successful. *Science*, **237**, 143–149.

Rothman, K. J. (1976). Causes. *American Journal of Epidemiology*, **104**, 587–592.

Rothman, K. J. and Greenland, S. (1998). *Modern Epidemiology*, 2nd ed. Philadelphia, PA: Lippincott Williams & Wilkins.

Sacher, G. A. (1977). Life table modification and life prolongation. In: Finch, C. E. and Hayflick, L. (Eds.). *Handbook of the Biology of Aging*, pp. 582–638. New York: Van Nostrand Reinhold Company.

Sacher, G. A. and Trucco, E. (1962). The stochastic theory of mortality. *Annals of the New York Academy of Sciences*, **96**, 985–1007.

Schatzkin, A. (1980). How long can we live? A more optimistic view of potential gains in life expectancy. *American Journal of Public Health*, **70**, 1199–1200.

Schneider, E. L. and Brody, J. A. (1983). Aging, natural death, and the compression of morbidity: Another view. *New England Journal of Medicine*, **309**, 854–856.

Schönemann, P. H. (1997). On models and muddles of heritability. *Genetica*, **99**, 97–108.

Schwartz, S. and Susser, E. (2006). The myth of the heritability index. In: MacCabe, J., O'Daly, O., Murray, R. M., McGuffin, P., and Wright, P. (Eds.). *Beyond Nature and Nurture in Psychiatry: Genes, Environment and their Interplay*, pp. 19–26. London: Informa UK.

Stearns, S. C. (1976). Life-history tactics: A review of the ideas. *Quarterly Review of Biology*, **51**, 3–47.

Stearns, S. C. (1992). *The Evolution of Life Histories*. New York: Oxford University Press.

Stoltenberg, S. F. (1997). Coming to terms with heritability. *Genetica*, **99**, 89–96.

Strehler, B. L. and Mildvan, A. S. (1960). General theory of mortality and aging. A stochastic model relates observations on aging, physiologic decline, mortality, and radiation. *Science*, **132**, 14–21.

Surbey, M. K. (1994). Why expect a horse to fly? *Canadian Psychology*, **35**, 261–267.

Susser, M. and Susser, E. (1987). Indicators and designs in genetic epidemiology: Separating heredity and environment. *Revue d'Epidemiologie et de Santé Publique*, **35**, 54–77.

Sutherland, J. E. and Costa, M. (2003). Epigenetics and the environment. *Annals of the New York Academy of Sciences*, **983**, 151–160.

Sutter, J. and Tabah, L. (1952). La mortalité, phénomène biométrique. *Population (French Edition)*, **7**, 69–94.

Tanzi, R. E. (1999). A genetic dichotomy model for the inheritance of Alzheimer's disease and common age-related disorders. *Journal of Clinical Investigation*, **104**, 1175–1179.

Taylor, H. M., Gourley, R. S., Lawrence, C. E., and Kaplan, R. S. (1974). Natural selection of life history attributes: An analytical approach. *Theoretical Population Biology*, **5**, 104–122.

Taylor, P. (2006). Commentary: The analysis of variance is an analysis of causes (of a very circumscribed kind). *International Journal of Epidemiology*, **35**, 527–531.

Tu, E. J. and Chen, K. (1994). Changes in active life expectancy in Taiwan: Compression or expansion? *Social Science & Medicine*, **39**, 1657–1665.

Turkheimer, E. (2000). Three laws of behavior genetics and what they mean. *Current Directions in Psychological Science*, **9**, 160–164.

Turkheimer, E. (2011). Commentary: Variation and causation in the environment and genome. *International Journal of Epidemiology*, **40**, 598–601.

Turkheimer, E. and Waldron, M. (2000). Nonshared environment: A theoretical, methodological, and quantitative review. *Psychological Bulletin*, **126**, 78–108.

van Asselt, K. M., Kok, H. S., van der Schouw, Y. T., Peeters, P. H., Pearson, P. L., and Grobbee, D. E. (2006). Role of genetic analyses in cardiology. Part II: Heritability estimation for gene searching in multifactorial diseases. *Circulation*, **113**, 1136–1139.

VanderWeele, T. J. and Hernán, M. A. (2006). From counterfactuals to sufficient component causes and vice versa. *European Journal of Epidemiology*, **21**, 855–858.

Vaupel, J. W. (1988). Inherited frailty and longevity. *Demography*, **25**, 277–287.

Vaupel, J. W. and Carey, J. R. (1993). Compositional interpretations of medfly mortality. *Science*, **260**, 1666–1667.

Vaupel, J. W., Carey, J. R., Christensen, K., Johnson, T. E., Yashin, A. I., Holm, N. V., et al. (1998). Biodemographic trajectories of longevity. *Science*, **280**, 855–860.

Vaupel, J. W., Manton, K. G., and Stallard, E. (1979). The impact of heterogeneity in individual frailty on the dynamics of mortality. *Demography*, **16**, 439–454.

Verbrugge, L. M. (1991). Survival curves, prevalence rates, and dark matters therein. *Journal of Aging and Health*, **3**, 217–236.

Vineis, P. and Pearce, N. E. (2011). Genome-wide association studies may be misinterpreted: Genes versus heritability. *Carcinogenesis*, **32**, 1295–1298.

Visscher, P. M., Hill, W. G., and Wray, N. R. (2008). Heritability in the genomics era — concepts and misconceptions. *Nature Reviews Genetics*, **9**, 255–266.

Vita, A. J., Terry, R. B., Hubert, H. B., and Fries, J. F. (1998). Aging, health risks, and cumulative disability. *New England Journal of Medicine*, **338**, 1035–1041.

Vitzthum, V. J. (2003). A number no greater than the sum of its parts: The use and abuse of heritability. *Human Biology*, **75**, 539–558.

von Mises, R. (1936). La distribution de la plus grande de n valeurs. *Revue Mathématique de l'Union Interbalkanique*, **1**, 141–160.

Vreeke, G. (2006). Commentary: The attainability of causal knowledge of genetic effects in complex human traits. *International Journal of Epidemiology*, **35**, 531–534.

Wachter, K. W. (1999). Evolutionary demographic models for mortality plateaus. *Proceedings of the National Academy of Sciences of the United States of America*, **96**, 10544–10547.

Wahlsten, D. (1994a). The intelligence of heritability. *Canadian Psychology*, **35**, 244–260.

Wahlsten, D. (1994b). Nascent doubts may presage conceptual clarity: Reply to Surbey. *Canadian Psychology*, **35**, 265–267.

Wallace, D. C. (1967). The inevitability of growing old. *Journal of Chronic Diseases*, **20**, 475–486.

Warner, H. R. (2004). Current status of efforts to measure and modulate the biological rate of aging. *The Journals of Gerontology Series A: Biological Sciences and Medical Sciences*, **59**, B692–B696.

Weibull, W. (1939). A statistical theory of the strength of materials. *Ingeniörs Vetenskaps Akademiens Handlingar*, **151**, 1–45.

Weibull, W. (1951). A statistical distribution function of wide applicability. *Journal of Applied Mechanics*, **18**, 293–297.

Weiss, K. M. (1993). *Genetic Variation and Human Disease: Principles and Evolutionary Approaches*. Cambridge: Cambridge University Press.

Weitzman, D. and Goldbourt, U. (2006). The significance of various blood pressure indices for long-term stroke, coronary heart disease, and all-cause mortality in men: The Israeli Ischemic Heart Disease Study. *Stroke*, **37**, 358–363.

Wexelman, B. A., Eden, E., and Rose, K. M. (2013). Survey of New York City resident physicians on cause-of-death reporting, 2010. *Preventing Chronic Disease*, **10**, 120288.

Wick, G., Berger, P., Jansen-Dürr, P., and Grubeck-Loebenstein, B. (2003). A Darwinian-evolutionary concept of age-related diseases. *Experimental Gerontology*, **38**, 13–25.

Wiley, J. A. and Camacho, T. C. (1980). Life-style and future health: Evidence from the Alameda County Study. *Preventive Medicine*, **9**, 1–21.

Williams, G. C. (1957). Pleiotropy, natural selection, and the evolution of senescence. *Evolution*, **11**, 398–411.

Williams, G. C. (1999). The Tithonus error in modern gerontology. *Quarterly Review of Biology*, **74**, 405–415.

Willis, B. L., Gao, A., Leonard, D., DeFina, L. F., and Berry, J. D. (2012). Midlife fitness and the development of chronic conditions in later life. *Archives of Internal Medicine*, **172**, 1333–1340.

Wilson, D. L. (1994). The analysis of survival (mortality) data: Fitting Gompertz, Weibull, and logistic functions. *Mechanisms of Ageing and Development*, **74**, 15–33.

Witten, M. (1989). A quantitative model for lifespan curves. *Age*, **12**, 61–68.

Zuk, M. (2013). *Paleofantasy: What Evolution Really Tells Us about Sex, Diet, and How We Live*. New York: W. W. Norton & Company.

AUTHOR INDEX

Abernethy, J. D., 10, 226
Abramowitz, M., 175, 226
Abrams, P. A., 49, 65, 226
Ackermann, M., 48, 226
Adamovic, D. D., 158, 226
Adams, C. S., 238
Adelman, R. C., 136, 226
Aguilera, O., 88–91, 226
Aickin, M., 50, 53, 227
Albin, R. L., 49, 227
Alfaro, B., 237
Allis, C. D., 233
Al-Samarrai, T., 127, 227
Alvarez, H., 234
Andersen, P. K., 119, 227
Andrew, M., 241
Andrew, T., 240
Andrews, H., 237
Aparicio, A., 231
Archer, M. A., 48, 241
Arepalli, S., 234
Arking, R., 237
Aspelund, T., 228

Ault, A. B., 144–5, 239
Austad, S. N., 4, 36–7, 39, 47–8, 56, 126, 227, 232, 236–7, 240

Bachrach, C. A., 233
Bailey, R. C., 100, 227
Baker, G. T., III, 136, 138, 227
Barendregt, J. J., 62, 228
Barker, D. J. P., 86, 227, 238
Barlow, R. E., 7, 12, 15, 53, 137, 227
Barrès, R., 90, 227
Barton, N. H., 38, 45–7, 49, 55, 239
Bateson, P., 233
Baudisch, A., 173, 227
Beaglehole, R., 238
Beard, R. E., 9, 59, 64, 70, 227
Beaty, T. H., 235
Beedle, A. S., 232
Belinsky, S. A., 80, 227
Bell, J. T., 89, 227
Benford, G., 241–2
Ben-Shlomo, Y., 85–6, 228, 236
Berger, P., 244

SUBJECT INDEX